Client-Centered Exercise Prescription

SECOND EDITION

John C. Griffin, MSc
George Brown College

HUMAN KINETICS

Library of Congress Cataloging-in-Publication Data

Griffin, John C.
    Client-centered exercise prescription / John C. Griffin. -- 2nd ed.
        p. ; cm.
    Includes bibliographical references and index.
    ISBN 0-7360-5495-2 (soft cover)
    1. Exercise therapy. 2. Exercise--Psychological aspects. 3. Physical fitness--
Psychological aspects. 4. Personal trainers.
        [DNLM: 1. Exercise. 2. Physical Fitness. 3. Exercise Therapy. QT 255 G851c 2006] I.
Title.
        RM725.G75   2006
        615.8'2--dc22

                                                            2005029040

ISBN-10: 0-7360-5495-2
ISBN-13: 978-0-7360-5495-9

The Web addresses cited in this text were current as of November 7, 2005, unless otherwise noted.

Acquisitions Editor: Michael S. Bahrke, PhD; **Developmental Editor:** Elaine H. Mustain; **Assistant Editor:** Lee Alexander; **Copyeditor:** Julie Anderson; **Proofreader:** Erin Cler; **Indexer:** Marie Rizzo; **Permission Manager:** Dalene Reeder; **Graphic Designer:** Nancy Rasmus; **Graphic Artists:** Angela K. Snyder and Denise Lowry; **Photo Manager:** Sarah Ritz; **Cover Designer:** Keith Blomberg; **Photographer (cover):** Mary Griffin; **Photographer (interior):** Mary Griffin with direction and guidance from Helen Boyd, **Art Manager:** Kelly Hendren; **Illustrators:** Keri Evans; Keith Blomberg; Paul To, figure 5.4; Marge Pavich, figure 5.8; Michael Richardson, table 8.8 figures 1, 2, 6; **Printer:** Sheridan Books

We thank the George Brown College Fitness Center in Toronto, Canada, for assistance in providing the location for the photo shoot for this book.

Printed in the United States of America   10   9   8

The paper in this book is certified under a sustainable forestry program.

Human Kinetics
Web site: www.HumanKinetics.com

United States: Human Kinetics
P.O. Box 5076
Champaign, IL 61825-5076
800-747-4457
e-mail: humank@hkusa.com

Canada: Human Kinetics
475 Devonshire Road, Unit 100
Windsor, ON N8Y 2L5
800-465-7301 (in Canada only)
e-mail: info@hkcanada.com

Europe: Human Kinetics
107 Bradford Road
Stanningley
Leeds LS28 6AT, United Kingdom
+44 (0)113 255 5665
e-mail: hk@hkeurope.com

Australia: Human Kinetics
57A Price Avenue
Lower Mitcham, South Australia 5062
08 8372 0999
e-mail: info@hkaustralia.com

New Zealand: Human Kinetics
P.O. Box 80
Torrens Park, South Australia 5062
0800 222 062
e-mail: info@hknewzealand.com

To my wife, whose dedication, integrity, and thoughtfulness embellish the lives of those around her

Mary

To my son, whose strength and ingenuity create quality in life

Jay

To my daughter, whose passion and physical prowess seem endless

Laura

To my parents, whose unconditional love continues to be my support and strength

Gord and Ruth

Contents

Reproducible Forms vi
Preface vii
Acknowledgments xi
Introduction xii

PART I   Foundations of Client-Centered Exercise Prescription

1   Activity Counseling Model   3

What Is the Activity Counseling Model? 5 • Introduction to the Model 5 • Step 1: Establish Rapport 6 • Step 2: Gather Information 10 • Step 3: Work With Stages of Change 19 • Step 4: Establish Strategies for Change 28

2   Client-Centered Motivation   41

Motivation and Adherence 42 • Motivational Strategies 42 • Case Studies 52

3   Principles of Client-Centered Assessment and Prescription   59

Client-Centered Assessment 60 • Client-Centered Exercise Prescription 68 • Prescription Guidelines for Health, Fitness, and Performance 71 • Ensuring Balance and Safety 77

4   Client-Centered Assessment   83

Cardiovascular Assessment 85 • Body Composition Assessment 87 • Musculoskeletal Assessment 89

5   Exercise Analysis, Design, and Demonstration   115

Anatomical Analysis of Exercise 117 • Biomechanical Analysis of Exercise 125 • Client-Centered Exercise Design Model 134 • Client-Centered Exercise Demonstration Model 139 • JAM Charts 145

PART II   Client-Centered Exercise Prescription

6   Client-Centered Cardiovascular Exercise Prescription Model   153

The Cardiovascular Prescription Model 154 • Case Studies 182

7   Client-Centered Resistance Training Prescription Model   193

Principles of Client-Centered Resistance Training Prescription 194 • The Resistance Exercise Prescription Model 203 • Case Studies 208

8   Client-Centered Muscle Balance and Flexibility Prescription Model   215

Muscle Balance 216 • Client-Centered Flexibility Prescription 220 • Client-Centered Muscle Balance Prescription 228 • Case Studies 233

9   Client-Centered Weight Management Prescription Model   243

What to Tell Your Clients 244 • Unique Role of Exercise in Weight Management 252 • The Weight Management Prescription Model 256 • Case Study 262

PART III   Design Issues for Injury Recovery and Prevention

10   Preventing and Treating Injuries   273

Causes of Soft Tissue Injury 274 • Understanding Soft Tissue Injuries 278 • Treating and Preventing Overuse Injuries 283

11   Exercise Prescription for Specific Injuries   293

Plantar Fasciitis 294 • Achilles Tendinitis and Tendinosis 296 • Shin Splints 298 • Patellofemoral Syndrome 300 • Hamstring Strain 302 • Low Back Pain 305 • Rotator Cuff Tendinitis (Impingement Syndrome) 314

Credits   319
References   320
Index   328
About the Author   339

Reproducible Forms

FORM	PAGE
Inventory of Lifestyle and Activity Preferences	18
What Do You Want?	21
Focus on Lifestyle	22
Stages of Change Questionnaire	30
Decision Balance Summary	31
Objective-Setting Worksheet	38
Self-Contract	45
Relapse Planner	49
FANTASTIC Lifestyle Checklist	61
RISK-I	63
Physical Activity Index (PAI)	65
PAR-Q & You	66
Strength and Endurance Testing	93
Field-Based Assessments of Flexibility and Muscle Tightness	98
Segmental Postural Assessment: Lower Body	107
Segmental Postural Assessment: Upper Body	108
Segmental Postural Assessment: Spine	109
Exercise Demonstration Model Checklist	141
Exercise Diary—Multipurpose	178
Recovery Heart Rate Progress Chart	180
Cardiovascular Prescription Card	192
Resistance Training Prescription Card	213
Joint Stress Questionnaire and Observations	221
Muscle Balance Prescription Card	230
Prescription Card for Weight Management	264
Pain Questionnaire	285
Risk Control Checklist	292

Preface

The second edition of *Client-Centered Exercise Prescription* substantially expands prescription theory and applications and is easy to use as a resource or as a primary course textbook. This edition maintains the previous edition's emphasis on the individual client and broadens the usual scope of books on this subject from exercise prescription alone to activity counseling, design modification, exercise demonstration, muscle balance assessment, injury prevention, and follow-up monitoring. New also are seven models that present the skills involved in counseling, prescription, and working with clients. Each model acts as a template that provides a menu of options for each decision. The theory and application required for making informed, client-centered decisions are provided following each model. These models cover the client-centered approach to

- activity counseling,
- exercise design,
- exercise demonstration,
- cardiovascular exercise prescription,
- resistance training prescription,
- muscle balance and flexibility prescription, and
- weight management prescription.

What Does "Client-Centered" Mean?

Like the first edition, the second recognizes that exercise prescription is about helping people adopt, enjoy, and maintain an active lifestyle. How well we help our clients do this is the true measure of our success. Having knowledge of exercise sciences, having technical skills, and having a fit body do not guarantee success in one-on-one training. Thus, this text continues to feature an unusually personalized approach for anyone who prescribes exercise: It takes clients off the assembly line and establishes them as the center of decision making. You will discover that **counseling** is a central concern of this book. I do not intend to suggest that the personal fitness trainer should be a psychological therapist. I use the term to refer simply to the art of listening intently to client feedback and modifying the program appropriately. It is not a simple art, but it is essential to develop if one is to be the best trainer possible. This art is also achievable, and this text makes clear in many ways and on many levels how this type of activity counseling can be learned.

As in figure P.1, the prescription process is a journey taken by the personal fitness trainer and client along a road leading to a uniquely tailored and progressive program of activity. Each stage of the journey has its own set of client-centered outcomes. This book will guide you, as an exercise specialist or personal trainer, in what questions to ask, what interventions to use, and what decisions to make along the way. This text challenges you to provide far more than a list of exercises. It will guide you through the stages of training, each characterized by "counseling"—that is, carefully listening to client feedback and modifying the path as necessary in response.

The three stages of this ongoing journey are

1. activity counseling and needs assessment,
2. personalizing prescription, and
3. program demonstration and follow-up.

The first stage of the journey begins with an inquiry from someone who needs help. Every time we take on a client, we encounter a new set of circumstances, a new personality, a new history, and a new journey. The first challenge in stage 1 is to get a clear picture of the client's history, needs, and hopes for achievement. This picture will develop, and perhaps change, as our relationship progresses. Determining the client's level of commitment to change will help you

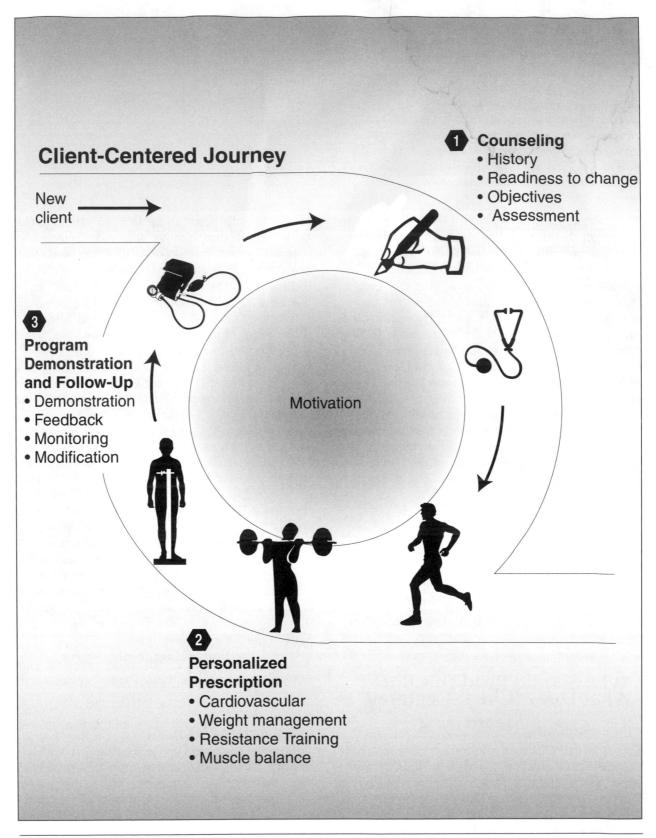

Client-Centered Journey

New client →

1 Counseling
• History
• Readiness to change
• Objectives
• Assessment

3 Program Demonstration and Follow-Up
• Demonstration
• Feedback
• Monitoring
• Modification

Motivation

2 Personalized Prescription
• Cardiovascular
• Weight management
• Resistance Training
• Muscle balance

Figure P.1 The three stages of prescription model are (1) counseling and assessing needs; (2) personalizing prescription by matching your client's needs; and (3) demonstrating, monitoring, and modifying as necessary.

know how to help her or him move to the next level. The counseling must challenge the client to create clear priorities for measurable and progressive objectives. More detailed information is gathered through the selective assessment of physical fitness. Without some physiological parameters to set prescription factors or monitor progress, we can only use broad guidelines that are not specific to our client's needs.

The second stage is the design process in which we select appropriate exercises, from a wide menu of choices, according to how they fit our client's goals. We can prescribe exercise programs to produce three potential outcomes: increased general fitness, performance improvements, or health enhancement. A variety of training methods allow us to match specific benefits to specific clients. The client's own preferences and availability of equipment will also influence our prescription. The details of the personalized exercise prescription are based on two main criteria: the physiological rationale and the needs of the client.

In the third stage, clients need to see the exercises demonstrated and then try them with some expert feedback. The exercise may need to be modified or the dosage reset. The follow-up program demonstration, along with the type of monitoring designed into the program, can strongly affect the client's motivation and self-esteem and ultimately determine the client's adherence to the program.

Parts I and II of the book follow these three stages. Part III looks at prescription situations that merit special consideration. It focuses on exercise prescription for clients recovering from or having a history of orthopedic injury, and it contains many new exercise designs for stretching and strengthening.

Who Should Read This Book?

In recent years, a number of factors have encouraged a shift to more client-centered exercise prescription. First, understanding of the effects of physical activity on human health has advanced and has increased the knowledge and skill base for exercise specialists, which has increased the demand for competent practitioners. Second, training has undergone a technological revolution, and the interface of client with machine, as well as training methodology using machines, requires close supervision. Third, fitness consumers want specific results, more choices, and guidance about

where and how to exercise; they also want service along with prescriptions. Fourth, personal fitness trainers are growing in numbers and are establishing new employment opportunities in private, clinical, and community sectors.

As one of these professionals—perhaps you are a clinical kinesiologist, a personal trainer, a strength training coach, or a fitness specialist in a private or community setting—you no doubt recognize the scarcity of available resources. This text is written for you. Physical therapists, athletic trainers, chiropractors, professors, and physical educators will also benefit from it. This text draws on applied exercise physiology, the art of counseling, and personal experience to provide skills that will help you prescribe and administer safe, effective, and enjoyable activities for your clients. Practical examples, applied models, and background scientific knowledge make the text well suited for undergraduate health and fitness courses such as Physical Activity, Health, Biophysical Sciences, or Theory of Conditioning and Training Methods. The text may also be used in conjunction with a traditional exercise physiology or exercise science course. It provides

- a bridge between industry practices and recent literature;
- a reliable method of matching client priorities with appropriate prescription factors; and
- specific examples, models, and case studies that demonstrate the skills of prescription.

A critical career step for many fitness employees and exercise science students is a personal training certification. *Client-Centered Exercise Prescription, Second Edition,* is a primary resource for candidates preparing for the Canadian Society for Exercise Physiology's Certified Personal Trainer (CSEP-CPT) certification practical and written examinations. It provides comprehensive treatment of the theory and applications covering more than 90% of the competencies needed for the CSEP-CPT and spans most of the requirements of other American and Canadian personal training certifications. The text will help you develop your confidence with the application of the knowledge and skills and contribute to your success on the certification exams.

Of particular note are several learning aids that you will find throughout the text. At the start of each chapter the expected competencies are listed. This edition also includes a "CPT Focus" icon, which marks elements that are closely related to the CSEP-CPT certification competencies. Greater emphasis is given to sequenced learning, starting from a prescription model and proceeding to a case sample that includes detailed design justifications from a physiological and client-centered perspective. Many chapters contain "Backgrounders," which are summaries of the scientific basis of the applied material. "Links" highlight matching client priorities with appropriate prescription applications. Each chapter is summarized with the important highlights. The text also contains many forms and charts you will find useful to copy and have at hand for direct use; an extensive list of recent and applied research in the references;

and exercise photos with instructions formatted to make them easy to photocopy and hand out to clients as take-home visual and textual aids.

Client-Centered Exercise Prescription, Second Edition, is a front-line resource that will help you focus on the individual in creating your initial prescriptions and in following up with service excellence. Whether used for learning the essentials of exercise prescription and personal training or preparing for a certification examination, *Client-Centered Exercise Prescription, Second Edition,* is a valuable reference.

Acknowledgments

My personal gratification from the work on this text was much greater with the involvement of my family and friends. Mary, my talented wife, emerged as the primary photographer capturing wonderful images of Michael Anobile, my daughter, Laura; my sister, Gail Collins; and my good friend, John Villiers.

I would also like to acknowledge my students over the years at George Brown College and in particular the models for this text: Rey Carroll, Marci Gurcharn, Faith Jones, Tammy Juco, and Shanique Small.

Early in the writing phase, a dedicated colleague, Dr. Tracy Gedies, contributed significantly as a manuscript reviewer. Finally, my experiences with Human Kinetics during both editions have been a delightful learning environment thanks to an outstanding developmental editor, Elaine Mustain.

Introduction

The best salespeople tell us that the first step in making a sale is to find out what consumers need or perceive themselves as needing. Similarly, a big part of what we do is to help clients "buy into" their exercise. If we act merely as experts, our success will be limited. Preaching the merits of fitness can create a frenzy of activity in our clients that can die out just as quickly as it began. Our first job is not to preach—it is to listen. We must hear what the people we are serving say to us. Our clients need our attention and our guidance, especially at the beginning of their commitment.

Recently, I invited a colleague to present a guest lecture on counseling skills for exercise prescription to my students at George Brown College. After I introduced her, she said, "For the next 15 minutes, I am your client." This was followed by a very long and awkward silence. Finally, a student said, "But we don't know anything about you." Of course, that was the whole point! Very quickly the floodgate of questions opened, and the students and the guest were well on their way.

Clients constitute the starting point of the prescription and training process. Rather than trying too early to design a solution, we must help our clients empower themselves by working with them to identify and develop their underused potential. Program designs are not ends in themselves. Our role is to formulate the right questions and choices and to provide the pros and cons from the clients' perspective and to help them develop the skills to become independent exercisers. We cannot help anyone we do not understand. So we must listen before we talk, keep listening, and remember that the journey to helping clients has many options for rerouting and that the map is in our clients' hands.

All too often in our exercise prescription, we limit ourselves by selecting or designing exercises that only suit the equipment we have in the facility or that follow traditional fitness components (e.g., strength or aerobics) rather than real client concerns. By taking a client-centered approach, we partner with our clients during the counseling stage to collect information or assess their personal interests and needs. In this way, we are better able to effectively and precisely prescribe exercise that addresses the complex issues that each client presents, such as fatigue, aches, tightness, joint pain, lack of energy, and body image.

Each client represents a new journey. Even if the choices are similar, the perspective of each client is different. This difference creates the challenge and the joy of exercise prescription and exercise-centered health care. It calls for us to become skilled not only in the science but also in the art of exercise prescription, and it is the reason why we all must be client-centered.

PART I

Foundations of Client-Centered Exercise Prescription

Many new clients start out with the best of intentions but quickly find that change is difficult. They find reasons to avoid their daily workout or their session at the gym. They may want to exercise more or lose weight, but when the day is full and stressful, it is hard to tie up the laces and head out. So people get discouraged and perhaps, as in the past, feel as though they tried and failed again. Although they believe they want to change their lifestyle to include more activity, somehow the shift doesn't happen.

The problem is that these clients have not even reached the point of being ready to adopt regular exercise. Activity and exercise are vague terms to them. Their idea of what is involved and even what they really want to achieve may not be well formed in their minds and is far from concrete. For these clients, before you can even consider designing an exercise prescription, you must change how they think about exercise. Your focus should be not only on fitness improvement (such as weight loss or improved strength) but also on a heightened awareness of personal fitness benefits and their own confidence that they can succeed. For example, discussing how far or how fast a client walks should emphasize the encouraging point that walking provides stress relief and higher energy levels; when walking is a regular habit, positive health benefits will accrue.

But success with such clients is more than a matter of enthusiasm and pep talks. To motivate them, you must, in the first stage of your journey, create a rapport in which your clients learn to trust you and develop confidence in your competence. Such rapport will free clients to discuss frankly both their present situation and their vision of the future. It will also allow you to help them clarify their experiences so they can better understand themselves.

The techniques you use for discovery and self-exploration will vary with the client's personality, but they will always include effective questioning and probing to determine his or her needs, wants, and lifestyle. The areas where a need and a want coincide and lifestyle is compatible are the areas of the greatest potential for success. Understanding your client's history through intelligent and empathetic listening will enable you to set priorities and formulate an effective motivational strategy.

In the first stage of the journey, we encounter a new set of circumstances, a new personality, a new history, and perhaps a new set of obstacles. To motivate our clients, we can use the change process strategies, presented in chapter 2, that are appropriate at each stage of change. This will help your clients recognize the personal relevance of the message and understand how it fits with their personal needs. The counseling must challenge the client to create clear priorities for measurable and progressive objectives. More detailed information is gathered through the selective assessment of physical fitness, allowing us to set prescription factors specific to our client's needs.

In preparation for personalized exercise prescription, we must be able to analyze various exercises, sport skills, and work tasks. Chapter 5 outlines a process for both anatomical and biomechanical analyses of exercise. Anatomical analysis allows us to select or modify the exercise by recognizing the joint movements, muscles used, and types of contraction. Applying biomechani-

cal principles can optimize exercise benefits for our clients and at the same time attend to their limitations through biomechanical alterations of the exercise. A final safety check can identify high risk in the design and later in the execution. This analysis allows us to tailor an exercise to suit our client's specific needs. The person-to-person demonstration of an exercise combines our counseling skills and technical knowledge, allowing us to teach and modify each movement.

This is the foundation of client-centered exercise prescription, and part I will give you the tools to build it.

Activity Counseling Model

Chapter Competencies

After completing this chapter, you will be able to demonstrate the following competencies:

1. Apply the four steps of the Activity Counseling Model.

2. Apply strategies, skills, and tools to establish rapport with your client.

3. Apply strategies, skills, and tools to gather client information.

4. Apply strategies, skills, and tools to work effectively with the stages of change.

5. Apply strategies, skills, and tools to effect behavioral change toward a more active lifestyle.

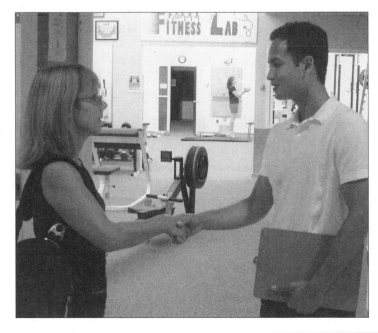

It was my first year teaching at the college. I had completed my graduate work, was running a fitness consulting business, and was up for any challenge when it came to designing conditioning programs. The word traveled quickly around the college that we were setting up a new employee fitness program, and before the doors were open I had received many calls, one from a staff member in the admissions office. Suzanne was in her mid-40s who wanted some help but was too self-conscious to go to the fitness center. With a naive desire to help, I jumped into the case. I explained that we start with a series of assessments, and then I would interpret the data and design a home program for her. The home program sounded fine, but Suzanne didn't want anything to do with the assessment. Although preprogram assessment was a standard approach I had always used with my practice and it was the procedure that I was teaching my students, I told Suzanne that I would still design a program. During our first meeting, she seemed as cautious as I was impetuous. The meeting was brief but I came out with the impression that she wanted something that was short, was easy to do at home, and would help her lose weight and tone her upper body. Armed with this I worked that night on what I thought was an effective program that combined skipping with a series of biomechanically modified exercises designed to tone her body. She was apprehensive about using any equipment so I designed several creative movements lifting soup cans to strengthen her arms. The next day, I went to her area at lunch to demonstrate the exercises. She was unable to participate but I enthusiastically went through each exercise for her. Her response seemed ho-hum, but I had classes and just left the program card with her. About 2 weeks later I ran into Suzanne coming into work and asked her how the program was going. She discreetly pulled me over and explained that she had incontinence after giving birth to three children and that jumping up and down was not something she could do. As for the soup can lifts, they were hurting her shoulder. After two sessions she stopped doing the program. Even more disheartening were her comments that nothing seemed to work for her and, despite my offer, she did not want a new program. I knew that I had failed Suzanne and vowed from that point to serve my clients more than simply design programs.

Recently, we were having an open house for an expansion of our employee fitness center and one of my staff introduced me to Marg, a woman from our college's human resources department who had called earlier for a private meeting. She had told my colleague that she was hypertensive and overweight and had been sedentary since her college days, 20 years earlier. I was concerned that she did not want to come to the center, but I wanted to support any desire to become more active. We talked about her past experiences that she saw as failed opportunities. As we continued, several doors were opened as she shared her feelings about gyms, embarrassments, and more recent health concerns. I knew it was important to gain her trust and reinforce the benefits of following through on these early intentions. Marg's last medical exam had given her a bit of a scare and she was looking for the connection between exercise and her high blood pressure. Despite some progress, she was still not comfortable exercising in the center with students and other fit staff. I walked away from that first meeting with a sense that we had connected and that Marg had a renewed hope of reaching her goals. Subsequent meetings over the next few weeks were shorter, but each seemed to bring us closer to determining what Marg wanted to do and getting a commitment from her. Our program was planning its annual hike and I invited Marg to come along. It was a comfortable setting, she now knew some of our staff, and I assured her that there were routes for all levels. She accepted the invitation and walked with one of our senior students. By the end of the day, Marg had linked up with her new friend as her personal trainer! Marg hired our student (graduate) over the summer and now is being trained by a new student with regular attendance in the fitness center.

What made the difference between Marg's success and the failure to affect Suzanne's health and quality of life? Both women had similar histories, health problems, and anxiety about public exercise. In both cases a sincere effort was made to help. Why did Marg eventually take responsibility for her health and become an enthusiastic convert to fitness? The difference was in the focus, which always remained on Marg's well-being. With Suzanne, I was preoccupied with assessment, prescription, and getting on with the exercise regime before establishing a commitment. There was little rapport, critical pieces of information were not gathered, her activity intentions were not clear, and my prescription did not meet her needs.

What Is the Activity Counseling Model?

This book is about taking the "client-centered" approach. This approach involves more than having the knowledge and skills as an assessor or program designer. In fact, it involves more than caring and wanting to help. But if you can use these characteristics as part of a client-centered approach, then you will be able to experience constant and rewarding success. We are always challenged to find ways to help our clients whether they are young athletes, professional people, community members, or seniors. Fitness programming often feels like an endless pursuit of the newest techniques and latest equipment. However, with the client-centered approach, your success will come from integrating the mosaic of applied experiences in this text with the unique physical, emotional, and social needs of each client. This book will allow you to put together the client-centered models and skill sets needed to help your clients achieve personal satisfaction and success.

Your job as an "activity counselor" is to help clients take charge of their own exercise regimens. You help them pursue their own objectives, whether they are an active lifestyle, recovery from injuries, or better athletic performance. By careful listening and questioning, you encourage your clients to tell their stories. You gather sufficient information and assemble a history for each. The value of the final prescription depends on how well you empower clients to set priorities for their actions—priorities that will satisfy their needs and wants within the limitations of their lifestyle. This kind of structured activity counseling can make a difference. Recent studies have shown that those receiving exercise counseling were more likely to report positive behavioral changes and increases in exercise duration (Duffy and Schnirring 2000). The benefits of counseling interventions have been well documented in the health care field (Sotile 1996). Several similar counseling models are based on fundamental problem solving (Wheeler 2000). For more than a decade, the Canadian physical activity, fitness, and lifestyle approach (Canadian Society for Exercise Physiology [CSEP] 2003) has been used to train thousands of fitness consultants using a multiple-step counseling strategy.

Introduction to the Model

The Activity Counseling Model developed in this text is based on four steps:

1. Create a rapport that allows openness to new information.
2. Determine your clients' degree of commitment to change.
3. Help your client set action-oriented objectives that will enable her to visualize where she wants to be.
4. Use strategies for behavioral change that are designed to increase your client's perceptions of personal control and are specifically client-centered.

The Activity Counseling Model retains the rapport-building and information-gathering steps from earlier similar models (CSEP 2003; Wheeler 2000) but expands on the skills and tools for each step. The stages and strategies for change become a focal point for the client's behavioral change. Physical assessment and activity planning steps, although part of the strategy that is built from the counseling, are not core elements in the process of behavioral change. Thirty years of clinical, consulting, and teaching experience have led me to the undeniable conclusion that this four-step Activity Counseling Model is simple to use, natural in its progression, and effective in providing a framework for activity counselors.

 The counseling steps shown in table 1.1 provide a framework that will enable you to change your clients' activity behaviors. As you develop the skills and tools listed in the table and taught in this chapter, you will receive the direction and confidence you need to achieve each step and develop productive relationships with your clients.

In this chapter, we will use the following scenario to work through the steps of the Activity Counseling Model demonstrating the skills and tools that you would use.

Counseling Scenario

Carol, a 42-year-old female client (CL), has come to you, the fitness professional (FP), to start an exercise program. She has not been successful in sticking with a program in the past. The client is concerned about her weight and has some back stiffness. Her doctor has encouraged her to be more active and presented no restrictions to increased activity. Carol works 9 to 5 in a human resources department and has a husband and two children, ages 10 and 12.

Table 1.1   Counseling Skills and Tools

Counseling steps	Counseling skills and tools
Step 1: Establish rapport • Be receptive and responsive • Outline the counseling process • Discuss the client's reason for attending	Active listening skills Supportive communication Nonverbal skills Counseling styles
Step 2: Gather information • Examine past, present, and future • Identify needs, wants, and lifestyle • Determine barriers	Questioning skills *Inventory of Lifestyle and Activity Preferences* Client profiling (learning and personality style) Needs (basic requirements) Wants (preferences, interests, expectations) Lifestyle (daily routines) tools and questionnaires
Step 3: Work with stages of change • Understand stages of change • Determine your client's stage of change • Match your client's stage of change	*Stages of Change Questionnaire* Summarizing and clarification Determining value by examining options *Decision Balance Summary* (pros and cons)
Step 4: Establish strategies for change • Select transtheoretical model strategies • Maximize benefits from the client's perspective • When goal setting, use measurable objectives	Goal and objective setting Self-talk, cognitive restructuring *Relapse Planner*

Step 1: Establish Rapport

Periodically, dialogues between the fitness professional (FP) and Carol (CL) will appear that illustrate material that has just been discussed. Although these dialogues are abbreviated compared with an actual dialogue, they will still demonstrate how you might apply the material that precedes them in a real-life setting.

Counseling Step1: Establish Rapport

Tasks

- Be receptive and responsive
- Outline the counseling process
- Discuss the client's reason for attending

Counseling skills and tools

- Active listening skills
- Supportive communication
- Nonverbal skills
- Counseling styles

Counseling is a client-centered process that leads to new behaviors. Building on a foundation of caring, rapport, and comfort, we help clients commit to changing their habits. We keep our clients at the center of this process by listening more than we talk and by encouraging them to learn from their own experiences. Counseling is an opportunity to help clients develop more options—to lead clients to open new doors, throw off chains, and stretch!

Strategies for Establishing Rapport

Our first objective is to put our client at ease and develop a comfortable working relationship. In establishing this rapport, be receptive and responsive while outlining the counseling process and discussing the reasons for attending.

Be Receptive and Responsive

For your client to make a lifestyle change, she must first examine her existing lifestyle for areas of desired change. She is most likely to do so when she feels comfortable with you. Establish rapport from the onset by being open, receptive, and responsive. Be aware of your impact on your client at all times. Sheer enthusiasm may show your level of dedication, but if your client is quiet and easily intimidated, your enthusiasm can create more harm than good.

A friendly welcome is essential. When you first meet, avoid pressure of any kind and start a short chat about an area of mutual interest (e.g., home, work, children, sports). As part of being receptive and responsive, you must learn to

- prepare the environment,
- show that you care, and
- establish credibility.

- **Prepare the environment.** Try to have people fill out most forms before they arrive. Showing new clients around your facility may help them relax, increase their comfort zone, and take the counseling out of the traditional office setting. Your clients will be poorly focused if their basic needs for comfort are not met. When you are ready to sit down together, be sure there is good lighting, appropriate temperature, good air flow, and comfortable chairs (avoid a desk). As appropriate, familiarize clients with various facilities, equipment, washrooms, and club procedures.

- **Show that you care.** Accepting your clients as they are makes it easier for them to accept themselves and therefore to change. Being sensitive to their concerns and demonstrating sincere interest will build trust. Your clients will be able to tell whether you care about making a difference. Desmond Tutu once said, "A person is a person because he recognizes other persons." Listening well shows that you care.

- **Establish credibility.** Without sounding boastful, explain your qualifications and experience. Not only does this establish your own credibility, it also provides your clients with confidence and shows them what expertise there is to draw on. For example: "You mentioned some previous back stiffness. . . . I had an opportunity to be part of the Healthy Back program staff at the YMCA while finishing my kinesiology degree. . . . I'm looking forward to helping you with that problem."

Outline the Counseling Process

Clients want to know what they are "letting themselves in for." When they can see the complete picture, it helps them focus and pace themselves. Outline what will be done and why. Organize your message into successive steps with particular emphasis on the essential aspects. Briefly describe options and choices clients will have throughout the program. Show them a copy of a sample questionnaire, assessment form, or prescription. Allow

enough time for questions. Try to link the answers to clients' particular situations and don't move on until you are sure they are satisfied with the explanation. Avoid rushing through this stage.

Discuss Clients' Reasons for Attending

In the first few minutes, avoid discussing health and fitness concerns in any detail. Once you have explained the counseling process, ask clients why they are there and what they hope to change. Some clients may elaborate and possibly continue to talk about physical problems or other barriers. When clients speak about themselves to you, they start a process of commitment to you and are more inclined to trust you.

Sample Dialogue for Establishing Rapport

Now that you have learned important ways of establishing rapport, and mistakes to avoid, look at this opening conversation between Carol (CL) and her personal fitness trainer. Note how the fitness professional (FP) communicates being receptive, responsive, and caring and how she is nonjudgmental, encouraging, and informative about how they will work on Carol's issues together.

FP: Hi, Carol. It's nice to meet you. How are you this morning?

CL: Well, pretty good. . . . I'm here to give it another try.

FP: The fact that you are here is a great start. And don't worry that you have to "get up and do" right now. Today we will just get to know each other a little better and explore how I can help you be successful this time around.

CL: Will I have to be tested today?

FP: Not at all! Let's just chat about your goals, any changes you may want to make, and any concerns that you have.

CL: You may have your hands full. . . . I haven't done very well in the past.

FP: Don't worry about that. We'll take another look at why those changes that you want to make are important and we'll work together to help you reach those goals. What is it that has you so concerned that you aren't going to stick with the program we develop together?

CL: I work with people all day and by 5 o'clock it's all I can do to get home, make dinner, and have a little time with my family.

FP: That really does sound full. It may be all the more reason to keep you healthy! And I'm sure that we can find some great benefits for you personally as well.

CL: That sounds good.

FP: I understand you have two children . . . so do I. What types of activities do you do as a family?

Skills and Tools for Establishing Rapport

Recently I accompanied a friend to an initial therapy session. The therapist began by saying that she wanted to start by building trust. On the drive home my friend said, "Did she think that I would fully trust her after one meeting?" This led me to think about my own expectations when counseling. My goal is to establish an affinity or rapport with my client. At times, this is a challenge that demands attentive behavior and a listening style that respects his feelings and clarifies his message; empathy and support must always be provided.

Counseling Step 1: Establish Rapport

Tasks

- Be receptive and responsive
- Outline the counseling process
- Discuss the client's reason for attending

Counseling skills and tools

- Active listening skills
- Supportive communication
- Nonverbal skills
- Counseling styles

Nonverbal Skills

Nonverbal skills involve your own "attending" behavior and your ability to perceive your client's nonverbal messages. Effective attending does two things: It tells clients that you are with them, and it puts you in a position to listen. Posture and gestures may be starting points that show you are interested. Egan (1990) suggested a series of nonverbal skills that are summarized by the acronym SOLER:

S: Face the client **squarely.** You may be at a slight angle—what is important is the quality of the attention. Remember, a **smile** can go a long way!

O: Adopt an **open** posture. Avoid crossed arms or legs, as they are seen as defensive postures.

L: At times **lean** toward the client. Leaning forward shows involvement, whereas leaning backward may be interpreted as a lack of interest.

E: Maintain good **eye contact.** The level of reluctance or comfort may be revealed by the consistency of eye contact.

R: Be **relaxed.** Your being natural helps put the client at ease.

These are only guidelines, because your clients differ individually and culturally.

Reading your client's nonverbal communication can increase rapport and improve the effects of your listening. Watch the whole body, not just the face and eyes. Hand gestures, body movement, the use of touch, and the way the person occupies space can be very expressive. For example, recently I had a daughter-and-mother session using a Theraball. As I was demonstrating I noticed that the mother was very tactile, sitting and moving on the ball and experimenting with different shifts in body position. The daughter was slow to even sit on the ball, and she kept her hands crossed on her thighs. I discovered after the session that the training was definitely the mother's idea and that building rapport with the daughter would be somewhat more difficult.

Observe shifts in your client's body posture, facial expressions, vocal tone, or rate of speech, particularly in response to your questions. Are the verbal and nonverbal messages telling you the same thing (Jones 1991)? A client may say that he understands how to start the treadmill, but squinting, perplexed looks, and cocked head provide another message when he is standing on the treadmill. Of course, you must check the accuracy of your interpretation with the client and avoid jumping to conclusions. Also be aware that just as you are watching your client's nonverbal cues, he will be watching yours.

Active Listening Skills

Asking good questions is useless if you are not actively listening. The following skills will make you a more effective listener.

- **Adopt the appropriate listening style.** Adopt a style of listening to fit the situation and content of the message being conveyed. For example, if your client just wants to get something off her chest, adopt a passive style and act as a sounding board. If your client is describing her first workout with a new program, listen actively, placing equal emphasis on both what and how things are said.

- **Check the feeling.** Repeat or reflect a client's feelings. Match her depth of meaning, whether light or serious. Give clues that you are trying to be empathetic. For example, a client recovering from a motor vehicle accident or a work-related injury may harbor pent-up feelings that emerge during her exercise rehabilitation. You might say, "The time it has taken to recover from your injury must be hard for you." You should not assume that you know accurately how a client feels, of course, but you should acknowledge feelings and communicate empathy. Verifying feelings and not assuming immediately that you understand can build trust and reduce negative feelings.

- **Check for clarity or accuracy.** Clarifying is an attempt to verify your understanding of what your client is saying. "It sounds like you are concerned with . . ." and "I'm a little unsure about . . ." are useful phrases for clarifying. Restate the client's basic ideas, emphasizing the facts. Although restatement is a check for factual content, it also can encourage the client to continue with her thoughts. For example, you might say, "Uh-huh, so it sounds like it's hard to find time with your new schedule. Is that right?" A check like this is also valuable as a method of summarizing major ideas and feelings at the end of a session. It pulls important ideas and facts together and may offer a springboard for further discussion. Try to use the client's own words and phrases: "Let's see now, I think I heard you saying that . . ."

Clarify, Don't Interpret

Clarification involves exploring your clients' feelings as well as behaviors. By clarifying emotions, you help clients understand their emotions. You need to catch the meaning of a message without interpreting or analyzing the meaning. The following two responses illustrate this difference:

CL: The XYZ Club said they would do a fitness assessment and design a personalized program for me. They took a few measurements and gave me the same program card as everyone.

FP response 1: Do you feel cheated and angry that they have not provided the services they promised?

FP response 2: So you think you were ripped off for your money and feel embarrassed that you were taken in by the club.

Response 1 reflects what the client said and asks for clarification of the client's feelings. By clarifying the client's feelings, you have begun to establish empathy and are in a better position to understand what the client wants. Response 2 may be true, but it is not what the client said and may not be an accurate interpretation of how she feels. It is critical that the client feels understood, not analyzed.

Supportive Communication

Supportive communication preserves the trust and positive relationship between you and your client while discussing any issue. It is a two-way process that allows you to empathize with your client and appreciate her uniqueness. Supportive communication avoids top-down conversation and rigid predetermined personal agendas. This aspect of active listening is far more than robotic head bobbing and deadpan "yeahs" and "uh-huhs." It involves selecting the appropriate response once you figure out the purpose of the conversation.

For example, if you need more information about your client's back stiffness, use a "probing" response. "Does your back stiffness affect daily activities or give you any problems when you sleep?" If the client describes a continual ache in her low back while at work, show empathy without deflecting the conversation to you. "When the ache is nonrelenting, it sounds like it can affect your whole day." Advising your client is a good coaching technique, but avoid giving advice as a first response. For example, if the client requests what equipment is best for burning calories, ask at least one more question before advising.

Sometimes clients will come to you because there is a discrepancy between what they want to be and what they are. Their goals may not be realistic or attainable. In that case, do not condemn or suggest by words or body language that the client is unrealistic. Instead, listen carefully to your client, recognizing that a helping role is necessary. Never judge the merits of what your clients say in terms of good or bad, right or wrong, relevant or irrelevant. The following exchange took place between one of my student trainers and a member of our employee fitness program:

Member: Well, the knee is still a little sore. The exercises are good, but I played hockey with my children over the weekend and it flared up again.

Student: That's the problem, isn't it? Why don't you stick to your program and forget the hockey?

This might well be sound counsel, but the student responded in his "advice-giving mode," with little empathy and no acknowledgment of the person's feelings. A better approach for the student would have been this:

Student: Do you think there is a way we can modify your play to avoid the flare-up, or is rest the best at this stage? I am pleased to hear that the exercises are good. Keep it up!

Accepting your clients as they are makes it easier for them to accept themselves and therefore to change. Being sensitive to their concerns will build trust and show genuine interest. Listening well shows that you care.

Counseling Styles

Personal characteristics and attitudes or beliefs about fitness and lifestyle are the basis for the counseling style that naturally evolves. By recognizing different counseling styles, you can respond more appropriately to different clients in different situations. A skilled personal fitness trainer will be able to use the appropriate counseling style depending on the client, his needs, and the situation. Following are some counseling styles:

• **Preacher.** The preacher often delivers mini-lectures on healthy behaviors, describing to the client what she should be doing. A judgmental lecture will ruin the establishment of any rapport, but the endorsement of positive choices and practical advice may be an effective way to respond to a client's question.

• **Director.** The director gives instructions or specific prescriptive guidance. The design and demonstration of the exercise prescription are an appropriate use of this style. This style does not exclude slipping into the counseling role to get a client's input.

• **Educator.** An educator provides relevant information about health and fitness to facilitate decisions about behavioral change. When providing written material, keep the information short and readable and make sure your client is interested in receiving it.

• **Counselor.** A counselor uses a collaborative problem-solving approach to help clients make informed decisions. This will be the style of choice most often throughout counseling. As new issues and interests evolve during training, this is also an effective style to implement action plans and change strategies.

Counseling a Client to Develop Options

Don, an automotive worker and avid lacrosse coach, suffered a heart attack during a father–son game. At first, he was devastated, feeling that his identity and role in life had been taken away. Feelings of "Why me?" progressed to frustration and helplessness. Medical and corporate counseling helped Don readjust to a modified work environment; however, his doctors set lacrosse out of bounds. Then a lacrosse friend of Don's provided some "counseling" advice. He had Don take a closer look at different roles he could take on with the team. He helped Don discover that his years of experience were invaluable as a strategist and advisor and that being on the floor was not the only option for a coach. His friend also introduced Don to an exercise specialist who showed him how to build his cardiovascular stamina and monitor his exertion levels and symptoms. Today, Don is co-coaching and providing a service to the team that goes beyond what he provided before the heart attack.

Step 2: Gather Information

In this age of information, we have made great gains in storing and retrieving data, but little advance in our skills or techniques for effectively gathering client information. What do we ask about and in what order? How do we deal with barriers or lifestyle issues as they arise? We need some refined questioning skills that are suited to the learning and personality styles of our clients. We also need tools to collect and prioritize needs and preferences and to understand our clients' lifestyles well enough to anticipate areas of integration.

Counseling Step 2: Gather Information

Tasks

- Examine past, present, and future
- Identify needs, wants, and lifestyle
- Determine barriers

Counseling skills and tools

- Questioning skills
- *Inventory of Lifestyle and Activity Preferences*
- Client profiling (learning and personality style)
- Needs (basic requirements)
- Wants (preferences, interests, expectations)
- Lifestyle (daily routines) tools and questionnaires

Strategies for Gathering Information

The initial consultation with a client is one of the most challenging aspects of personal training. The purpose of this session is to gather information about the client that will help you design a safe and appropriate exercise program and motivation strategy. Getting clients to talk about themselves is one thing; asking the right questions is another.

Where do you start? You are usually faced with a limited period of time and a daunting task of finding out "all about" your client! Counseling skills and tools like effective probing techniques and interview questionnaires can be very effective (see next section). However, some structure to the collection of information can reduce your anxiety about the session, save time, and provide more complete information. There are two effective methods: (1) past, present, future, and (2) needs, wants, lifestyle. Either method of approaching information gathering can stand alone, but merging the two methods is the most comprehensive and client-centered approach.

Past, Present, Future Approach

Begin by asking your client about past exercise and activity. The objective here is to understand your client's interests, physical aptitude, and skills. For example, if your client tells you that she has felt awkward exercising and has never done anything except walking and some cycling, this might indicate that the prescription should begin at a basic level. With little sport background, she may have issues with coordination and dynamic balance. Further questioning may reveal that she has avoided some physical activities because she was embarrassed by her body. Try to glean information about her feelings during discussions about past activities. It would not be surprising if this bias continued to the present.

Questions about what your client is doing at present will provide information about the quantity, intensity, and type of exercise you should prescribe. For example, the client may state that she is involved regularly with various types of exercises but still has a high body fat level. You need to know if she is exercising adequately to create a negative caloric balance and lose weight. Appropriate questions can help you determine how and where to start the exercise prescription.

A future-oriented line of questioning may reveal specific information about the direction that the program should take. What does your client want to get out of his program, and how much time and effort can he put into the program? Notice what makes your client's eyes light up; this will help you design the motivation strategy.

Needs, Wants, Lifestyle Approach

Needs are not the same as wants (Trottier 1988). **Needs** originate in human biology and in the human social condition. In the case of our clients, needs are basic requirements related to an injury, a specific weakness in a fitness component, a health risk factor, or some other personal situation such as participation in a sport or a problem with motivation. **Wants** are desires to meet these needs in specific ways or perceptions of value for things that may not be related to needs at all. Wants often determine our clients' choices about how to address their needs; wants, of course, are influenced by social forces. **Lifestyle** includes time, facilities, partners, travel, and employment. The areas of overlap—where a need and a want coincide and the lifestyle is compatible—are the areas of the greatest potential for success. It is on these overlapping areas that we should focus.

Figure 1.1 depicts the client history as a Venn diagram showing the overlap of three primary areas of that history: needs, wants, and lifestyle.

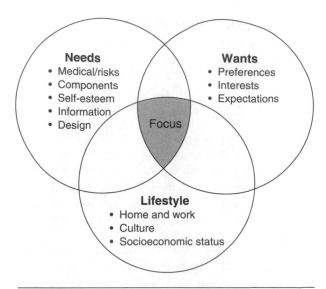

Figure 1.1   The areas with the greatest potential for success are where needs and wants coincide with a compatible lifestyle.

Types of Needs

Client needs may be related to medical, high risk, educational, or motivational factors; needs also can be defined by results of fitness assessments, by lack of self-esteem, or by special designs necessitated because of physical limitations.

- **Medical needs.** A questionnaire can identify medical issues and help determine if you need clearance from a health care specialist. Gather information on past medical history, present symptoms, medications, and existing medically prescribed limitations to exercise. Clients may be quite general in their comments ("I'd like to feel more healthy or have more energy"), or they may be specific ("My doctor says I have to lower my blood pressure and reduce my cholesterol"). If clients believe that exercise will produce the desired health effects and they are willing to commit to realistic goals, these health needs will be effective motivators.

- **High risk needs.** Always evaluate coronary heart disease risk factors such as smoking, high blood pressure, obesity, inactivity, and poor diet. Age, previous injuries, or low back pain may present special limitations. Risk factors can be identified with specific screening tools such as PAR-Q and RISK-I, with follow-up clearance from a physician obtained with the use of PARmed-X (see chapter 3).

- **Educational or informational needs.** Whether a client actually changes his lifestyle often depends on well-timed sharing of information. This need for information may emerge from a conversation. For example, a client tells you that

he joined a health club, tries different pieces of equipment each time he goes, and is disappointed that he hasn't seen results after five visits over the last 3 weeks. This client may need information about what he can realistically expect from exercise. In addition, literature is readily available concerning exercise and chronic conditions such as diabetes or asthma, and a compendium of medications is a valuable resource. Referrals to clinics specializing in hyperlipidemia, hypertension, or obesity can provide credible supplements to exercise guidance. If you do not have appropriate information for a particular condition or situation, know when and where to refer your client.

- **Special motivational needs.** Depending on their reasons for participation and their stage of change, clients may have specific motivational needs. Your strategies can include self-testing, logging, supervision, and support systems. I recently had a client who returned to exercise after almost 15 years. At that earlier time he had religiously followed the Cooper aerobics point-based exercise system and wanted to use it again with the new equipment in our facility. Using the physiological value of an "aerobic point," I prescribed a program of cardiovascular cross-training that allowed him to continue using a system of motivation with which he was comfortable.

- **Fitness needs.** A fitness assessment can indicate your client's fitness component needs. However, if you first determine the client's priorities—before doing the fitness assessment—you will be able to select only those test items that relate to those priorities. The prescription model is flexible, allowing you to loop back and verify needs through selective assessment. No matter when it is done, fitness assessment is a vital source of information for both writing the prescription and monitoring progress.

- **Self-esteem needs.** Good self-esteem can help people adopt more healthful lifestyles. Physical self-esteem may include how a client feels about his appearance, his perception of personal skill levels, or his realistic expectations of an ideal self (CSEP 2003). Counseling should encourage the continuation of healthy habits and develop an awareness of the value of changing high-risk behaviors. This assistance will improve overall self-esteem. Avoid setting standards for clients that are not realistic or are judgmental, such as looking like someone with an ideal body build. Self-esteem traps like these can prevent clients from enjoying the intrinsic aspects of activity. Motivation to continue physical activity usually comes from the sheer pleasure of the experience. But positive feelings about oneself as an active, fit person can also be powerful motivators.

- **Special design needs.** Special design needs may include these:

  - Specific equipment (e.g., special shoes or orthotics needed for running)

  - Focus on a specific sport or skill for training (e.g., energy systems and anatomical demands)

  - Limitations of the venue or facility (e.g., lack of resistance equipment in a home program, requiring biweekly visits to the Y)

What Is a Want?

Wants relate to clients' preferences. Wants may include what your clients enjoy, their special interests, or their expectations or aspirations. Marketing trends and other societal influences shape your clients' wants, which in turn will affect the way you address their needs.

To focus on your clients' wants, you need to examine their activity preferences, interests, and expectations. The questionnaire titled *What Do You Want?* (p. 21) will assist with this important function.

- **Activity preferences.** You may want to present clients with a list of possible activities and ask them to check which ones they most enjoy. They may also enjoy a particular method of training, type of equipment, training partner, or location.

- **Special interests.** Clients may be interested in something old or new, a specific challenge, or background information.

- **Expectations.** The desire for a more muscular body or one with less fat brings huge numbers of people to fitness clubs and exercise specialists. But be careful not to encourage the pursuit of the fashion industry ideal. The desire to change body image and appearance can be positive, but you must exploit that desire responsibly by helping your client establish realistic goals.

Sample Dialogue for Clarifying Needs and Wants

FP: Now that we have had a chance to chat about your past activities and the things that you are doing right now, tell me, Carol, exactly what you want to get out of your program. Do you have any specific expectations?

CL: Well, I want to lose some weight, tone up, and just have a little more energy.

But somewhere in the future I would like to be able to run a long distance, maybe a marathon, with my son—he's really interested in running.

FP: That's really exciting! Let's talk about the marathon in just a moment but first, are there any areas of your body that you want to tone up?

CL: Certainly my trunk and thighs are my problem areas for flabby muscles and fat. My back is often tight too, probably because of work.

FP: Are your thighs and back weak or do they tire easily, or do you believe the muscles are not toned?

CL: It is partially an appearance thing but I think my back could benefit from some stronger stomach muscles. What do you think?

FP: That's pretty perceptive. Your trunk should benefit from strengthening and building some muscular endurance in your abdominals but we'll also plan some stretching for your back for some relief.

CL: Good.

FP: I see that you have written on the *Inventory of Lifestyle and Activity Preferences* that you want a structured plan that you can do on your own.

CL: Yes, that may be best with my schedule.

FP: Carol, you also mentioned that you would like to get a treadmill to make things a little more convenient.

CL: Will the treadmill help me tone up and reduce my weight?

FP: Certainly in combination with your exercises and meal plan you will notice a difference. Walking on the treadmill will be a good calorie burner. It will also address a couple of your other goals by helping condition your legs and being a first step toward running with your son.

CL: This is exactly what I am looking for. I'm looking forward to getting started.

FP: That's great, Carol. I'm excited too!

In this dialogue, the client revealed her fitness goals and areas of greatest concern. It gave the client a forum to discuss expectations and speak further about herself. By asking some probing questions, the fitness professional was able to discover more detail for the eventual prescription and some underlying motivations. Finally, the rapport from step 1 was further reinforced.

Determine Barriers

It has probably happened to many of your clients. Despite best intentions, their new fitness plans began to fade after a few months. Their Pilates instructor moved, their bike broke down, or they had an injury and they never started up again. We need to understand barriers to exercise and strategies that will enable our clients to overcome these barriers. Barriers can be internal or external.

External barriers are the product of our environment and lifestyle. Socioeconomic status, age, and culture can affect external barriers. Check your client's personal external barriers:

- No convenient facilities
- Financial limitations
- Significant work demands
- Significant family demands
- No support from family or friends
- Inclement weather
- Injury or medical problems
- Lack of free time
- Lack of interesting programs
- Lack of child care
- Lack of transportation

Now, encourage your client to ask himself some introspective questions:

- What stands in my way? What are my potential barriers and how will I meet them?
- How much do I want this? Do I believe that this is important in my life?
- Where is my support?
- What does success mean to me? How will I know when I have accomplished my objective?

Convenience Brings Compliance

Marie, a new employee, learns of a small fitness center in her new company. She almost never used her previous club membership because of its inconvenience. She wants to "tone up" and lose some weight, but the center at her job has only resistance machines and one bike, and cycling holds limited attraction for her. She has slightly elevated blood lipids and some motivational needs. Where do her needs, wants, and lifestyle overlap?

Working out at her place of employment should ensure better compliance. A "workout buddy" would provide additional support. This client will benefit from a special program design. If the machines using large body parts are set up in a circuit with low resistance and high reps (see chapter 9 description of circuit training) and every other station is designed as an aerobic calisthenic, the training results should include weight loss, increased muscular endurance, and reduced blood lipids (Goldfine et al. 1991).

The obvious part of convenience is proximity; that is, the fitness center was right there. We often do not pick up on things that could be convenient in our lives. Marie knew the center had potential, but at first glance it was not obvious how the equipment would suit her needs. It became the challenge of the health and fitness professional to overcome barriers, design a plan, and shape the environment to satisfy the client. Marie's needs, wants, and lifestyle may change, but for the time being she feels good about her start in the corporate fitness center.

Internal barriers are personal thoughts, perceptions, and feelings about exercise and ourselves that may prevent us from being active. Despite a desire to become fit, those starting a program may be deterred by intimidation, physique anxiety, or lack of self-esteem and self-efficacy. Clients attempting to maintain an exercise routine face other barriers to exercise maintenance: lofty goals, perceived lack of time, and boredom (Kimiecik 2000). You need to help clients recognize and deal with whatever interior barriers they may have. Table 1.2 describes how the barriers manifest themselves in the client's behavior and some strategies for overcoming the barriers.

Table 1.2   Internal Barriers and Coping Strategies

Internal barriers	Strategies for overcoming barriers
Intimidation and embarrassment are frequently quoted as reasons for not joining health clubs, especially for those who are overweight or out of shape.	Adopt a one-on-one approach for personal training. Start with a lifestyle approach to behavioral change. Discuss exercise barriers, goal setting, and other client concerns.
Physique anxiety is a concern about visibility and judgment of one's body.	Avoid the use of mirrors. Be sensitive in how you dress and speak to anxious clients. Focus on their positive physical points.
Self-esteem is how positive a client feels about herself. Self-efficacy refers to a client's belief in her ability to complete a goal.	Choose a level at which the client can be successful. Take time to teach and demonstrate carefully. Provide personal attention and sincere positive feedback, encouragement, and follow-up (e.g., e-mail can be an effective follow-up).
Outcome objectives get clients started but are too long-term to maintain motivation. Clients need to shift their focus to the process of daily activity.	Set short-term goals for each exercise session (e.g., maintain excellent form in last 2 reps of each set). Monitor regularly, and assign subsequent progressive increases (e.g., increase resistance by 10% when reps have gone from 8 to 12).
Perceived lack of time is most often mentioned as the major barrier. We must help clients see exercise as a higher priority for their allocation of time.	Work with clients to set priorities. Examine the inactive parts of your client's day to see if an activity can be substituted or integrated (e.g., walking instead of driving).
Boredom is common with activities that are continuous and repetitive. We must incorporate variety and change.	Try different equipment; Therabands and Swiss balls are cheap alternatives. Use digital displays and personal progress reports to keep interest high.

Elements of a healthy lifestyle include a positive attitude toward self and others and a love of life. If these positive attitudes are missing, the client faces serious internal barriers. Circumstances such as economic status, educational background, cultural or ethnic factors, and home or work environment are external barriers that may make it difficult to adopt a healthy lifestyle. You must develop a sense of empathy and good problem-solving skills to find practical ways to help clients overcome both internal and external barriers so they can change their lifestyles.

Sample Dialogue for Dealing With Barriers

FP: Carol, tell me about the difficulties you have had sticking to an activity regime.

CL: Well, the goal usually looks good at the start. I say that I want to lose a certain amount of weight and they tell me how long and how often I need to exercise.

FP: Why do you think that approach doesn't work for you?

CL: It's not so much that it is hard work. It is just so long before I see any improvements.

FP: Absolutely. We all need some regular feedback and encouragement. Without losing sight of those long-term goals months away, let's work out some short-term goals for each week.

CL: I won't be able to lose much weight in a week.

FP: That will come if you keep yourself motivated with other benchmarks, like monitoring the number of steps you take with a pedometer.

CL: Can I count the steps that I put in at work?

FP: Exactly. That's the idea. Something that keeps you engaged in activity even when you don't think that you have the time!

Skills and Tools for Gathering Information

The type and timing of questions can make or break a counseling session. Listen carefully to your client's issues and gather additional information about her wants, needs, and lifestyle. The clearer the profile we have of our client, the better the information and support we can provide.

Counseling Step 2: Gather Information

Tasks

- Examine past, present, and future
- Identify needs, wants, and lifestyle
- Determine barriers

Counseling skills and tools

- Questioning skills
- *Inventory of Lifestyle and Activity Preferences*
- Client profiling (learning and personality style)
- Needs (basic requirements)
- Wants (preferences, interests, expectations)
- Lifestyle (daily routines) tools and questionnaires

Questioning Skills

Questionnaires, inventories, and checklists can increase the efficiency of counseling. They may be filled out in advance, allowing time during the counseling to discuss and clarify the most relevant information. See pages 61 *(FANTASTIC Lifestyle Checklist)* and 18 *(Inventory of Lifestyle and Activity Preferences)* for sample questionnaires. Develop the techniques of questioning detailed next.

- **Open or broad question strategy.** Start questions with a broad framework, narrowing to specifics later. For example, "Where do you see your fitness and health needs in the next few years?" Open-ended questions are used to gather information and are increasingly effective as your client feels more comfortable with you. Use them to learn how your client thinks about something. For example, "I'd like to hear more about your past experience with health clubs," or "How did you come to be involved in old-timers baseball?"

- **Closed or narrow question strategy.** After obtaining general information, use a series of narrow questions to focus the client's attention on a specific topic. Closed-ended questions provide detailed information, verify accuracy, and clarify understanding. They may help the client recall facts or choose options from a list. For example, "You mentioned that you wanted to start weight training—would you prefer free weights, machines, or calisthenics?" Closed-ended questions are also effective in getting agreement or commitment. For example, "How many days per week do you think you can devote to this part of your prescription?" Be careful, however, not to overuse narrow questions, lest the conversation become too centered on your concerns rather than on the client and her concerns.

- **Probing strategies.** Probing techniques help your clients think more deeply about the issues. When initial responses to questions are superficial, use probing questions to prompt clients to provide more information, meaning, critical awareness, or reflective thinking. Listen carefully, then proceed from "where the client is at." Acknowledge previous responses before presenting the next probe. There are several types of probes:

  - Clarification. These probes ask for more information or meaning. "Can you give me an example of . . . ?" "What do you mean by muscle tone?"

  - Critical awareness. These probes analyze, justify, or evaluate a response. They usually deal with values and attitudes. "Why do you think that is the best way to get in shape?" "How does the old diet compare with the new one?"

  - Perception. The intention of these probes is to anticipate a cause and effect or probable consequences. "If you sprinted without warming up, what do you think would happen?" "How do you think you would feel if . . . ?"

  - Refocusing. Often the discussion needs to shift back to the main issue. "How does that relate to your fitness goals?" "That's right, and how can that time be managed to allow . . . ?" (Orme 1977).

- **Softening a question.** Questions can be threatening. Use of a lead-in statement can soften the impact of an open-ended question, particularly if clients are being asked about their values or lifestyles. For example, "There has been a lot written recently about the effects of smoking—how do you feel about your own smoking habits?" or

"Many people have trouble starting an exercise program—what would help motivate you?" Note that the softening statements that introduce the questions are in the third person.

Conversations During Personal Training Sessions

Asking questions during a personal training session can be challenging. Try to keep questions brief. Often a client will bring up a problem or issue during the workout. In this case, your questions and dialogue should follow a process similar to the Activity Counseling Model but should be suited to an intermittent format flowing between or during exercises.

Focus on the client's issue, listen carefully to what he has to say, and encourage him to elaborate on details that will help you later. Gather specific information on barriers to change and what he has tried or might try to alleviate the problem.

Determine his thoughts on how important the issue is and what would be different in his life and workout if it were resolved.

Work with your client to establish what needs to happen, determine who or what can help him, and start to formulate an action plan.

For example, during a warm-up stretch, Carol mentions to her trainer that she has booked a massage. Seeing an opportunity to probe further, her trainer asks what motivated that decision. Carol talks a little more about the stiffness she often has in her back. Still gathering information, the FP asks if the stiffness is the result of an injury or a chronic problem. At this point, the FP is starting to process the information. Depending on her answers, he may refer Carol, perform a postural assessment, or introduce a stress reduction technique. This illustrates that the more you know about your client, the better able you are to support her.

Inventory of Lifestyle and Activity Preferences

This inventory (p. 18) helps people identify their three most important lifestyle needs from a list of 35 suggestions. It is an excellent counseling tool to help your clients identify activities that will satisfy these three needs. When Carol came to her trainer, she wasn't sure what activities would be best for her. They talked about barriers in the past and what the future might look like.

Together they filled out the *Inventory of Lifestyle and Activity Preferences* and identified three lifestyle needs: to have a structured activity, to improve her health, and to be time efficient. Good tools and some skillful questioning can help at the early stages of an action plan. If your client's prescription comprises activities she has chosen and considers important to meeting her lifestyle needs, her chances of long-term compliance will be significantly improved.

Client Profiling (Learning and Personality Style)

Unlocking the mysteries of how people think and learn will help you be more effective with your clients. The clearer the "profile" you have of your client, the better the information and support you can provide at the most appropriate times. Two areas of profiling that present opportunities for better understanding of what is needed to change behavior are preferred learning style and personality style.

- **Preferred learning style.** By keeping in mind the preferred learning style of your client, you can decide the best method to demonstrate an exercise, teach a monitoring technique, explain test results, introduce a new piece of equipment, and much more. If you select an approach that does not match the learning style of your client, you run the risk of moving at the wrong pace, providing too little or too much information, and generally not making a useful connection with your client regardless of earlier rapport. See *How Does Your Client Learn?* for one good way to understand your client's learning style. Once you have determined that, here are ways you can match each style:

  - Applying the information to individual situations: "Up until now, to gauge how hard you were working, I would palpate your heart rate. By wearing this heart rate monitor, you can have that information whenever you want. Even during the hard interval training, you could use that information to judge your recovery."

  - Learning by observation: "The watch that I have on is a new heart rate monitor that we can use. By presetting these controls, we can set the target zone. I'll show you, when I go below that zone . . . that is the sound of the buzzer that prompts me to speed up."

Inventory of Lifestyle and Activity Preferences

Lifestyle needs

I feel it is important to me to

___ like the people I'm with.

___ be in a group.

___ be independent.

___ get to know other people well.

___ meet many new people.

___ be a leader.

___ feel confident.

___ learn something.

___ be in pleasant, attractive surroundings.

___ be alone.

___ have a structured activity.

___ be able to do things at the last minute.

___ follow rules.

___ be praised.

___ have fun and enjoy myself.

___ release frustration.

___ release energy.

___ have common interests with other people.

___ improve my health.

___ be able to contribute something to a group.

___ have other people like me.

___ be physically active.

___ use my imagination.

___ create something.

___ find the activity challenging.

___ feel safe and secure.

___ try something new and different.

___ be myself.

___ use my talents.

___ improve myself and my skills.

___ accomplish something.

___ relax.

___ spend time with my family.

___ take a risk.

___ enjoy the outdoors.

Once you have checked the lifestyle needs that are important to you, list the three most important and identify which activities would most probably satisfy these needs.

Lifestyle needs	Activity preferences
1.	
2.	
3.	

From *Client-Centered Exercise Prescription, Second Edition,* by John C. Griffin, 2006, Champaign, IL: Human Kinetics. The Canadian Physical Activity, Fitness & Lifestyle Approach: CSEP-Health & Fitness Program's Health-Related Appraisal and Counselling Strategy, 3rd Edition © 2003. Reprinted with permission of the Canadian Society for Exercise Physiology.

- Learning by knowing the theory: "This heart rate monitor displays the updated average of the last five beats. It's good during exercise but for a person like you with such a low casual heart rate, it may be misleading at rest or light exercise. Why don't we keep a chart comparing the monitor and palpation in different situations?"

- Learning by doing: "Check out this new heart rate monitor. Try it for a few workouts and let me know what you think and how it works for you."

Often as we move from one client to the next, we catch ourselves explaining, demonstrating, or counseling using the same methods and style that we used for the earlier clients. It is natural to fall back to the comfort level of our own preferred style. Catching yourself is a great start; it means your intention is to be truly client-centered. If you sense that your client is having difficulty following something or is showing signs of frustration, think about your client's preferred learning style and try to match it.

How Does Your Client Learn?

Here is an exercise you can do with your client to determine his learning style:

"The new computer you ordered has just arrived. After you take it out of the box, what do you do?"

- Rely on past experience with a similar computer.
- Call my friend over to get some instruction and a good start on what I should be doing.
- Read the manual carefully and figure out the problems that emerge.
- Set it up, plug it in, and start playing.

If the client elects to rely on past experience, he prefers to learn by applying the information to individual situations. If he calls his friend, he prefers to learn by observation. If he reads the manual carefully, he likes to learn by knowing the theory. And if he just sets up the computer and starts playing, he prefers learning by doing.

- **Personality style.** Identifying a client's personality style can help you understand how she sees and reacts to things. If you effectively adapt to her style, it will make her feel more comfortable and trusting. This will go a long way toward helping reach her objectives. Being client-centered involves adapting to others' needs. In a counseling setting, use your listening skills (Step 1) to determine the client's predominant personality style.

Of course, most people combine their styles somewhat, but the value of this profiling is that it will help you choose a strategy that will be effective with each client (Prukop 1997). Table 1.3 presents treatment strategies for three common personality styles.

Wants, Needs, Lifestyle Tools

You may get ample information about your client's wants and needs if you start with an open-ended question such as, "Tell me about your favorite activities." But many people need a bit of help to recall even what is important to them. So unless you are completely convinced that your client has "revealed all," you can use the forms *What Do You Want?* and *Focus on Lifestyle* (p. 22) to check and gather additional information about your client's wants, needs, and lifestyle.

Step 3: Work With Stages of Change

Early discussions should clarify what clients hope to gain or learn and why they are there. Determining their level of commitment to change will help you move them to the next level of readiness to change. One effective way to work with a client's readiness to change is to think in terms of the five "stages of change" postulated by Prochaska et al. (1992).

Strategies for Working With Stages of Change

Emerson once said, "One who lacks the courage to start is already finished." This is a motivational quote and an apparent truism but falls short of explaining human behavior. People start things when they are ready to start. Our role is to recognize how close they are to initiating a

Table 1.3   Personality Styles and Treatment Strategies

Personality style	Client characteristics	Treatment strategy
Technical	Systematic Analytic Questioning Organized Reflective Theoretical	Explain pros and cons of choices Be accurate Allow time—moderate pace Provide tangible evidence (educate) Follow up
Sociable	Friendly Attentive Supportive Amiable Relationship-oriented Demonstrative	Address the whole person Maintain relaxed and moderate pace Be a partner in the change Be a good listener Make eye contact Invite feedback
Assertive	Leader Controlling Pragmatic May be competitive May be energetic Opinionated	Be stimulating Increase pace, once successful Be businesslike May need to limit options but incorporate input Find the client's dreams or hidden agenda

Counseling Step 3: Work With Stages of Change

Tasks

- Understand stages of change
- Determine your client's stage of change
- Match your client's stage of change

Counseling skills and tools

- *Stages of Change Questionnaire*
- Summarizing and clarification
- Determining value by examining options
- *Decision Balance Summary* (pros and cons)

change in behavior. Once we determine their stage of readiness, we can provide the appropriate type of counseling support.

Understand Stages of Change

The stages of change describe the motivational readiness of clients. These stages are as follows:

1. **Precontemplation**—Not intending to make changes
2. **Contemplation**—Considering a change

3. **Preparation**—Making small changes or ready to change in the near future
4. **Action**—Actively engaging in the new behavior
5. **Maintenance**—Sticking with the behavior change

Here are more detailed descriptions of these stages. Chapter 2 provides specific motivational strategies for each stage:

1. **Precontemplation stage.** A client comment at the precontemplation stage may be, "Exercise may be fine for young people but I'm too old to start." Your strategy here should be to increase his awareness of the importance of appropriate exercise at any age. Here is a typical conversation between a precontemplative client (CL) and a fitness professional (FP):

FP: I'm really happy to meet you, and I'm sure that I can help you achieve the goals that brought you here.

CL: Frankly, I'm only here because my wife made me come. I figure we can talk for a bit and then I can get out of here and back to my armchair.

FP: Oh. Well, OK. Then I guess we'd better have that conversation! So, were you active when you were younger?

What Do You Want?

Activity Preferences

What type of training activity (e.g., jog, cycle, hike, ski) do you prefer? _____

What method of training (e.g., interval or continuous) do you prefer? _____

Do you prefer group or personal training? _____

Do you enjoy competitive or noncompetitive activities? _____

What type of location do you prefer? _____

What is your favorite type of equipment? _____

What aspects of a past prescription did you enjoy? _____

_____

Is there anything in your type or level of current activity that you want to maintain? _____

_____

Special Interests

Do you have any current or past skills that you want to pursue? _____

_____

Do you want more information or resources on particular activities, health, or lifestyle topics? _____

_____

Do you definitely want to avoid anything? _____

_____

Are you interested in accomplishing something specific or being challenged? _____

_____

Are you looking for something new or some variety in your prescription? _____

_____

Expectations

Do you have any objectives that are particularly important? _____

_____

How will we know when you have reached your objective (be specific about measurable areas of improvement)?

_____

Are there major behaviors that you wish to change (e.g., eating habits)? _____

_____

Do you have expectations for changes in a medical condition? _____

_____

Do you have any performance or sport-specific expectations? _____

_____

Do you want to know your status or improvement with respect to population standards or in comparison with your own previous efforts? _____

_____

Can you set priorities for your expectations? _____

_____

From *Client-Centered Exercise Prescription, Second Edition,* by John C. Griffin, 2006, Champaign, IL: Human Kinetics.

Focus on Lifestyle

One way of increasing activity is by altering daily routines to encourage more exercise. Ask your client questions that will indicate which of the following aspects of her lifestyle you can target to provide the best prescription. Use the following list to record appropriate notes and check off the ones you can target for modification.

___ current work routine

___ current leisure routine

___ most convenient times

CL: Oh, yes. I was always involved in sports and activities in the neighborhood.

FP: Why were you so active at that time?

CL: Well, it was fun and the better shape I was in, the more competitive I was in sports.

FP: That's great! Sounds like being active suited your goals at that time. For that matter, having fun at any age is a worthwhile goal.

CL: Yes, but I can't still do those activities, and why would I want to?

FP: Good question. You certainly aren't training for the Olympics, but the training effects from even light exercise at your age can be very substantial. Your interests have changed, but activity can help you reach new goals.

CL: Yeah, sure. Can it help my tired feet or give me more energy?

FP: It can do that, and the experience you've gained since your youth can help you shape your activity to get what you want from it. Let me tell you a bit about what it can do. . . .

2. **Contemplation stage.** The most common excuse of contemplative clients is, "I know I should exercise, but I just don't have time." Help the client examine things that will keep her motivated; discuss what might make it hard for her to stick with exercise. Your goal is for her to decide for herself that the gains outweigh the losses. Here is another typical conversation between such a client and her personal fitness trainer:

CL: I just never seem to have enough time to take up a regular fitness program.

FP: I'm amazed at how much you accomplish in a day. You are very organized.

CL: Sometimes I feel like too many things are pulling in too many directions.

FP: You seem to enjoy much of what you do.

CL: Yes, I just need more hours in the day and more energy to last.

FP: Well, I can't change the hours in a day, but with your skill for time management, I think we could come up with a strategy for rejuvenation. You already have your priorities well established—a convenient activity break can actually help you meet your commitments.

CL: You've got my ear and 20 minutes of my time. . . .

3. **Preparation stage.** The preparation stage may include two different types of clients: those who are making their first serious attempt to incorporate enough regular physical activity in their lives to improve their health, and those who have tried before and failed:

- "I play baseball once a week but I think I'll start doing more," may be a comment from a client in the preparation stage who is trying "serious exercise" for the first time. Now you must seek a commitment. Booking an assessment at this stage may still be too threatening: Rather, schedule a consultation to find out what the client really wants to achieve, and establish short-term goals like learning a baseball warm-up routine or getting a few stretches for an old groin pull. A check-off log incorporated into the prescription reinforces every positive action taken in the early activity stages.

- Another client at this stage may be like our 42-year-old mother of two from our counseling scenario. She appears to have made an initial commitment although she has had some unsuccessful attempts in the past. Probe for the true measure of success she expects from her efforts, because any changes she may have attempted in the past probably have not met these criteria. Provide opportunities for her to believe in her ability to make change. Frequent contacts and simple encouragement in the first 30 days are extremely important. Keep your own journal of contacts and comments you have with all your clients. Your care and attention will impress them when you can recall earlier conversations.

4. **Action stage.** The client in the action stage may be a new club member who says, "I started 6 weeks ago at three to four times a week but I'm not working out as often now. Perhaps I need a personal trainer?" This client has made some very positive actions and needs to hear praise.

5. **Maintenance stage.** Once at the maintenance stage, your clients must work to prevent relapse and to consolidate their gains—especially if they are involved in rehabilitation (Sotile 1996). Remind these clients of their prior state of health, and encourage activities that might help their transition from clinical exercise to active lifestyle: Increase their awareness of an exercise technique, for example, or of a method for self-monitoring.

Determine Your Client's Stage of Change

Table 1.4 lists some characteristics of the different stages of change. Watch your clients for these characteristics to help you determine their stages of change. Just as with any New Year's resolution, your client's degree of commitment can fluctuate and she may fall back to a preparation rather than an action stage. Even when using the *Stages of Change Questionnaire* (see p. 30), you can't always be sure that your client's self-reported level

is correct. You may also be misled by the apparent determination of her speech. Sometimes planning specific time slots and discussing what must change to open up that slot can avert this problem. Regular contact in the early stages seems to be the best method of maintaining adherence and helping clients move through their stages of change.

Match Your Client's Stage of Change

Once you know your client's stage of change, you can choose strategies that are effective for that specific stage. Becoming client-centered requires that you match your frame of reference to that of your client. We will discuss in detail how to do this in chapter 2. For the present, simply consider the following examples, which will give you an idea of what it means to match your client's stage of change.

- **Precontemplation.** Consider one of my clients, Gerry, who was rehabilitating from a motor vehicle accident and had not previously been active. He had never considered what regular exercise would be like and had taken no voluntary steps toward doing it—the "cons" to regular exercise outweighed the "pros" in his mind. If I had simply assigned him an exercise prescription, I would have set him up for failure. Recognizing that he was at a precontemplation

Table 1.4   Stages of Change: Characteristics

Stage	Characteristics
Precontemplation	Has no intention to change Has low awareness Never considered it Believes that cons outweigh pros
Contemplation	Intends to change in next 6 months May be ambivalent May have low self-confidence
Preparation	Intends to take action in next 30 days Is making some small changes May have tried in past year
Action	Has changed behavior in last 6 months Has a high risk of relapse Needs support—challenging time mentally Is changing beliefs and attitudes
Maintenance	Continues program 6 months or more Has high confidence Has learned strategies to deal with lapses to prevent relapse May not get further support

or contemplation stage, I knew that he had not yet made a commitment to take action. I knew that no matter how appropriate a plan is, if it is presented at the wrong time, it won't be heard. If I moved too quickly or sent Gerry off on his own, a trust relationship might never develop. I wanted to be there at the right time, so I made sure that I was predictably reliable for every session. I worked at helping him over his negative perceptions, always looking to highlight his personal benefits. I knew my goal was about creating positive feelings about his sessions as much as it was about continued rehabilitation. Providing positive feedback merely for his attendance at the sessions and giving encouragement for reaching even a small goal showed Gerry that his behavior was worthwhile and acceptable. Then one day a gear mechanism on one of the pieces of equipment was malfunctioning and he saw me struggling with it. Without hesitation, Gerry fixed it in no time. Praise soon came from other patrons and staff. This small equipment repair episode gave him a feeling of empowerment based on his knowledge of mechanics. This positive experience played a pivotal role confirming in Gerry's mind the relationship between his rehab effort and feeling better. Gerry still comes in once a month or on call to do my fitness equipment maintenance and we always have a workout together.

• **Preparation.** Another client was considering an increase in her physical activity but seemed to be putting it off because of a lack of self-confidence. If I had presented her with a program featuring a wide variety of activities and detailed self-monitoring, I probably would have scared her off. She was at the preparation stage: Small changes were within her abilities, but large, complex changes would have set her back. Working together, we established a step-by-step plan that helped build her confidence.

• **Action or maintenance.** Josie felt great about one of her newer clients, Tony. Tony had been working hard under Josie's direction and was starting to meet many of his short-term goals. Josie looked forward to working with Tony but knew he could easily do the workouts on his own and should move into a maintenance stage.

"Tony, I wanted to take a few minutes today and review your progress."

"Yeah, it's great! I feel like a new man."

"Tony," Josie continued, "you certainly know what you are doing with each workout and I'm sure you can handle working out on your own from this point on. Congratulations."

Tony pulled back awkwardly, apparently not as pleased with the graduation. "Well . . . ya know I really like working out with you," Tony said with doubt in his voice.

"I like training with you, too," explained Josie, "but I thought you wanted to eventually be independent."

"I did say that, Josie, but I've made such good progress with you, I'm not sure if I can do that on my own."

Josie realized that the transition was moving too rapidly for Tony and that she may have left him with the feeling that she did not want to continue on with him. "Tony, why don't we work toward that goal a little more slowly," Josie suggested. "Why don't we work out together twice a month and see how that goes?"

A gradual smile came across Tony's face. "I'll still have a chance to touch base with you but I think that might just work. Thanks for the confidence, Josie."

Find out what your clients know, think, and feel about physical activity before actively engaging them in exercise. The more information you discover about your clients, the better able you are to determine the right combination of strategies for them. You can help your clients move from one stage to another most effectively if you understand what stages they are in and devise your strategies with them accordingly.

Skills and Tools for Working With Stages of Change

Clients are often at different points in their desire to commit, which often changes with the introduction of a new activity or component of fitness. Many long-time athletes have a difficult time adopting regular exercise routines. Similarly, avid runners who know that they should be doing some upper-body resistance work are struggling on either side of the preparation stage even though they have been maintenance runners for years. In such cases, you must use counseling skills and tools that will help your clients either adopt or maintain their new behavior.

Counseling Step 3: Work With Stages of Change

Tasks

- Understand stages of change
- Determine your client's stage of change
- Match your client's stage of change

Counseling skills and tools

- *Stages of Change Questionnaire*
- Summarizing and clarification
- Determine value by examining options
- *Decision Balance Summary* (pros and cons)

Use Stages of Change Questionnaire

The Canadian Society for Exercise Physiology (2003) has developed a *Stages of Change Questionnaire* designed to establish the stage of motivational readiness of clients (see p. 30). The questionnaire identifies five stages of change corresponding to the number of the statement selected.

Use Summarizing and Clarifying as Tools for Change

You must define the important issues for your client and her intentions to change. You can help identify her willingness to commit to these priorities by using the summarizing and clarifying techniques discussed on page 9. In the following dialogue between Carol and her trainer, notice how the fitness professional uses the summarizing technique to recognize Carol's frustration and even despair about her condition and her past experiences and then introduces hope into the situation in his response:

In our scenario, the client, Carol, has described to the fitness professional a number of unsuccessful attempts at regular exercise. At this point, she is quite pessimistic.

FP: Let's take a look at what we have so far. After almost 20 years of serving the public first, your body and health are feeling the toll. Your experiences in school with physical education and sports were not positive and at times embarrassing. In the last 3 years, you have joined two different health clubs that appeared to welcome you initially, but there was little follow-up assistance. You want to look and feel better, but you appear to have little support.

CL: (Pauses.) Not a rosy picture, but that about sums it up. Maybe I wasn't thinking straight for a while, but until lately, I haven't wanted to stop and look at my situation. Maybe the time has come for a serious change. I do feel anxious that I need to turn things around.

FP: One way of doing that is to take a look at what you have accomplished and enjoyed in the last few years. Let's work together on a general vision of where you would like to be, and we can build on these things as we create some short-term objectives.

You can see that the trainer not only used summarizing to state the facts but also suggested an approach to turn things around one step at a time. This helped refocus the client's feelings.

The first challenge, then, is to get your clients to clarify the issues before them; the second is to move them toward committing to appropriate plans of action. The process of clarification can help them determine what needs to be changed and get ready to move forward. Here is another sample dialogue in which the exercise professional uses clarification to set the stage for commitment. In our scenario, the client, Carol, talks to her personal fitness trainer about her difficulties with her weight.

CL: My problem is that I am overweight. I just don't like how I look.

FP: How does this make you feel?

CL: I'm frustrated with myself and embarrassed. . . . It just makes me so angry because I do more to watch my weight than a lot of my skinny friends!

FP: Carol, you sound disappointed by the results of your efforts to lose weight.

CL: Yeah . . . but I don't know what to do about it.

FP: The causes of overweight are different for different people. Could you tell me why you think you have put on the weight?

CL: Well, I don't think I eat that badly, but I've never been very active. So I think maybe my avoidance of exercise is the main reason.

FP: So you're suspecting lack of exercise as a major culprit in your gaining weight, but you also know that regular exercise causes you some difficulty. Any examples of an attempt that has gone astray?

CL: Yes, I bought an exercise bike last year and used it regularly for 3 weeks, but after about 6 weeks it was out in the garage. I got bored easily, and the seat was very uncomfortable.

FP: You want to do something about your weight, but stationary cycling didn't keep your interest. The club has spin classes during the winter or you could cycle outdoors when the weather is good. Would either of those work, since they'd probably solve the boredom problem?

CL: I don't think so. I think I'd rather give my seat a bit of a rest!

FP: OK, then. Besides biking, what sort of other exercise choices do we have?

CL: Well, I don't like sports and jogging seems difficult right now, but I like to walk if the scenery is pleasant or I'm with a friend. I'm pretty much a homebody in the winter except to walk the dog, but I like to garden in the nicer weather. I have been thinking about buying an exercise video.

FP: Carol, those are great ideas! We've come a long way. That is a good list that we can work from. Which do you think are the most likely choices from that list that you can see yourself doing on a regular basis?

Notice how the personal fitness trainer established early trust by avoiding judgment and premature advice. The trainer's reflective listening, probing, and clarifying helped the client get a clearer picture of the problem. The trainer then moved into the analysis step of decision making. We leave the pair as they are about to select the best combination of options (priorities) and the most effective strategy for achieving those priorities. Chapter 2 will expand on techniques for motivating clients to act.

Determine Value by Examining Options

Value is determined by your clients, not by you. Value is the consumers' estimate of the service's capacity to satisfy their needs and wants. Most exercise specialists know well the positive effects of exercise. But clients select their program priorities based on the benefits they see from their own perspective ("What does it do for me?" [Weylman 1995]). The challenge is knowing how to describe effects of exercise in a way that will clearly demonstrate how those effects will fill the clients' needs and wants while not introducing negative factors into their lives (such as interfering with family life or being terribly inconvenient). Three steps that will increase your chances of doing this are to identify options, rank the options, and lead the client to commitment.

- **Identify options.** A client wants to develop a flatter stomach and increased muscular support for a low back problem, all in a home program (lifestyle). After brainstorming with the client, you present her with the following prescription choices:

  - Perform sit-ups.
  - Reduce body weight and body fat.
  - Stretch muscles that pull the back into lordosis.
  - Join an aerobics or aquafit class specializing in abdominal work.
  - Use a video that teaches abdominal exercises or prevention of low back problems.
  - Perform a variety of abdominal strengthening exercises.
  - Practice sitting abdominal exercises at her work desk or standing exercises at the bus stop.
  - Do a short routine before bed each night.

- **Rank the options.** The next step is to weigh or rank the options. You can eliminate some options immediately because they are impractical or do not meet criteria required by the client. Your client may discard the aquafit class suggestion, for example, because it cannot be done at home. Working with your client, rank the rest of the options according to interest, time, and availability, which are the features of any given option. One way to help rank the options is to list the personal benefits of any given feature. Try using a simple chart (see table 1.5) to describe the benefits of any given feature.

• **Lead the client to commitment.** Finally, help your client commit to an action based on the analysis—select the highest priority, the best combination of options, and the most effective strategy for your client. For example, the client described here may choose to work out at home with a prescription that includes stretching the back muscles, performing a variety of abdominal strengthening exercises, and doing some aerobic work to burn calories. You can also provide a list of appropriate home videos to provide variety in the workouts.

Cautionary Note

At this crucial point of commitment and implementation, a host of things can happen to challenge this rational process. Many clients demonstrate ambivalence by stating that they can see why they should exercise but the costs of making that change are a significant deterrent (Prochaska 1994). You can work positively with this ambivalence if you guard against these potential pitfalls:

- Skipping or ignoring the analysis stage and moving quickly to a decision.

- Allowing the client to fall into "defensive avoidance" (Egan 1990), that is, rationalizing a delay in choice or commitment: "Yeah, that sounds good but I'll have to wait until this busy time at work is over."

- Letting the client seize on a comfortable short-term option. For example, "OK, that first step was new walking shoes. . . . I can do that at the end of the month when I get paid. I love to shop!"

- Suggesting a course of action more because it is highly recommended or popular than because it is suitable for the client.

- Pushing before the client is ready to change a lifestyle habit.

- Allowing the client to translate the decision into action half-heartedly. For example, "I'll probably get started sometime next week."

Use the Decision Balance Summary

The earlier discussion about personality styles indicated that some approaches to counseling may work better for some clients than others. The *Decision Balance Summary* (CSEP 2003) is a tool to help clients weigh the pros and cons of changing their activity behavior. The client who is analytical and technical should respond very well to this approach. It allows clients to consider the potential benefits and costs not only for themselves but for family and others around them. Decisions will be realistic and informed after clients weigh the gains and losses anticipated from physical activity.

Figure 1.2 is an example of how you might fill out the *Decision Balance Summary* as you and Carol, the client in our scenario, discuss the pros and cons of her becoming active.

Step 4: Establish Strategies for Change

We must help our clients establish which of their concerns should be dealt with first. To set those priorities, begin with your client's concerns, not

Table 1.5   Describing the Benefits of a Prescription Feature

Feature	Benefits
The prescription is designed to suit the space and equipment within your home.	Suits your busy schedule Saves time, because you don't have to wait for equipment or commute Is less expensive in the long run Will produce desired results Provides a personalized approach Allows you to circuit train
The prescription includes using exercise videos for education and leadership.	Requires less reading or attending special classes on back care Helps you understand your body and how to move it correctly Can be performed any time Is less expensive after several uses Provides motivation through music and visuals

your strengths. Although health issues need attention, unless you choose manageable problems that can show improvement, you may be setting your client up for failure. Once you have established priorities, help your client translate these into action and provide visualization of a future outcome. This should be a fun process that moves your client from theory to reality. Skills and tools for establishing strategies for change include how to write a good objective and the effective use of a self-contract, self-talk, self-efficacy, and the *Relapse Planner* (chapter 2, p. 49). Some of the skills and tools to establish change are only mentioned in this chapter, because they are all motivational tools for promoting or restoring commitment—and that is a subject that needs an entire chapter to itself (chapter 2).

Counseling Step 4: Establish Strategies for Change

Tasks

- Select transtheoretical model strategies
- Maximize benefits from the client's perspective
- When goal setting, use measurable objectives

Counseling skills and tools

- Goal and objective setting
- Self-talk, cognitive restructuring
- *Relapse Planner*

Strategies for Change

Strategies for change are not simply a list of recommendations. The strategies are the final product of a progressive narrowing exercise. After pertinent information has been gathered and the stage of commitment established, you help your client set his priorities. Then looking to the future, you and your client envision goals. With further focus and specific measurability, the exercise culminates in working objectives tailored to your client.

Set Priorities for Change

Your client has come for guidance and consultation. She has expectations but wants you to help develop a plan that will produce results. What is most important? What should you tackle first? What will make a difference in her life? Our clients usually have several concerns, and we must help them establish which is to be dealt with first. You must use all the listening and questioning skills discussed earlier if you are to understand your clients' true priorities and discern what action should be taken first.

The following three principles can serve as guidelines to help you set those priorities: Begin with client concerns, choose manageable issues that can show improvement, and highlight the client's health concerns.

1. **Begin with client concerns.** Do not confuse what is important to you with what is important to your clients. Not everyone places the same priority on fitness that you do, and you cannot expect all of your clients to immediately buy into your enthusiasm for exercise.

Begin with the concerns (needs, wants, or lifestyle issues) that the client sees as important. You may believe that her focus should be broadened, but beginning at this point will send an important message: "Your interests matter to me." For example, a sedentary client with elevated blood lipids wants to start a weight training program to tone up. You soon see that she is more interested in her appearance than in the health issue. So for the present, you address the client's chief concern: With appropriate prescription precautions and monitoring, she begins light weight training. Later you will look for opportunities to address the lipid problem. Or if an overweight office worker comes to you with hypertension, stress, and muscular tension, you may discover as you gather information that you need to address his work environment before becoming too specific with an exercise prescription.

2. **Choose manageable issues that can show improvement.** Although you neither can nor should try to force your clients to adopt your views about what their priorities should be, it is your job to show your clients the benefits of certain choices. If clients are skeptical or fearful, give them information and encouragement to see the issues in focused, realistic, and concrete ways. If you help them picture the benefits of relatively undemanding strategies and imagine what things would be like if they were to use those strategies, such clients will often adjust their priorities. If you can help a hesitant client buy into a simple prescription, the reinforcement he experiences may empower him to attack more difficult tasks. Clear and measurable results that show up early in the training can magnify commitment. Intervention and monitoring provide feedback and help the client to focus on his gains. This can sometimes be more difficult for clients who have multiple

Stages of Change Questionnaire

Physical activity can include such activities as walking, cycling, swimming, climbing stairs, dancing, active gardening, walking to work, aerobics, and sports. Regular physical activity is 30 min of moderate activity accumulated over the day, almost every day, or vigorous activity done at least three times per week for 20 min each time.

Here are a number of statements describing various levels of physical activity. Please select the one that most closely describes your own level:

(Please pick one)

I am not physically active and I do not plan on becoming so.	1	2	3	4	5
I have been thinking about becoming physically active, but I haven't done anything about it yet.	1	2	3	4	5
I am physically active once in a while, but not regularly.	1	2	3	4	5
I have become involved in regular physical activity within the past 6 months.	1	2	3	4	5
I participate in regular physical activity and have done so for more than 6 months.	1	2	3	4	5

(Answer if not currently active.)

I was physically active in the past, but not now.	Yes	No

From *Client-Centered Exercise Prescription, Second Edition,* by John C. Griffin, 2006, Champaign, IL: Human Kinetics. The Canadian Physical Activity, Fitness & Lifestyle Approach: CSEP-Health & Fitness Program's Health-Related Appraisal and Counselling Strategy, 3rd Edition © 2003. Reprinted with permission of the Canadian Society for Exercise Physiology.

Decision Balance Summary

Gains from physical activity (to self, family, and others)	Losses from physical activity (to self, family, and others)
Strategies (to maximize gains)	**Strategies (to minimize losses)**

From *Client-Centered Exercise Prescription, Second Edition,* by John C. Griffin, 2006, Champaign, IL: Human Kinetics. Modified from *The Canadian Physical Activity, Fitness & Lifestyle Appraisal: CSEP's Plan for Healthy Active Living.* Published by the Canadian Society for Exercise Physiology, 2003.

Gains from physical activity (to self, family, and others)	Losses from physical activity (to self, family, and others)
I may finally lose those extra pounds that I put on after my last child. My energy levels should increase. I will be a less stressed, happier person for my family.	I may miss transporting my kids to some of their events. I may hurt my back. My husband may have to prepare dinner if I work out after work.
Strategies (to maximize gains)	**Strategies (to minimize losses)**
Although some of your gains will be physical and some psychological, it looks like both are dependent on being regular. Keep a calendar posted at home with the dates and times of anticipated workouts clearly marked. (Don't be hard on yourself if you miss some!)	Take your husband out for dinner this week and talk to him about how important this is to you and that you recognize and appreciate his extended role. Your family is obviously an important part of any change that you make and maintain. Perhaps you can organize something the whole family can do together on weekends like hiking, biking, or skating. We will avoid back fatigue in every workout.

Adapted from Canadian Society for Exercise Physiology, 2003.

Figure 1.2 Carol and her trainer weigh the pros and cons of becoming more active.

tasks in their lives or for those who may be overwhelmed with new or busy challenges. The story of Jay, a teenage athlete suffering from tiredness, describes one of these situations.

Jay, a Young Athlete

Jay, a young athlete, was brought to me by his parents. He was part of an active family with a very full agenda. I had worked with Jay's hockey team the previous year, and his parents knew that I worked one-on-one with many young athletes. Jay enjoyed sports, but his parents had noticed some fatigue and anxiety about meeting all his obligations, including doing homework and spending time with friends. They asked if I would try to help improve his energy level and what they called a waning attitude.

My first conversation with Jay was about how he managed all the demands on his time. I identified the areas where he was doing well and also those that showed a lack of self-discipline. Jay wanted to please everyone: his parents, teachers, and coaches. As the demands increased, he found himself overwhelmed and feeling like he was not meeting anyone's expectations. I explained that it is hard to set things aside temporarily to allow focus on an immediate concern, yet that skill is the cornerstone of setting priorities. He agreed to try.

Jay and I pulled out a large calendar and listed all the things he had to do for the next 2 months. Then we went back over each one and tried to give it a priority rating of 1, 2, or 3. This was not easy, because Jay initially saw everything as a priority 1! We made sure to include all the 1s and managed to drop a few of the 3s. Jay maintained the monthly calendar and continued not only to list all his sports activities and school assignments but to add blocks of free time where he scheduled to spend time with his friends. He enjoyed "checking off" accomplishments and seeing progress.

I gave Jay's parents a list of symptoms of overtraining for which they were to be watchful. They also agreed to assist Jay during the busy times to focus on the higher-priority activities and to celebrate any and all accomplishments. Jay decided to play hockey for a less demanding team, which provided not only more time but a psychological break. He continues to use his calendar to record important dates and assignments, and the last time I called, he was out with his friends!

3. **Highlight the client's health concerns.** Consider seriously any health issues the client wants to change. Determine the client's primary goal: general fitness, performance-related fitness (e.g., for athletic competition), or health-related fitness (chapter 3). If he is open to modifying his behavior in any health-related area, cautiously seize the opportunity. He may expect immediate and tangible results, however, so educate him while still sympathizing with his impatience. Careful screening will reveal any cardiovascular or metabolic problems the client may have. If necessary, work closely with other health care practitioners and consider other lifestyle issues (e.g., diet, reducing stress, eliminating smoking) along with the exercise prescription. Many clients with fitness or performance goals have a limiting musculoskeletal problem. Determine the stage of the injury, its seriousness, and the original or ongoing cause. Address this hurdle first or at least in parallel with other prescriptions. Chapter 11, "Exercise Prescription for Specific Injuries," is a valuable resource for such clients.

Benefits of Alternatives

DeBusk and colleagues (1990) examined an alternative to the traditional prescription. They showed that three 10 min jogging workouts a day, 5 days a week for 8 weeks at moderate intensity, increased $\dot{V}O_2$max by 8% in healthy middle-aged men. Another group who performed a standard 30 min jogging workout increased their $\dot{V}O_2$max by 14%. This shows that more vigorous exercise is not necessary for initial conditioning in more sedentary clients.

Set Goals

Goals are broad, general (usually long-term) statements that describe overall intentions. They translate priorities into action and specify a future outcome.

Importance of Goals

Working with your clients to write their goals down, you clarify your own thinking and make sure that you are using the same vocabulary as your clients. The act of writing down goals sometimes triggers a design idea that opens up new ways of approaching a problem.

Helping clients develop goals can have a number of advantages (Egan 1990):

- It can focus attention. Clients with clear goals are less likely to engage in aimless behavior, such as walking down a row of weight machines wondering which one to try.
- Setting goals mobilizes energy and effort. It is not just a mental exercise but often arouses in clients a need to act.
- Setting goals seems to increase persistence. Clients with clear goals work harder and don't give up as easily.
- Setting goals motivates clients to search for strategies to accomplish them.

Kyllo and Landers (1995) performed a meta-analysis involving 36 studies on goal setting in sport and exercise. They found that moderately difficult goals led to greater improvement than goals that were too easy or too difficult. These authors reported that critical variables for success included

- specifying goals,
- setting both long- and short-term goals,
- allowing individuals to participate in setting their own goals, and
- making goals public.

Types of Goals

Goal setting can enhance performance but it needs to be implemented properly to maximize its benefits. Implementation begins with the realization that there are different types of goals:

- Outcome goals focus on final results. For some clients, the result may involve weight or size. With athletes, it may be the outcome of a competitive event such as winning a game or beating an opponent on the squash ladder.
- Performance goals focus on improving a personal best and are usually independent of others' performance. Examples include reducing your time to complete a circuit, improving a 1RM lift, or bettering your 10K time. Performance goals should be broken down into smaller units, each still measurable but short enough to provide regular positive reinforcement.
- Process goals focus on behaviors during training or competition. This may include a client's form or technique during a series of lifts or stretches or the maintenance of core stability throughout an abdominal workout. Completing a behavior (e.g., an exercise session) means immediate success. Process

goals can be very effective especially when it is difficult to see regular measurable performance-type improvements (e.g., changes in weight or fitness).

Process goals improve performance more quickly than do longer-term performance goals and are associated with lower anxiety, greater self-confidence, and improved concentration (Tod and McGuigan 2001).

Move Beyond Goals to Measurable Objectives

The vagueness of many goals makes them easy to ignore. "I'm going to become more active this year" is a common New Year's resolution, yet it rarely leads to action. People need specificity. Ask the question, "What will you be doing or what will be different when you make the change?" The answer may be, "I'm going to spend 3 days a week in an exercise class at my health club and ride my bike to work each day." Notice how specific this statement is. It describes a pattern of behavior that will be put in place, not a vague concept of greater activity.

Creating Useful Objectives

A goal is often defined by a series of objectives that break the strategies down into a number of distinct and sometimes progressive steps. Here are some sample objectives:

Goal: To learn more about my personal diet.

Objectives:

1. To attend a weekly seminar this semester and keep a binder of all the course notes.
2. To have my diet analyzed before and after the course and calculate the improvements.

Goal: To improve my ability to work with free weights.

Objectives:

1. To attend a second program demonstration session next week with my exercise specialist to get personal feedback.
2. To ask my friend, who has more experience, to be a training partner 1 day per week.
3. To keep a training log that records my performance and my subjective feelings of improvement.

Recently, I had a client whose history, assessment results, and priorities centered around her cardiovascular improvement. Her goal was "to feel less tired and to last longer when doing aerobic activities." Her objectives were

- to complete 10 walk–jog sessions within 3 weeks at her training heart rate,
- to increase the length of each session (duration) by 10% each week, and
- to monitor her feelings of fatigue at the end of each aerobic session and at the end of each day with an overall outcome of increased energy by the end of 3 weeks.

Note that each objective proposes clearly defined steps and describes the desired outcome of the goal more precisely. Objectives are action-oriented. They tell how well and under what conditions the outcome should be performed. Working in small, measurable chunks gives people frequent successes in the journey to their goal, empowering them and feeding their enthusiasm and persistence in reaching the long-term goal.

SMART Objectives

A simple technique used to create and evaluate objectives is the SMART system (CSEP 2003). In this system, exercise objectives have five characteristics: specific, measurable, attainable, realistic, and timed. Francis (1990) recommended that the term **attainable** be replaced with the term **action-oriented** because both **attainable** and **realistic** are so similar as to be redundant and because **action-oriented** is an important characteristic of an effective objective. Thus, we have the modified SMART system to include objectives that are

- specific,
- measurable,
- action-oriented,
- realistic, and
- timed.

• **Specific.** Objectives should be clear and specific enough to drive action. Effective use of questioning, probing, and paraphrasing can help your client articulate the level of specificity he needs to act. If a client whose objective is to get in shape does not state for what reason or in what component areas, she makes it impossible for you to prescribe an exercise program—let alone be client-centered. By contrast, the objective of "running 40 min nonstop" is a specific and measurable outcome.

• **Measurable.** For most clients, being able to measure progress is an important incentive. Moreover, if the objective is not specifically measurable, how will the client know when it is accomplished? Always have your clients ask

themselves, "What will I be doing or what will be different when I make the change?" You can gauge progress on some objectives through measuring and others by rating or describing the desired outcome clearly:

- You can easily measure changes in cardiovascular fitness, body composition, strength and endurance, flexibility, posture and muscle balance, and performance-related fitness. Conducting fitness assessments and providing periodic evaluations are two important motivational strategies known to improve exercise compliance (Francis 1990).

- It is difficult to objectively quantify a goal such as, "To feel better about exercising." One suggestion is to construct a rating scale from 1 to 10, with 1 representing the poorest and 10 the best (Clark and Clark 1993). The client estimates where on the scale he thinks he is at a given time and logs any trends.

- Another method is to describe, in advance, what is meant or implied by the objective. For example, your client who wants to feel better about exercise might verify this accomplishment if he looked forward to each workout, saw activity as a break in the day, enjoyed the social aspect of the activity, and felt much more relaxed and energized after exercise. If you can't quantify, measure, rate, or otherwise describe an objective, then you should forget it, because your client will never be able to attain it!

• **Action-oriented.** The cornerstone of an effective objective is the specific activity or exercises that will accomplish the objective. It is not a detailed prescription, but the client must be able to visualize what she will be doing. "I want to start doing some exercise" is a nonspecific activity, whereas, "Within six months, I will be running 3 miles in less than 30 min at least four times a week" is a specific outcome that your client can visualize. To check your objectives, look for the verbs; they are the action words and should reflect the activity needed to accomplish the outcome.

• **Realistic.** Many people quit exercising because they are disillusioned when their program fails to accomplish the anticipated results. The exercise objective might have been unrealistic to begin with. An objective is realistic if

- the resources necessary for its accomplishment are available (exercise noncompliance is often related to inconvenience of location or inaccessibility of equipment),
- it is under the client's control (her genetic background may never allow her to look like a thin fashion model), and
- it has a high priority for the client (it is something your client wants to do because it will satisfy her most important needs in a way that accommodates her lifestyle) (Egan 1990).

An objective is most realistic when these three elements coincide. Objectives are unrealistic if they are set too high, but they are inadequate if they are set too low. They must be relevant to the goal, painting a manageable picture of what success looks like while challenging the client.

- **Timed.** A timed objective provides a powerful motivation for following an exercise program. To set realistic target dates, consider each objective from a time perspective. An objective can be long-term (months) or short-term (perhaps within a day). Losing 25 lb in 4 months may be realistic, but a short-term objective of losing 1.5 lb per week may seem more manageable. Short-term objectives, successfully completed early in your client's program, can start a cycle of challenge and achievement that enhances his self-confidence.

Select Strategies Appropriate for the Client's Stage of Change

In the earlier stages, you should concentrate on building self-confidence and motivation and highlighting benefits specific to your client. Provide all possible kinds of feedback that can increase positive emotions and help resolve any problems created by change. In step 3 we discussed how crucial it is that you recognize and match your client's current stage of change. Chapter 2 will discuss how selecting strategies to match that stage of change will motivate her and promote commitment, and it will describe the appropriate strategies for each stage.

Sample Dialogue for Establishing Strategies for Change

Here is another sample dialogue in which the exercise professional continues to focus and provide specific measurability, which culminates in working objectives tailored to Carol, the client.

FP: Now that we have had a chance to chat about your past activities and the things that you might like to do, tell me, Carol, exactly what do you think your weekly commitment could be?

CL: Well, until the weather gets a bit warmer and I can work in the garden, I know that I could walk the dog every day.

FP: Great start, and it fits into your daily pattern of activities. How fast does the dog go and how long are the usual walks?

CL: She tugs me along as fast as I can go with very few stops! I usually do kind of a double loop that takes about 20 min and sometimes on the weekends I'll go down to the creek for 30 to 40 min but it is a bit slower.

FP: Carol, can you see yourself doing a brisk 20 to 25 min walk with the dog Monday through Friday and two extended 30 to 40 min hikes down to the creek each week?

CL: Oh yeah. My husband will appreciate me taking over that chore and I think that I will enjoy getting outside. Is that in addition to my program?

FP: Actually, that will be a big part of your aerobic exercise prescription and a significant objective in itself. I'm glad it sounds realistic.

Skills and Tools for Establishing Strategies for Change

Strategies to facilitate personal behavioral change can be initiated in the counseling session. There are tools that can help support the various stages of change such as setting objectives, self-contract, self-talk, encouraging self-efficacy, and using the *Relapse Planner* (chapter 2, p. 49). Listen carefully to your client's issues, because a tool may not work with one client but will with the next.

Set Goals and Objectives

Goals are like looking at a painting from a distance; you get an overall impression of the image and colors. However, any details about the painting, its style, and technique will only come with more specific examination; this is much like the progression from a goal to an objective. Review the following definitions and checklists to assist you in writing goals and objectives.

Counseling Step 4: Establish Strategies for Change

Tasks

- Select transtheoretical model strategies
- Maximize benefits from the client's perspective
- When goal setting, use measurable objectives

Counseling skills and tools

- Goal and objective setting
- Self-talk, cognitive restructuring
- *Relapse Planner*

 ### How Do You Write an Effective Goal?

A goal is a clear, broad statement of intention. It is a start to making a behavioral change. Write each client priority as a goal statement that includes an action verb, as in the following examples.

- To lose weight and body fat.
- To improve my poling action in cross-country skiing.
- To reduce my blood pressure.

Try this simple checklist to judge the quality of each of your client's goals:

___ Is it a broad statement based on a single priority?

___ Does it describe the client's intentions?

___ Is it easy to understand?

___ Is it good for the client's overall health?

How Do You Write a Good Objective?

Objectives make goal statements a reality by providing specific directions. They are precise statements of specific commitments to produce measurable results. The structure of an objective includes

- outcome—what your client will do and how success will be measured, and
- activity—the actions taken to accomplish the outcome.

Here's an example of a good objective: "to run three days a week, adding 5 min to the length of my run each week, until I am running 40 min nonstop." The activity is running 3 days a week. The successful outcome is being able to run 40 min straight.

Setting objectives can take as little as 10 min and can improve your client's awareness of her "future vision." Remember the SMART system of creating objectives, which include the five criteria: specific, measurable, action-oriented, realistic, and timed. Use SMART to help clients develop objectives that have some probability of success. For one client, this may mean focusing on being clear and specific. You may help one client devise a way to measure improvement and another to develop realistic time frames. Most clients need some help with at least one of the five criteria. SMART not only helps to devise objectives but also provides a menu for intervention.

Use the SMART criteria as a checklist to evaluate the following objectives.

___ specific

___ measured

___ action-oriented

___ realistic

___ timed

Goal: To improve my cardiovascular fitness.

Objectives:

1. To walk briskly in the evenings for 40 min, four days per week.

2. To monitor weekly my walking time and heart rate over a measured distance and to have my cardiovascular (CV) fitness remeasured at 3 and 6 months—targeting a 10% increase every 3 months.

Objective 1:

S ___ Walk for CV fitness improvement

M___ 40 min, 4 days/week

A ___ To walk briskly

R ___ Accomplishment has been demonstrated repeatedly in research and in personal experience; time commitment and resources such as walking shoes must be confirmed.

T ___ Ten percent improvement every 3 months for one-half year

Objective 2:

S ___ Monitor the walk for CV fitness improvement

M ___ Monitor heart rate over a measured distance and CV reassessments

A ___ Monitor duration and intensity (heart rate)

R ___ A 10% increase every 3 months is valid for the prescription.

T ___ Weekly monitorings are short-term checks, and the 3- and 6-month reassessments are longer-term benchmarks.

The *Objective-Setting Worksheet* on page 38 is designed to guide the process of setting objectives following the SMART criteria.

Use Proven Motivational Strategies

A number of motivational strategies can help clients through various stages of exercise adoption. Each of these should be used appropriately as your client's stage of change varies. Self-contracts can be used to help clients commit themselves to their choices and specific exercise objectives. Perhaps the most important factor in commitment, however, is the client's own belief that she is capable of committing to her goals and objectives. Two excellent strategies for helping a client embrace this belief are encouraging self-talk and promoting self-efficacy. Self-talk or cognitive restructuring involves thinking about a situation in a new way and serves as a vehicle for making perceptions and beliefs conscious. With practice, we can help our clients develop more positive ways of thinking that will support a regular activity pattern. It is important to help our client develop the confidence to act by tapping into opportunities to facilitate self-efficacy. This is extremely important in the early stages of exercise adoption and critical in its role of confronting barriers. Self-efficacy is one of the strongest predictors of exercise behavior. However, relapse is almost inevitable, and you should be prepared for it. When small lapses occur or if new challenges arise, discuss tactics for countering them and use the *Relapse Planner* (chapter 2, p. 49) as an important tool for motivating the client to address them. Chapter 2 will discuss all of these motivational strategies and tools in greater detail.

Objective-Setting Worksheet

Goal 1: _____

Objective 1: _____

_____

Fill in the specifics of how the objective fulfills each SMART criterion.

___ Specific

___ Measured

___ Action-oriented

___ Realistic

___ Timed

Objective 2: _____

_____

Fill in the specifics of how the objective fulfills each SMART criterion.

___ Specific

___ Measured

___ Action-oriented

___ Realistic

___ Timed

Objective 3: _____

_____

Fill in the specifics of how the objective fulfills each SMART criterion.

___ Specific

___ Measured

___ Action-oriented

___ Realistic

___ Timed

From *Client-Centered Exercise Prescription, Second Edition,* by John C. Griffin, 2006, Champaign, IL: Human Kinetics.

Highlights

1. **Apply the four steps of the Activity Counseling Model.**

   The Activity Counseling Model involves four steps: rapport, information, commitment to change, and strategies for change. In this model, the primary objective when counseling about activity is to create a rapport that allows openness to the gathering of information. Only then can you determine your client's degree of commitment to change and help her set action-oriented objectives that will enable her to visualize where she wants to be. You must use strategies for behavioral change that are designed to increase your client's perceptions of personal control and are specifically client-centered.

2. **Apply strategies, skills, and tools to establish rapport with your client.**

   Your first objective is to put your client at ease and develop a comfortable working relationship. In establishing this rapport, be receptive and responsive while outlining the counseling process and discussing the reasons for attending. The goal is to establish an affinity or rapport with the client. This demands attentive behavior and a listening style that respects feelings and clarifies your client's message. Although the appropriate counseling style for a given client should be used, empathy and support should always be provided.

3. **Apply strategies, skills, and tools to gather client information.**

   The fundamental purpose of the initial consultation with a client is to gather information about the client that will help you design a safe and appropriate exercise program and an effective motivation strategy. Counseling skills and tools like probing techniques and interview questionnaires can be very useful. Structure your approach to reduce your anxiety about the session, gather all pertinent information, and make the best use of time. There are two effective methods: (a) past, present, future and (b) needs, wants, lifestyle. Either method of approaching information gathering can stand alone, but a merger of the two methods will be most comprehensive and client-centered. The type and timing of questions can make or break a counseling session. Listen carefully to your client's issues and gather additional information about her needs, wants, and lifestyle. The clearer the profile of your client, the better the information and support you can provide. As well, you must develop a sense of empathy and good problem-solving skills to find practical ways to help clients overcome both internal and external barriers so they can change lifestyles.

4. **Apply strategies, skills, and tools to work effectively with the stages of change.**

   Early discussions should clarify what clients hope to gain or learn and why they are there. Determining their level of commitment to change will help you know how to help them move to the next level of readiness to change. One effective way to work with a client's readiness to change is to think in terms of the five "stages of change" postulated by Prochaska et al. (1992). The stages of change describe the motivational readiness of clients:

   1. Precontemplation—Not intending to make changes

   2. Contemplation—Considering a change

   3. Preparation—Making small changes or getting ready to change in the near future

   4. Action—Actively engaging in the new behavior

   5. Maintenance—Sticking with the behavior change

   Once you know your client's stage of change, you can choose strategies that are effective for that specific stage (chapter 2). The challenge is knowing how to describe effects of exercise in a way that will clearly demonstrate how those effects will fill the clients' needs and wants while not introducing negative factors into their lives (such as interfering with family life or being terribly inconvenient). Three steps that will increase your chances of doing this are to (a) identify options, (b) rank the options, and (c) lead the client to commitment.

5. **Apply strategies, skills, and tools to effect behavioral change toward a more active lifestyle.**

   We must help our clients decide which concern to deal with first. To set those priorities, begin with your client's concerns, not your strengths. Health concerns need attention, but you must also choose manageable issues that can show improvement. Goals translate priorities into action and provide visualization of a future outcome. Objectives take a vague concept of activity outcome and make it "SMART." They describe a pattern of behavior that will be put in place that is specific, measurable, action-oriented, realistic, and timed. Skills and tools for establishing strategies for change include how to write a good objective and the effective use of a self-contract, self-talk, self-efficacy, and the *Relapse Planner* (chapter 2, p. 49). Strategies for change are not simply a list of recommendations. The strategies are a final product from a progressive narrowing exercise. After pertinent information has been gathered and the stage of commitment established, you help your client set their priorities. The exercise culminates in working objectives tailored to your client.

Client-Centered Motivation

2

Chapter Competencies

After completing this chapter, you will be able to demonstrate the following competencies:

1. Apply motivational strategies to help clients through various stages of exercise adoption.

2. Use the change process strategies that are appropriate at each stage of change.

3. Help clients commit to their objectives.

4. Describe the role and provide examples of extrinsic motivation and apply motivational techniques that will reinforce intrinsic change to healthy behaviors.

5. Suggest some client-centered approaches to solving problems that will increase exercise adherence.

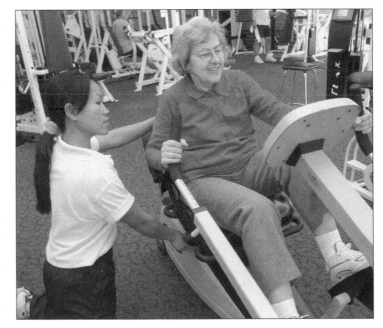

6. Apply appropriate client-centered motivating tactics learned in case study scenarios.

Each stage of change is different and each client unique, which creates the challenge of selecting a motivation strategy and support tools to help each individual when early enthusiasm wanes. We can cajole, encourage, or threaten, but in the long run clients become active only because they think it is good for them. They will stick with an activity because they enjoy it and believe they are achieving something. The heart of effective motivation is learning what drives a particular client at a particular time.

Motivation and Adherence

Forty to sixty-five percent of new clients will drop their exercise regimens within three to six months time. This despite virtually every member acknowledging the positive effects regular activity will have on their lives—both physically and mentally. A puzzling paradox. (Annesi 2000, p. 7)

Annesi's observation is both powerful and discouraging, and it highlights how crucial it is that we learn how to motivate clients. The good news is that working with personal trainers can increase exercise adherence by 40% over 24 weeks (Pronk et al. 1994).

In chapter 1, you learned to ask the following questions about each client:

- What are the client's goals?
- Is the client motivated intrinsically or extrinsically?
- What is the client's stage of change?

Once you understand these things about your client, how do you proceed? In this chapter we explore in detail how to work with clients to keep them motivated, following their priorities and objectives within the context of their lifestyles.

Motivational Strategies

The counseling skills and tools outlined in the previous chapter include a number of strategic plans to help clients through various stages of exercise adoption. Use each of these appropriately as your client's stage of change varies. This chapter elaborates on some of those strategies briefly presented in chapter 1 and presents new ones.

Motivational Strategies and the Stages of Change

Living in the developed world discourages physical activity, leading many people to exert as little physical effort as possible. Drive; don't walk or bike or run. Buy a robotic vacuum cleaner; don't push the old-fashioned kind. Watch basketball on television; don't play the game yourself. And on and on. Many people are aware that they should be physically active but have never been able to overcome their inertia.

Table 2.1 lists the change processes that are most likely to increase motivation at each stage of change; specific strategies to encourage the appropriate change process are listed in the next column. (Refer to *Definitions of Change Process*, p. 43, if you are unsure of what the listed change processes mean.) For example, if you have a precontemplative client, raise her consciousness of the importance of activity for her health. By informing her, conversing with her, and emphasizing the specific benefits she could experience from activity, you are likely to move her to the next level: contemplating the idea of becoming active. Look through the skills and tools presented in chapter 1 and identify which can be used to implement each strategy. For example, you can

- inform her by using the assessment tools and discussing the results and their implications with her,
- facilitate dialogue by using a tool like the *Decision Balance Summary* (chapter 1, p. 31), and
- use active listening skills combined with questioning skills to help her understand the specific benefits she can experience.

Relapse is almost inevitable, and you should be prepared for it. You must help the client resume the process of change through simple, short-term objectives, because his confidence will be bolstered by the success that comes with small changes. Match his current stage (he will have regressed!) with a stage in table 2.1, think about the change processes that are necessary to move him forward again, and use the strategies associated with those change processes. To help lessen the chances of relapse, don't let new enthusiasts skip a stage, lest they miss a mechanism of support and be less successful in the long run. Success requires stage-to-stage transitions. The challenge is to match your strategy with natural progression through the stages of change.

Table 2.1   Strategies for Change Process

Stage	Client behavior	Change process strategy	Counseling strategies
Precontemplative	Is somewhat aware of the message	Consciousness raising	Increase awareness of importance. Start a dialogue. Increase "pros" for activity.
Contemplative	Is aware and interested in the message Recognizes the problem	Consciousness raising Contingency management	Increase intention to action by addressing ambivalence, highlighting personal benefits, and building self-confidence. Create an understanding and acceptance.
Preparation	Identifies a course of action Is ready to take action	Consciousness raising Contingency management Self-liberation	Help client plan (e.g., set date, location). Focus on the "pros." Strengthen self-confidence. Provide helpful resources (knowledge and skills).
Action	Makes a decision to implement a course of action Tries the activity Makes short-term adoption	Contingency management Self-liberation Helping relationships	Teach client how to deal with lapses. Promote social support. Deal with lapses; reevaluate next action step. Provide encouragement.
Maintenance	Makes long-term commitment Achieves permanent lifestyle change	Helping relationships Counterconditioning Stimulus control	Refine and add variety to program. Prepare in case of relapse. Provide support in maintaining behavior to prevent relapse.

By understanding your client's stage of change, the change process appropriate to that stage, and the strategies that will facilitate change, you will help your client recognize the importance of fitness and how it meets her personal needs. This recognition is the beginning of motivation.

Definitions of Change Process

- **Consciousness raising** happens when the unconscious becomes conscious. Individuals become aware of new alternatives and there is increased information about self and health. Consciousness raising may be brought about by changes in environment (e.g., a new bike path or employee fitness center) or a change in a stage of life. It usually requires education and feedback.

- **Contingency management** is a self-evaluation that involves reinforcement made contingent on behavior. It depends on the individual's value of the particular consequence. We can help the client assess the impact of current or future behaviors. For example, by questioning, we may find that clients believe that if they were to take a yoga class, they would be less stressed and more productive.

- **Self-liberation** is the belief one has the power to change her own life, which is based on the sense of self-efficacy. If my client believes that she can strengthen her ankle after injury, her thoughts and actions will increase her commitment to change.

- **Helping relationships** are provided by caring, understanding, and committed trainers, especially in the areas of acquiring skill and achieving self-efficacy. From the client's perspective, this process involves accepting support and trusting others.

- **Counterconditioning** is a strategy that involves changing one's response to particular stimuli. The objective is to counteract old habits and to reinforce new habits. For example, you can help your client change his thinking so that the break between classes that used to trigger a trip to the cafeteria becomes instead a signal for a walk to the local park.

- **Stimulus control** involves changing one's environment to minimize negative stimuli. This involves recognizing, controlling, or avoiding anti-exercise stimuli; an example is to avoid turning on the television until one has worked out (Brooks 2000).

To motivate these people, we can use the change process strategies that are appropriate at each stage of change. For example, as the precontemplative person becomes aware of the message about activity and health, she moves to a level of comprehension where she recognizes and understands the problem. You will be most effective here by using a consciousness-raising interaction with the client as outlined in table 2.1.

Motivation and Commitment

You can expect resistance from your clients when they need to make decisions and when they need to move from discussion to action. Making decisions and moving into action involve a commitment of the client's physical and psychological resources. This involves both the initial commitment to exercise objectives and an ongoing commitment to the full strategy. The client should attempt to make steady progress toward the objectives; however, after a lapse, the client must get back on track and move forward.

Several factors that we can control can help our clients commit to, then follow through on, their objectives:

- **Ownership.** Make sure the objectives are the client's, not yours. Jogging is still one of the most popular suggestions for a start-up activity. However, it also has the highest attrition rate—particularly when it was someone else's choice. If you work through the forms *What Do You Want?* and *Focus on Lifestyle* (pp. 21-22) with your client and pay close attention to the results, you will be able to offer activity options that came from the client, not you.

- **Options.** Provide a choice of activities that can produce similar training results. The *Energy Deficit Point System* (chapter 9, p. 253) groups activities with similar caloric costs. These activities are virtually interchangeable in an exercise prescription.

- **Reinforcement.** Encourage any action taken toward the client's objective. Teach clients how to monitor themselves (chapter 6), because this

will show them their progress and help build self-confidence. Even during an exercise demonstration, recognize the things your client is doing well.

- **Appeal.** Look for ways to increase the appeal of the exercise program or to change the source of interest. A training partner, new exercises, a change of equipment, even a change of workout time can make the workout more pleasant.

- **Obstacle management.** Help clients see how to manage disincentives. One of the appeals of personal trainers is the expectation that they will help to remove obstacles or at least work around them. If your client tells you that he can't get started on his weight reduction program until work slows down, tell him that every calorie counts and help him find some active living habits like taking the stairs.

- **Challenge.** Help clients set objectives that are not just substantive but challenging. Small, measurable victories toward an objective can feed the drive to achieve. One of my clients was getting bored with the small gains in weight he was lifting, so I set up a recording chart that summed every pound he lifted. The totals accumulated quickly and soon he was lifting "tons."

- **Contracts.** Use contracts to help clients commit themselves to their choices. The worksheet on page 45 will help guide your clients through a self-contracting process of commitment to their exercise objectives (CSEP 2003).

Perhaps the most important factor in commitment, however, is the client's own belief that she is capable of committing to her goals and objectives, following through on that commitment, and reaching her goals. Two excellent strategies for helping a client embrace this belief are encouraging self-talk and promoting self-efficacy.

Encouraging Self-Talk

Any time you think about something, you are talking to yourself. Negative self-talk, such as making excuses for skipping exercise, is counterproductive. Positive self-talk can be used to focus attention, build confidence, modify poor habits, and increase energy. Your client may engage in negative thinking that interferes with his intentions to work out. When you sense that this is the case or when your client appears keen but repeatedly cancels, he may benefit from a technique to change his thoughts, called cognitive restructuring (Brehm 2003). Cognitive restructuring involves thinking about a situation in a new way and serves as a vehicle for making perceptions and beliefs conscious, which is the key to gaining cognitive control.

Self-Contract

1. My physical activity goal is

_____

_____

2. To achieve my goal, I need to change the following:

_____

_____

3. I am willing to do the following to make it happen:

_____

_____

4. Others will know about the change I am making when

_____

_____

5. I might sabotage my plan by

_____

_____

6. Therefore, my contract to myself is

_____

_____

7. Check-up dates:

_____

_____

Signed:

_____ Client

_____ Appraiser

From *Client-Centered Exercise Prescription, Second Edition,* by John C. Griffin, 2006, Champaign, IL: Human Kinetics. From *The Canadian Physical Activity, Fitness & Lifestyle Appraisal: CSEP's Plan for Healthy Active Living.* Published by the Canadian Society for Exercise Physiology, 2003. p. 8-47. Reprinted by permission.

Clients may have trouble sticking to an exercise program because of misconceptions that underlie their negative thoughts. Some may believe that exercise is a waste of time and that other things take precedence. This may be a subconscious belief that it is selfish to take care of yourself. Help these clients see that their health is a priority and that exercise is a good use of time. Teach them to talk back to this negative self-talk: "What can be more important than my health, and without good health how can I take care of my family?"

Other clients may avoid exercise because they feel too tired or believe that an exercise program adds to their stress. They may feel emotionally tired, and we need to help them discover how exercise can make them feel energized or revitalized. Help them construct reinforcing self-talk like, "I'll need the energy from this workout to get through that presentation this afternoon." Once underlying beliefs are clarified, clients can use a rehearsed positive self-talk to counter negative thoughts. With practice, we can help our clients develop more positive ways of thinking that will support regular activity.

We can use this technique in a number of ways. Many of our clients have developed unsafe movement habits by the time they reach us. Self-talk can help them overcome the habit if you teach them to interject a mental reminder at a well-chosen time in the execution of the exercise. Sometimes all it takes is a single word like "squeeze" or "breathe" or a short phrase like "pinch those scapulae together" or "hold the core" to cue the movement behavior.

My editor provided a wonderful personal account of how this technique worked for her. "I used the self-talk strategy about 5 years ago. I talked to myself out loud primarily while walking to and from the bus—very early in the morning and then evening, so not many people were around to wonder about this woman talking constantly to herself! The topic of my self-talk was how great it was to have better eating habits. I would list all the new habits I wanted to have but would talk as if I already had them. I'd rhapsodize about how great it was not to be enslaved to food, how much more pleasant my encounters with food were, how empowering it was to eat slowly and savour small amounts of the food I loved instead of pigging out and then feeling fat and disgusted with myself. I didn't 'diet' at all. I simply found that after a few weeks of doing this, my habits began to change to be consistent with my self-talk. I lost 20 lb in the first year and have lost 15 more since then. I don't believe I would have been successful had I not, in the first few months, held these extensive 'conversations' with myself. Hearing the statements repeatedly out loud helped me remember, when tempted by an unhealthy eating choice, to challenge the poor eating habits that were so ingrained in my head. If I find myself slipping, I use the strategy again until I get back on track."

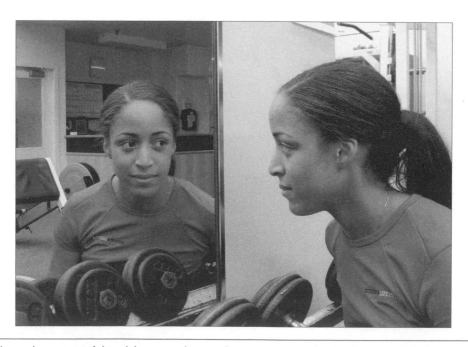

Positive self-talk can be a powerful tool for your clients who are trying to change their eating habits. Encourage them to talk positively to themselves about how they eat—they can even do this out loud whenever they use a mirror—provided there are no bystanders!

Negative self-talk is as destructive as positive self-talk is helpful. Thus, you must learn the technique of **reframing** to help clients avoid negative self-talk that can sabotage their motivation. For instance, reframe guilt about time away from the office as an earned time-out and an investment in future energy. Encourage your client to regard that minor muscle soreness as the stage before the important rebuilding phase. After a shortened workout, remind your client that the smallest good deed is better than the grandest intention.

Promoting Self-Efficacy

Dishman (1990) referred to an individual's self-efficacy as an ability to match behavior to behavior intentions in the face of competing external pressures. Self-efficacy is extremely important in the early stages of exercise adoption and critical in its role of confronting barriers. Self-efficacy is one of the strongest predictors of exercise behavior.

Six principle sources of self-efficacy have been identified (Ball 2001). Here they are, along with examples of how you can provide these to your clients:

1. **Performance accomplishment:** Look for opportunities to identify training successes to raise the level of self-efficacy.

2. **Vicarious experience:** Use techniques such as exercise demonstrations and your own personal example to help clients learn new skills.

3. **Verbal persuasion:** Use encouragement and verbal cueing to keep clients positive and focused.

4. **Imaging experiences:** Use imagery to build confidence. For example, during balance or proprioceptive tasks, ask your client to close his eyes and visualize full stability and flawless execution.

5. **Physiological states:** Some clients may associate an elevated heart rate with anxiety and perceived incompetence. Try to reframe it as a sign of readiness for performance.

6. **Emotional states:** Depression and low self-efficacy may accompany a client with an injury. Have her picture full function and then show some progress; she will feel more energized about rehabilitation and may experience enhanced self-efficacy.

We must help our clients develop the confidence to act by tapping into these opportunities to facilitate self-efficacy.

Planning for Relapse

Relapse is almost inevitable, and you should be prepared for it. By working through the *Relapse Planner* (p. 49) with your client in the early stages of his program, you may be able to minimize serious relapse. When small lapses occur, remind your client of the strategies you have already used. If new challenges arise, discuss them and add them, along with tactics for countering them, to the *Relapse Planner*. And if a major relapse occurs, use the *Relapse Planner* to motivate the client to address the problem.

Be sure that the client always has a copy of the most recent version of the planner, and encourage him to review it periodically. Always be positive and encouraging as you try to help your client overcome the tendency to drop out. Use statements like the following to help clients to deal positively and effectively with relapse: "I know you may feel discouraged, but it's normal for everyone to experience these setbacks. If we keep working together, we'll find that key or strategies that will work for you. So don't give up!"

Here are some examples of typical high-risk situations and some approaches that have worked in dealing with them:

High-risk situations

- People at work ask me to go for drinks after work, which is my usual workout time.

Suggested solutions

- Tell everyone my regular workout schedule so they'll consider it when they're choosing a time to go out.
- Join them later.
- Schedule a makeup time every week to cope with any unplanned changes.
- Restrict how many times a week I go out for drinks after work; if I do want to go out, schedule alternative workout times a couple of times a week.

High-risk situation

- I'm afraid to walk after work when it gets dark and rainy in the winter.

Suggested solutions

- Ask my friend to join me.
- Use the community "safe walk" program.
- Walk at lunch or only when it is daylight.

High-risk situation

- I can't jog or even walk briskly when my shin splints return.

Suggested solutions

- Get fitted for orthotics.
- Start cross-training or rest at the first signs of discomfort.
- Ask my trainer to prescribe some supplemental exercises to help prevent the onset of shin splints.

Despite all your efforts to help your clients overcome relapse (or inertia at the beginning of your work together), some of them may still have problems organizing their lives to support a more holistic, balanced lifestyle. For these clients, consider suggesting that they add lifestyle coaching to their repertoire of relapse-fighting tools. **Lifestyle coaching** is a collaborative effort where clients present a situation and then work with a coach to set goals, explore possibilities, remove barriers, and create an action plan that suits the client's needs and values. The coach's job focuses on providing support to enhance the skills, resources, and creativity that the client already has (Cantwell 2003). If your client is considering using a coach, give her the following tips:

- Select a coach very carefully, because the relationship between you and your coach is critical.
- Although the Internet is a good way to initially check for rates and any niche market specialists, rely on word of mouth from a reliable reference.
- Check credentials and experience.
- Ask a prospective coach to give you a complementary first session, which provides a great opportunity to judge the fit before you commit.

Using Extrinsic and Intrinsic Motivators

Many clients start exercise expecting rewards or outcomes such as weight loss, disease reduction, performance, or other health outcomes. If these changes do not happen quickly (and they generally do not), these clients may become discouraged or quit because their expectations are not being met. To prevent this from happening, you must become skilled at using extrinsic and intrinsic motivators. Extrinsic motivators are not essentially part of the goal: for example, the chance to win a monetary award by completing a fitness program at work. Intrinsic motivators are an essential outcome of something valued for its own sake: for example, exercising because you love how it increases your energy. Most clients must be kept motivated extrinsically long enough to experience the positive effects of activity that will give them the intrinsic motivation that is critical in maintaining long-term exercise (Kimiecik 1998).

Using Extrinsic Motivators

Extrinsic motivators are great to get people going. But the rewards and recognitions you use must be psychologically satisfying to your client. At my college, we have tried gift certificates, free personal training sessions, and even money. However, by asking clients directly, we found that they preferred either a recognition T-shirt that they would proudly wear in the center or their name up on the display. The concept that behavior that is rewarded is repeated appears to be true only if the extrinsic incentive is client-focused. Another example: We get a much more positive reaction to sending a card on the client's birthday than to sending a thank-you letter that is perceived as standard issue; both take the same effort and expense. Responsiveness to your client's needs means customizing the services and motivation you provide whenever possible. Better hotels and restaurants are masters at customized motivation. They will greet you by name, find your favorite table, or mention something thoughtful from the last visit. Each is an extrinsic motivator but because it is client-centered, it shapes our behavior and we return our patronage.

Clients who expect quick results (usually people just entering the action stage of change) are often so disappointed that they quit. Extrinsic motivators are crucial for these people. I have found that some of the extrinsic motivators in the following list can be effective:

- **Motivation through a phone call.** Call your client periodically. If he knows you will be calling, he may work out just so he can honestly tell you he did it.
- **Motivation through variety.** Get involved with clients to refine or add variety to their programs.
- **Motivation through music.** Find out what music your client likes and use it. This may help to prolong his energy during a cardiovascular workout.
- **Motivation through change.** Organize a novelty activity, perhaps with a new social group.

Relapse Planner

How confident are you that you'll keep doing your physical activity during the next three months?

Not confident at all	_____	1
Not very confident	_____	2
Somewhat confident	_____	3
Confident	_____	4
Very confident	_____	5

If your score was less than 4, complete the following exercise:

Many people have periods of inactivity. Sometimes these breaks can last for just a few days and sometimes a few years. Planning ahead for the tough times may help you stay active.

1. Have you ever had trouble keeping your physical activity going before? If so, write the reasons.

_____

_____

2. If you have had trouble, what has helped you get back on track (e.g., support from friends, joining a class, setting goals)?

_____

_____

3. What situations do you think would make it tough to keep your physical activity routine? How will you handle these situations to increase your chances of being successful?

_____

_____

High-risk situations   Solutions

_____

_____

_____

4. What will help you get started again if you do have a break? Write down your ideas.

Start-up strategies

_____

_____

From *Client-Centered Exercise Prescription, Second Edition,* by John C. Griffin, 2006, Champaign, IL: Human Kinetics. Reprinted, with permission, from *The Canadian Physical Activity, Fitness & Lifestyle Appraisal: CSEP's Plan for Healthy Active Living.* Published by the Canadian Society for Exercise Physiology, 2003.

- **Motivation through a partner.** Pair your client with a partner. If the partner is reliable, the ongoing commitment is very helpful. People are more likely to exercise if they know someone is waiting for them.

Developing Intrinsic Motivators

There is clearly a role for well-designed extrinsic motivators, but unless clients develop some intrinsic motivators, they're not likely to continue regular activity. People simply never reach the maintenance stage without intrinsic motivators. Wheeler (2000) reminded us that change must occur within the person (intrinsic change). To support this process with our clients, we must constantly reinforce facts and ways of thinking to ensure the following:

1. They are aware of the reasons and need for making changes.
2. They perceive the meaning and importance of the change.
3. They see that benefits for the change outweigh the costs.
4. They feel confident in their abilities to maintain new behaviors.
5. They have realistic outcome expectations and revisit them often.
6. They recognize that change takes time and effort.

These are elements that you must help clients grasp and remember if they are to achieve intrinsic motivation. The process is often an accumulation of experiences that come as the client stays with the program for a significant period of time—experiences that will tend to create intrinsic motivation. We can facilitate and support this process within our clients based on principles such as those just listed. Let's take a look at some motivational techniques and how they can reinforce intrinsic change.

- **Motivation through monitoring.** There is no better immediate and ongoing method of showing the benefits of a training program than well-designed monitoring of progressive improvement. Some clients will want to see concrete changes attributable to their fitness programs. For example, your client may want to see if his heart rate is decreasing with the same amount of work over a period of 2 months. Visually recording or plotting items that are monitored clearly shows clients the benefits of their efforts.
- **Motivation through increased knowledge.** Knowing good reasons for exercise and for correct diet may encourage your client to make additional changes in his lifestyle. In addition, some of your clients will be very interested in the technical side of the exercise process. Once I recognize that a client has a specific interest, I often bring in a related article or brochure and discuss how it relates to his situation.
- **Motivation through retesting.** If your client knows you will be retesting him in 3 weeks, this may encourage him to continue faithfully with the program. To move this from extrinsic to intrinsic, provide some guidance as to what is realistic; the test results can provide your client with confidence in his ability to reach outcome expectations.
- **Motivation through goal and program modification.** Set a time to update goals and reinforce the goals already achieved. Intrinsic rewards come from reaching goals and setting down more challenging prescriptions.
- **Motivation through supervision.** Through personal contact, a personal trainer or staff supervising within a facility can increase awareness and importance of regular activity. Your support can help build confidence and prevent relapse.

Improving Adherence With Effective Problem Solving

We assume that our clients have good intentions to start or maintain an exercise program. There will be times, however, when they discontinue the program for various reasons. They may have long periods of time when other priorities preclude regular physical activity, leading to feelings of guilt and a drop in self-esteem. Emphasize to these clients that they are not failures, and help them seize this opportunity to refocus on some start-up strategies. The *Relapse Planner* presented on page 49 is useful for those who have discontinued their regular activity (CSEP 2003).

When clients are not compliant with your exercise prescriptions, review their situation and behavior over the previous weeks in a nonthreatening manner. Listen carefully to what they tell you and try a rational problem-solving approach. Here is a process and some questions to ask:

- Does the program still seem like it is meeting your needs?

  (Establish whether the client clearly understands the link between your prescription and her goals. Have her priorities changed?)
- Is the prescription appropriate or are you having any problems with the exercises?

(Establish if the program is appropriate for her levels of fitness.)

- Are external barriers getting in the way of regular activity?

  (For example, establish if the program's time frame is realistic. Has there been a change in the client's work or home life?)

- What alternatives can get you back on track?

  (Musing on the issues identified, brainstorm some possibilities.)

- Considering the pros and cons of each alternative, what do you think is your best choice?

  (Help your client examine the choices, consequences, and personal benefits.)

- What do you think will help you stick with this program?

  (Establish a follow-up that is consistent with your client's preferred reinforcement system and establish strategies for commitment.)

Table 2.2 suggests some client-centered approaches to solving problems and increasing adherence.

Table 2.2   Effective Problem Solving to Improve Adherence

Client information	Problem-solving strategies
Overweight clients may have to struggle more and may have unrealistic expectations about what can be accomplished.	Be honest and help clients form realistic goals. Provide monitoring techniques that clearly show their progress. Avoid positive feedback that is undeserved, but look for opportunities for recognition of progress. Use social support systems such as "buddies" or a personal trainer if good rapport is present.
Clients need to be aware of the benefits and costs of their fitness program.	Help your clients list the benefits they hope to experience and also the inconveniences and difficulties they may encounter. Discuss how they will deal with these.
Smokers have difficulty sticking with exercise.	Give permission to feel winded and less energized after exercise. Avoid making smoking a big issue, but have literature available.
A client's personality problems or mood may affect attendance.	Don't assume that you are responsible for how your clients feel or for the fact that they often miss sessions because of mood disturbances.
Improvement of health is often given as a reason for initiating exercise.	Point out the specific health benefits that may be expected from their type of prescription. Use screening tools (e.g., PAR-Q or FANTASTIC Lifestyle Checklist) to assure clients that they are ready for exercise and increase their health-related awareness.
There are large differences in goals and activity for specific ages and sexes. In one study, competition was seen as a benefit for young men and health for young women, whereas health was seen as a barrier for older men and women (De Bourdeauhuij and Sallis 2002).	Emphasize to seniors that improved health should reduce that barrier. Use careful monitoring and appropriate prescription to keep activities manageable and safe.
Satisfaction with you as an exercise specialist is an important issue for many clients.	Seek your clients' input on many aspects of goal setting, techniques of training, variations in routines, and satisfaction. Give your clients feedback about their progress and solicit their feedback about your abilities as a trainer. Provide support and be available.
Clients often have trouble getting past common road blocks.	Consider the following responses, as suggested by Patrick and colleagues (1994): (a) If time is the barrier: "We're aiming for three 30-minute sessions each week. Do you watch a lot of TV? If so, maybe cut out three TV shows a week?" (b) If enjoyment is a problem: "Don't exercise. Start a hobby or an enjoyable activity that gets you moving." (c) If exercise is boring: "Listening to music during your activity keeps your mind occupied. Walking, biking, or running can take you past lots of interesting scenery."

I recall a female client, Marie, who worked outside the home and had two children, ages 6 and 8. She had a low estimation of her physical capabilities and had even expressed doubts about her need to exercise. She exercised with me two times a week for 3 weeks but did not work out at all during the fourth week. Her reason was that she had deadlines at work. On the weekend I happened to meet her in the neighborhood park. In an emotional confessional she gave me the following reasons for stopping her exercise program:

1. I want to exercise, but by the time 5:00 comes around, I am not able to leave. I have too many things left to do.

2. I don't have the time. I have too many other responsibilities: I work, I have to do grocery shopping, pick up the kids, take them to lessons, help with their homework, cook dinner, make lunches. . . . Get the picture?

3. It will take too long to make a dent in my weight gain. I am so heavy, why even bother?

Of the reasons Marie gave, what do you think is the main issue and how would you address it? Remember: Program adherence is not an all-or-nothing situation. We need to be flexible to allow for real life. Determine how you would respond to Marie, and then read *Convincing the Unconvinced*.

Convincing the Unconvinced

Marie was overwhelmed. Exercise seemed like just one more thing to fit into a busy day. Our six sessions were prescheduled and prepaid, and that, along with the motivation of having a training partner (me), was enough to get her started. But once those sessions were over, her enthusiasm fizzled. That Sunday afternoon we met and had a very open chat. She thought that the prescription was meeting her fitness needs and was at the appropriate level, but there were too many barriers in the way of making it a regular habit. I sensed that we needed to change the way Marie thought about her activity. She was more concerned about providing justification to me than she was about her own well-being. She had to reconnect with her original reasons for starting and the meaning and importance of making the change.

We spent a fair amount of time talking about the demands of her work and home life . . . and they were significant. We talked about some of the ways that she might get back on track and how the fitness benefits could outweigh the costs of committed time. But the real breakthrough came when we talked about her children. She truly wanted to be fit enough to be an active mom, but sheer "kid maintenance" was leaving her drained. So I said, "Why not take a break for 30 minutes every day with no kids, no work . . . time just for you to enjoy some activity!" Her eyes widened! "Think of it as an active minivacation. Line up your favorite music, forget about the task of weight loss, and just enjoy the time to yourself. Your relaxation and confidence will increase if you accept that change is a process, and although it takes time, there is every reason to enjoy the process." Marie's energy level increased over the weeks and although some of it was attributable to the physiological improvements, the commitment was caused by her frame of mind, realistic expectations, and refocus on a new reinforcement.

Case Studies

In the three case studies that follow, consider how you would apply appropriate client-centered motivating tactics. It may be helpful to think of yourself in three distinct roles—as a leader, a designer, and as an educator. **Leadership** involves the way in which you approach and support your client. **Design** includes developing creative programs, devising incentives, and meeting goals. **Education** relates to how you provide information in a client-centered way, how you engender feedback, and how you create autonomy in your client.

Case Study 1: Motivating a New Client

Trent was a young, single accountant who had just joined a local club. Audrey worked at the club as a personal trainer and met Trent for the first time during his appointment for an assessment. Audrey sensed some apprehension and so spent time listening carefully until Trent was more comfortable sharing his feelings.

Counseling and Assessment

"When people come to the center for the first time, Trent, they nearly always feel overwhelmed with the new equipment and protocols. I'll guide you through all of this, and we'll have a chance to talk about each stage of the assessment."

The assessment was a good time to build rapport through telling a personal story:

"I really can appreciate how hard it is to make the changes in your lifestyle that you'd like to make. There are a lot of obstacles. I've struggled with some of them myself. When I first came to work at this club, all the state-of-the-art machines were terribly intimidating. Just like in your line of work, I gradually added a few new pieces of equipment to my exercise 'portfolio' every day. I'll help you do the same, but we'll focus on the ones that are right for you. We'll start with more simple exercises using your own body weight, and each week we'll introduce a new piece of equipment. OK?"

Audrey's feedback during and after the assessment was both specific and encouraging.

A: I don't very often see someone as flexible as you in the shoulders, Trent—especially when you have such good strength in your pectoralis and other chest muscles.

T: I didn't realize that these tests provided that degree of detail.

A: Yes, in fact, your aerobic capacity places you in an above-average category. You scored better than 75% of other men your age.

T: That's encouraging, but I'm not about to run a marathon tomorrow.

A: Maybe not, but we'll set some smaller goals that will still be pretty challenging.

Trent had remarked on the professional quality of the test result information. Audrey was pleased at how the test results led to discussion about goals and possible outcomes. In addition to his exercise prescription, Trent was keen to get some squash lessons and to avoid the type of high-intensity running he remembered from 10 years earlier in high school.

T: About these goals: I hope you won't be like my high school physical education teacher—he was brutal!

A: Well, the good news is that you'll set your own objectives. I'll help you make them measurable, but the commitment will be to yourself.

T: I want to be able to finish a squash game as strongly as I start it.

A: That's both realistic and challenging. It will help us plan your exercise prescription, and if we monitor your perceived exertion during squash, we can keep track of your progress.

Because Trent was unfamiliar with the equipment, Audrey scheduled her time to be with him for his entire workouts during the first week. This gave her time to improve Trent's technical skills and to share many personal anecdotes about her own training. At the end of the week, Audrey presented Trent with a club T-shirt and her phone number and e-mail address in case of problems.

Overcoming Problems

Things went well for a few weeks, but Audrey started to notice that Trent was not working out as often. She set up a meeting and learned that Trent's new career was demanding and his commitment to his program was slipping. Recognizing how important the first 3 months of a new habit are, Audrey helped Trent set up an exercise diary with a copy for his office and one for his refrigerator at home. Audrey marked every Monday as a time that she would e-mail Trent to check in on the week to come. Trent appreciated a 10% discount incentive on his squash lessons that Audrey arranged if he checked in with her on his squash days. Trent gravitated toward the squash and started running

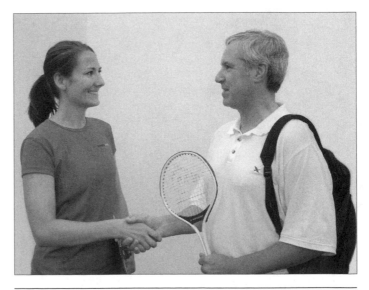

Because Audrey paid attention to and capitalized on Trent's developing interest in squash and gave him realistic and effective strategies for dealing with his overtraining tendencies, her work was key in helping him develop an active lifestyle.

on his own to build his stamina. Early in this running craze, Trent competed in a 10K run and came limping back to Audrey. Her approach was to design a running schedule and set more short-term objectives that allowed Trent to perceive progress in his program more easily. Trent found a squash partner and now, after 1 full year of club membership, he meets with Audrey every 4 months for a fitness assessment or a prescription update.

Questions to Think About

- How did Audrey's support of Trent change after the first few weeks?
- What adjustments to Trent's program did Audrey make when his commitment was slipping?
- How did feedback in the early encounters differ from that at the end of the year? Was the change necessary?

Case Study 2: Motivating an Intermittent Exerciser

Jane, a single mother of two, had a busy schedule that found her on and off exercise for many years. The community fitness center had asked Tony, a personal fitness trainer, to work with her because both still played some competitive baseball. Jane was just returning to the center after her second child and wanted to get in shape before the baseball season. Tony realized that Jane's yo-yo pattern occurred when exercise was crowded out by her

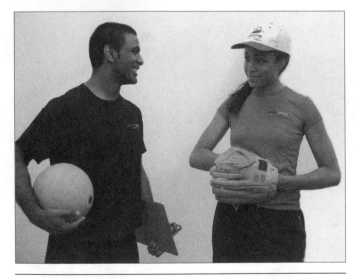

Tony helped Jane become active through targeted counseling based on their conversations: he enabled her to identify and deal with the guilt she felt about taking time for herself; showed her how to build exercise into her busy routine through active living; and introduced her to new and interesting exercise activities.

work schedule, home duties, or vacations. She also admitted that her exercise routine would take a downward spiral when she couldn't see any results, it wasn't fun, or it was boring.

Counseling and Assessment

"I know at times you don't see the type of progress you'd like, but you are very effective when you do work out more regularly. Everyone I work with goes through short relapses for various reasons. I appreciate that it's hard to make an ongoing commitment. I've struggled with this myself. We can take a look at your overall approach to an exercise habit."

Jane always believed that she was taking time from someone or something else when she exercised. Tony started their second meeting by discussing these feelings. He wanted to help Jane realize that slippage in attendance did not imply failure and that the time spent exercising would more than pay back benefits and quality of time to job and family.

"Jane, I've noticed how concerned you are about your family and about the time you spend away from them. I admire your devotion and care. They are rare qualities. Your support and encouragement are important. In working with many single parents, I've found it important to remember that the better care you take of yourself—physically and emotionally—the better you can care for the people you love."

He worked with Jane on some positive self-talk. They developed some questions that highlighted the benefits of regular workouts. Whenever Jane started to feel guilty about taking time to exercise, she reviewed these questions in her mind:

- "How does exercise make me feel later in the day?"
- "How do I feel after completing a workout that I originally had planned to skip?"
- "What are some of the positive feelings I get with a good workout?"

Dealing With Time Commitments

Tony's second approach tackled the problem of not enough time. He introduced Jane to the concept of **active living,** whereby, during hectic weeks, she could substitute walking to work, taking the stairs, and doing manual chores for her formal workout. Since Jane's exercise pattern was usually irregular (fewer than six workouts per month), Tony discussed the benefits of adding only a few more sessions per month and slightly increasing the intensity of her workouts.

Knowing that injury can be a major reason for dropping out, Tony adjusted her previous prescription and introduced some interesting cross-training variety in her new program. Subsequent progressions were regular and became more specific to baseball. Jane thought she now had the right attitude and approach to maintain a more regular, healthy, and balanced lifestyle.

Questions to Think About

- What leadership qualities did Tony demonstrate that were well-suited to helping Jane?
- Select one feature of Tony's exercise prescription and explain why it was appropriate for Jane.
- How did Tony influence Jane's attitude toward regular exercise?

Case Study 3: Motivating an Impatient Client

It occurs more often than you may think. You are scheduled to meet a client for the first time and within a few minutes you realize that his expectations are to get moving as soon as possible. The client may not say "let's get moving," but you read this in his nonverbal communication. This does not mean that you should discard the Activity Counseling Model (chapter 1) or that you necessarily have a problem. This situation only becomes a problem if you don't recognize and adapt to it. You should begin by being supportive, empathetic, and appreciative of the uniqueness of your client.

Counseling and Information Gathering

Clients "on the go" are often systematic, analytic, organized, pragmatic, energetic, and a leader in their own domains. Recognizing that, try treatment strategies that are businesslike, stimulating, and fast paced and that include the client's input.

Many clients may have spent a long time deciding to begin an exercise program, and now they want to get started right away. This will require that you reduce the initial time with the interview and exploration. After some essential counseling, engage the client in activity and integrate more information gathering and selected counseling strategies as the sessions progress. In fact, it is common that after the client begins activity, she experiences an increase in interest and a greater recognition of the benefits and enjoyment. Once a client starts to get "hooked," she is much more responsive to new information and suggestions.

The prescription process should be flexible, allowing you to loop back and verify needs through selective assessments after some lighter activity is initiated.

The initial consultation with a client will be more challenging with the hurried format. The fundamental purpose of this session is to gather information about the client that will help you design a safe and appropriate exercise program and motivation strategy. It is our task to help clients see the issues before them in more focused and concrete ways. Work together to come up with a few priorized objectives and then break the goals down into a number of distinct and sometimes progressive steps. Early discussions should clarify what clients hope to gain or learn and why they are there. Once you know your client's stage of change, you can choose strategies that are effective for that stage (table 2.1). Ensure that change occurs within the person (intrinsic). At any stage, try to help clients find the inner motivation so necessary to maintain physical activity.

A big part of commitment is not just setting clear objectives but also having awareness of the "why" behind the objective. Ask your client to explain how it felt when he was fit or how it might feel when he has achieved his objective. "Boarding effortlessly through the powder," "feeling strong and energetic," and "enjoying the morning sun on a bicycle ride" are all responses that make an emotional connection with the decision to be active. If you can help your clients make that connection and focus on that captured visualization, you've helped them take the first step to becoming intrinsically motivated.

FP: We've done the health history questionnaire and I think we can safely move on.

CL: Good. I'm anxious to get out on the floor. I'd like to do some free weights and the treadmill.

FP: I'm sure we can accommodate that request.

CL: Will we get at it today?

FP: What we can do today is get acquainted with some of the equipment and find out what level would be best for you to start at. Let's focus for a minute on your specific goals.

CL: I want to get back into running and build some muscle.

FP: You mentioned the charity 10K run in 4 month's time. We can set up a training schedule for that. Did you have a more specific objective for the weights? Why was this an area of concern?

CL: The running schedule sounds doable. As for the muscle work, I want to strengthen my abs. They are starting to look and feel flabby, and if I can make some improvements, I'll feel a lot better about my fitness and appearance.

FP: OK. If you are interested in trying some new techniques, I can show you a short ab routine on the Theraball.

CL: Hey, that sounds like more fun than sit-ups.

FP: Yes, but it is still a challenge. Next session I'll have some of these things documented on your program card, but right now let's move to the floor and we'll get started.

Safe and Snappy Prescription Guidelines

Ensure that all screening and health forms have been completed (see chapter 3). If no formal assessment has taken place, the initial activity should be a sample with a duration of about half the anticipated full prescription. Use the warm-up as an opportunity to see how the client reacts to light aerobic loads, basic body mechanics, and confidence. Monitor intensity and form, continuously looking for any signs of distress, discomfort, or imbalance. Keep the exertion levels moderate, below the level that you anticipate prescribing in the future.

With safety well established, focus on your client's enjoyment of the workout. Small apparatuses may be easiest and most fun to use. Many of these items are affordable and convenient for home use. Design a program that is dynamic and continuous. Mix an ample share of new and interesting exercises (see figure 2.1). Keep them simple, allowing for minimum teaching and maximum use. Stay close physically for both spotting and tactile cueing. Maintain a brisk pace with an organized series of exercises that hold the interest of your client. Use continuous verbal encouragement and positive feedback to keep the pace of the session high. Try to reinforce the client's objectives

and any emotional connection made earlier (e.g., "This should make those morning bicycle rides a little easier!").

Continue to watch your client carefully during the cool-down. Check with her as to how the workout felt physically and from an enjoyment perspective. Partner-assisted stretching can show some dramatic results at some joints and provide an opportunity to increase rapport. Important information gathering can happen at this point.

Monitoring on the Go

Monitoring in the hands of an informed personal fitness trainer is a very valuable tool. Monitoring can be passive, active, or interactive. As a passive activity it involves watching, observing, and tracking for a specific purpose; that is, to see something, you must be looking for it. You anticipate or expect a client to look or react in a standard manner with well-tolerated exercise. You also are watching the equipment and its function for safety and effectiveness. Active monitoring involves taking heart rate, monitoring perceived exertion, adjusting workloads, resisting or assisting partner exercises, and checking angles and alignments. Interactive monitoring requires a close and continuous communication with your client. Nonverbal cues may be as effective as spoken ones.

If you create standardized segments of your prescription, monitoring can be an effective alternative to formal assessment, which is very useful for this type of client. The information derived from monitoring provides personalized feedback and a basis for making changes or progressions in the program. Finally, the support, interest, and motivation provided by the monitoring are well suited to our systematic, pragmatic "on the go" client.

Questions to Think About

- Are there any safety issues that have been compromised by moving at this pace?
- During the dialogue, did it appear that the client was motivated? Extrinsically or intrinsically? How could you help him increase the awareness of his intrinsic changes?
- How does careful and selective monitoring allow the trainer to effectively deal with the impatient client?

Warm-up

Treadmill walk (monitor heart rate and perceived exertion)

2 min: light to moderate pace

3 min: moderate to brisk pace

2 min: continue with moderate to brisk pace or elevate by 3%

Final minute: Ease down and slow

Stretch: Front lunge (hip flexors)

    Chest to thigh (hamstrings)

    Wall stretch (gastrocnemius and soleus)

Workout

(1) Upper strength (tubing with handles):

    Narrow row (posterior shoulder and girdle)

      Lateral rotations (infraspinatus and teres minor)

      Biceps curls (on Bosu ball)

    Stretch: Mecca position (push, relax, reach)

(2) Strength and balance (Bosu ball round-up):

    Partial squat (quads, glutes, hams, lower leg)

    Push-up, two legs and one leg (chest, triceps, core)

    Stretch: Proprioceptive neuromuscular facilitation: Quads and hamstrings

(3) Core stability (Theraball):

    Bridge: roll out and back

    T-bridge side roll

    Stretch: Standing side reach and hold

Final stretch

Supine star, then pull knees to chest

Figure 2.1   Sample introductory workout.

Highlights

1. **Apply motivational strategies to help clients through various stages of exercise adoption.**

    The counseling skills and tools outlined in the previous chapter included a number of strategic plans to help clients through various stages of exercise adoption.

    By understanding your client's stage of change, knowing the change process appropriate to that stage, and choosing strategies that will facilitate the change process, you will help your client recognize the relevance of the message for herself and understand how it fits with her personal needs. This recognition and understanding are the beginning of motivation.

2. **Use the change process strategies that are appropriate at each stage of change.**

    To motivate people, use the change process strategies that are appropriate at each stage of change. For example, you should help the precontemplative person become aware of the activity and health message. You will be most effective here by using some form of consciousness-raising interaction with the client as outlined in table 2.1.

3. **Help clients commit to their objectives.**

Making decisions and moving into action require the client to commit physical and psychological resources. Several factors that we can control can help our clients commit to, then follow through on, their objectives: **Ownership:** Offer activity options that come from the client, not you. **Options:** Provide a choice of activities. **Reinforcement:** Provide encouragement. **Appeal:** Look for ways to make the workout more pleasant. **Obstacle management:** Help clients see how to manage disincentives. **Challenge:** Help clients set challenging objectives. **Contracts:** Help clients commit themselves to their choices.

Perhaps the most important factor in commitment, however, is the client's own belief that she is capable of committing to her goals and objectives, following through on that commitment, and reaching her goals. Two excellent strategies for helping a client embrace this belief are encouraging self-talk and promoting self-efficacy.

4. **Describe the role and provide examples of extrinsic motivation, and apply motivational techniques that will reinforce intrinsic change to healthy behaviors.**

Many clients start exercise expecting rewards or outcomes such as weight loss, disease reduction, better performance, or other health outcomes. If these changes do not happen quickly (and they generally do not), these clients may become discouraged or quit because their expectations are not being met. These clients may not experience activity for its own sake and thus miss the process of developing positive intrinsic experiences that are critical in maintaining long-term exercise. There is clearly a role for well-designed extrinsic motivators, but unless clients develop some intrinsic motivators, they're not likely to continue regular activity. To support this process with our clients, we must constantly reinforce the facts and ways of thinking to ensure the following:

- Clients are aware of the reasons and need for making changes.
- They perceive the meaning and importance of the change.
- They see that benefits for the change must outweigh the costs.
- They feel confident in their abilities to maintain new behaviors.
- They have realistic outcome expectations, which they think about often.
- They recognize that change is a process that takes time and effort.

5. **Suggest some client-centered approaches to solving problems that will increase exercise adherence.**

We initially assume that our clients have good intentions to start or maintain an exercise program. There will be times, however, when they discontinue the program for various reasons. They may have long periods of time when other priorities preclude regular physical activity, leading to feelings of guilt and a drop in self-esteem. Emphasize to these clients that they are not failures, and help them seize this opportunity to refocus on some start-up strategies. Review the situation and behavior of clients who are not compliant with your exercise prescriptions, listening carefully and trying a rational problem-solving approach. The problem-solving approach should reexamine priorities, prescription fit, external barriers, alternatives, personal benefits, and incentives. Table 2.2 suggests some client-centered approaches to solving problems and increasing adherence.

6. **Apply appropriate client-centered motivating tactics in case study scenarios.**

Three case studies applied specific client-centered motivating tactics for a new client, an intermittent exerciser, and an impatient client. The situation often demands distinct roles—as a leader, a designer, and an educator. **Leadership** involves the way in which you approach and support your client. **Design** includes developing creative programs, devising incentives, and meeting goals. **Education** relates to how you provide information in a client-centered way, how you engender feedback, and how you create autonomy in your client.

Principles of Client-Centered Assessment and Prescription

Chapter Competencies

After completing this chapter, you will be able to demonstrate the following competencies:

1. Be "client-centered" in your approach to assessment and prescription.

2. Use lifestyle appraisal tools to change behavior.

3. Screen your clients for risk factors and symptoms.

4. Select appropriate test items suited to the client.

5. Describe three potential outcomes of client-centered exercise prescription.

6. Identify guidelines for prescription for health-related fitness.

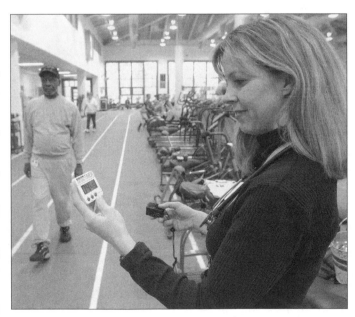

7. Identify guidelines for prescription for general fitness.

8. Identify guidelines for prescription for performance-related fitness.

9. Create a safe, balanced exercise prescription.

In client-centered assessment, we look for things our clients want to do that will satisfy their most important needs and complement or at least accommodate their lifestyles. Every client is at a different stage of readiness to make changes in his or her lifestyle (chapter 1). If we learn to view assessment in terms of stages, we deviate from two rather standard practices: (a) We do not perform assessments before establishing priorities, and (b) we do not use a predetermined battery of tests that cover most fitness components.

When prescribing exercise, you should use an approach to problem solving or a formalized decision flow that is appropriate for our discipline. We too often want to give our client the newest exercise or equipment we've seen, whether it is appropriate or not. When we formulate a client-centered prescription, we should make decisions by progressing through the issues systematically, making informed selections from a menu of options. As important as the individual exercises within a prescription may be, their chance for success depends on whether we have considered all options and made appropriate decisions.

Client-Centered Assessment

Both initially and on an ongoing basis, a client's exercise prescription should be validated by using the baseline values for components of fitness and using appropriate laboratory or field-based assessment tools. But also remember that first impressions are strong and lasting. If the first thing you do is probe and prod and induce fatigue, clients with low self-esteem may leave with less resolve to change than they had when they entered. Take sufficient time to establish clients' commitment, question them carefully, and focus on their areas of concern.

Health and Lifestyle Appraisal

We need to understand the links between physical activity, health, and physical fitness. It is preferable to assess a client's health status and lifestyle during the early phase of counseling, before other assessments. We also can use this information for preassessment screening.

The human body does not function optimally when it is abused. The major causes of disability and death are no longer infectious diseases but rather diseases of lifestyle. Behaviors that contribute to various chronic illnesses include alcohol and drug abuse, smoking, inappropriate diets, and insufficient physical activity. Elements of a healthy lifestyle include positive attitude toward self and others, ability to cope with stress, a zeal for life, and the practice of healthy behaviors. Early recognition of and empathy with our clients' lifestyles help us set priorities and plan well-rounded fitness programs.

A health risk appraisal, or, more positively, a health and lifestyle appraisal, may be a client's first step to behavior change. It may be just the extra nudge that a client preparing to take some action needs. Its greatest value is as a tool that leads to healthy lifestyle intervention. Inactivity is so common that we have a critical role to play as providers and promoters of health care. In the next sections we examine some useful lifestyle appraisal tools.

- **FANTASTIC Lifestyle Checklist**. This checklist (page 61) allows clients to understand the effects of various habits and attitudes on their health (Wilson and Ciliska 1984). Most lifestyle behaviors can be modified: activity, nutrition, tobacco or alcohol use, sleep, stress, and personality. The scoring system provides a straightforward interpretation of health benefits associated with behavior change. The structure of the checklist makes it easy to discuss results with clients. The checklist directs clients to their lifestyle areas that need attention and provides tips to help people make the appropriate changes.

- **RISK-I.** *Risk-I* (pronounced "risky") can be self-administered and involves selecting the appropriate numerical value in each of the risk categories on the chart (Canadian Society for Exercise Physiology [CSEP] 2003; Getchell and Anderson 1982; NIH, NHLBI 1998). The first five categories (age, family history, smoking, body mass index, and exercise) are risk factors for coronary heart disease. The last two categories (back and knees) are areas of musculoskeletal risk. You can use the total score, which represents overall risk, to screen clients for a medical referral. *RISK-I*'s application is broader than most tools because of the inclusion of musculoskeletal risk. Although the scoring is not precise, it opens the opportunity to talk to clients about a broad spectrum of issues that may need attention in their exercise prescription.

- **Physical Activity Index (PAI).** Physical activity and fitness reinforce each other. Just as the most fit people tend to be the most active, the most active are frequently the most fit, and the components of fitness are determined by patterns of habitual physical activity. Physical activity questionnaires can help determine the health

FANTASTIC Lifestyle Checklist

Instructions: Unless otherwise specified, place an 'X' beside the box that best describes your behavior or situation in the past month. Explanations of questions and scoring are provided on the next page.

Adapted with permission from the "Fantastic Lifestyle Assessments" © 1995, Dr. Douglas Wilson, Department of Family Medicine, McMaster University, Hamilton, Ontario, Canada L8N 3Z5

Family Friends	I have someone to talk to about things that are important to me	almost never	seldom	some of the time	fairly often	almost always
	I give and receive affection	almost never	seldom	some of the time	fairly often	almost always
Activity	I am vigorously active for at least 30 min per day (e.g., running, cycling, etc.)	less than once a week	1-2 times/week	3 times/week	4 times/week	5 or more times/week
	I am moderately active (gardening, climbing stairs, walking, housework)	less than once a week	1-2 times/week	3 times/week	4 times/week	5 or more times/week
Nutrition	I eat a balanced diet (see explanation, page 43)	almost never	seldom	some of the time	fairly often	almost always
	I often eat excess: (1) sugar, or (2) salt, or (3) animal fats, or (4) junk foods	four of these	three of these	two of these	one of these	none of these
	I am within _____ kg of my healthy weight	not within 8 kg (20 lb)	8 kg (20 lb)	6 kg (15 lb)	4 kg (10 lb)	2 kg (5 lb)
Tobacco Toxics	I smoke tobacco	more than 10 times/week	1-10 times/week	none in the past 6 months	none in the past year	none in the past 5 years
	I use drugs such as marijuana, cocaine	sometimes				never
	I overuse prescribed drugs or 'over the counter' drugs	almost daily	fairly often	only occasionally	almost never	never
	I drink caffeine–containing coffee, tea, or cola	more than 10 times/week	7-10/day	3-6/day	1-2/day	never
Alcohol	My average alcohol intake per week is _____ (see explanation, page 43)	more than 20 drinks	13-20 drinks	11-12 drinks	8-10 drinks	0-7 drinks
	I drink more than four drinks on an occasion	almost daily	fairly often	only occasionally	almost never	never
	I drive after drinking	sometimes				never
Sleep Seatbelts Stress Safe sex	I sleep well and feel rested	almost never	seldom	some of the time	fairly often	almost always
	I use seatbelts	never	seldom	seldom	most of the time	always
	I am able to cope with the stresses in my life	almost never	seldom	seldom	fairly often	almost always
	I relax and enjoy leisure time	almost never	seldom	seldom	fairly often	almost always
	I practice safe sex (see explanation, page 43)	almost never	seldom	seldom	fairly often	always
Type of behavior	I seem to be in a hurry	almost always	fairly often	fairly often	seldom	almost never
	I feel angry or hostile	almost always	fairly often	fairly often	seldom	almost never
Insight	I am a positive or optimistic thinker	almost never	seldom	seldom	fairly often	almost always
	I feel tense or uptight	almost always	fairly often	fairly often	seldom	almost never
	I feel sad or depressed	almost always	fairly often	fairly often	seldom	almost never
Career	I am satisfied with my job or role	almost never	seldom	seldom	fairly often	almost always

Step 1 Total the X's in each column → ☐ ☐ ☐ ☐ ☐

Step 2 Multiply the totals by the numbers indicated (write answers in box below) → 0 ×1 ×2 ×3 ×4

Step 3 Add your scores across bottom for your grand total → ☐ + ☐ + ☐ + ☐ = ☐ Grand total (see explanation)

(continued)

▼ A balanced diet:

According to Canada's Food Guide to Healthy Eating (for people four years and over):

Different People Need Different Amounts of Food

The amount of food you need every day from the four food groups and other foods depends on your age, body size, activity level, whether you are male or female, and if you are pregnant or breast feeding. That's why the Food Guide gives a lower and higher number of servings for each food group. For example, young children can choose the lower number of servings, while male teenagers can select the higher number. Most other people can choose servings somewhere in between.

Grain products	Vegetables & fruit	Milk products	Meat & alternatives	Other foods
Choose whole grain and enriched products more often.	Choose dark green and orange vegetables more often.	Choose lower fat milk products more often.	Choose leaner meats, poultry and fish, as well as dried peas, beans, and lentils more often.	Taste and enjoyment can also come from other foods and beverages that are not part of the 4 food groups. Some of these are higher in fat or calories, so use these foods in moderation.
recommended number of servings per day:				
5-12	5-10	Children 4-9 yrs: 2-3 Youth 10-16 yrs: 3-4 Adults: 2-4 Pregnant and breast-feeding women: 3-4	2-3	

▼ Alcohol intake:

1 drink equals:

		Canadian	Metric	U.S.
1 bottle of beer	5% alcohol	12 oz.	340.8 ml	10 oz.
1 glass wine	12% alcohol	5 oz.	142 ml	4.5 oz.
1 shot spirits	40% alcohol	1.5 oz.	42.6 ml	1.25 oz.

▼ Safe sex:

Refers to the use of methods of preventing infection or conception.

What does the score mean?				
85-100 Excellent	70-84 Very good	55-69 Good	35-54 Fair	0-34 Needs improvement

Note: A low total score does not mean that you have failed. There is always the chance to change your lifestyle—starting now. Look at the areas where you scored a 0 or 1 and decide which areas you want to work on first.

Tips:

❶ Don't try to change all the areas at once. This will be too overwhelming for you.

❷ Writing down your proposed changes and your overall goal will help you to succeed.

❸ Make changes in small steps towards the overall goal.

❹ Enlist the help of a friend to make similar changes and/or to support you in your attempts.

❺ Congratulate yourself for achieving each step. Give yourself appropriate rewards.

❻ Ask your physical activity professional, family physician, nurse, or health department for more information on any of these areas.

From *Client-Centered Exercise Prescription, Second Edition,* by John C. Griffin, 2006, Champaign, IL: Human Kinetics. Adapted with permission from the "Fantastic Lifestyle Assessments" © 1995, Dr. Douglas Wilson, Department of Family Medicine, McMaster University, Hamilton, Ontario, Canada L8N 3Z5.

RISK-I

Select the number that best describes your situation for each of the following and compare the total score for an overall rating.

	1	2	3	4	5	Score
Age	20s	30s	40s	50s	60s	
Family history	No known heart disease	One relative over 50	Two relatives over 50	One relative under 50	Two relatives under 50	
Smoking	Nonuser	User <5 yrs ago	<10/day	10-20/day	>20/day	
Body mass index	18.5-23	24-27	28-31	32-35 or <18.5	>35	
Exercise	Active >2 times/week	Active 1-2 times/week	Moderately active 1-3 times/ month	Stopped activity <3 months ago	Sedentary	
Back	Healthy	Minor problems in past	Aches occasionally or after activity	Problems in past or current discomfort	Frequent problems/ diagnosed condition[a]	
Knees	Healthy	Minor problems in past	Occasional pain after vigorous activity	Problems in past or current discomfort	Frequent problems/ diagnosed condition[a]	
					Total score	

Family history: Count parents, grandparents, brothers, and sisters who have had a heart attack or stroke.

Smoking: If you inhale deeply or smoke a cigarette right down, add 1 to your score.

Body mass index (BMI): This is a measure of body proportion and a better indicator of risk than just weight (CSEP 2003). It is the ratio of body weight (in kilograms) divided by the square of height (in meters).

Example:

Weight = 75 kg Height = 1.72 m

$$BMI = 75/1.72^2$$
$$= 75/2.96$$
$$= 25.3 \text{ (RISK-I score = 25)}$$

Interpretation:

Total score	Rating
7-10	Very low risk
11-15	Low risk
16-20	Average risk
21-25	High risk
26-30	Dangerous risk [a]
31-35	Extremely dangerous risk [a]

[a]Medical clearance necessary.

From *Client-Centered Exercise Prescription, Second Edition,* by John C. Griffin, 2006, Champaign, IL: Human Kinetics.

benefits of an activity (Tremblay et al. 2001). Appraisal tools such as the *FANTASTIC Lifestyle Checklist* or *RISK-I* may have identified lack of physical activity as a habit in need of change. Yet an intense cardiovascular appraisal may not be appropriate for some clients. The *PAI* (page 65) will help you assess the activities in which your client already participates.

For example, if your client exercises at a moderate intensity (3 points) for 40 min (5 points) four times per week (4 points), then her physical activity index is $3 \times 5 \times 4 = 60$. This "good" rating is a level of physical activity with considerable health benefits, such as lowering blood lipids, blood pressure, and body fat (Shephard and Bouchard 1994). You can administer the *PAI* periodically to show improvements and help motivate your client.

Screening

Provide an initial screening of your clients relative to risk factors and symptoms. Regardless of the type of preparticipation screening you use, information should be interpreted by the appropriate health care professional, and results should be documented (American College of Sports Medicine [ACSM] 2000). You can use information from the health and lifestyle appraisals (e.g., FANTASTIC *Lifestyle Checklist* and *RISK-I*) to classify and screen individuals by health status before exercise assessment or prescription.

PAR-Q and Personal Health History

Older individuals and people with high-risk symptoms should obtain medical permission before proceeding with vigorous exercise. All maximal exercise tests should include supervision by a physician.

The Physical Activity Readiness Questionnaire (*PAR-Q*) can help determine whether a client should provide a detailed medical history before entering an exercise program. You can use *PAR-Q* (see page 66) as a screening instrument both for submaximal aerobic assessment and for beginning moderate and progressive exercise programs (CSEP 2003; Shephard 1988).

PAR-Q helps to identify clients for whom certain physical activities might be inappropriate or who should receive medical advice concerning the type of activity most suitable for them. To ensure the validity of the test as well as to protect yourself legally, administer the *PAR-Q* without providing any interpretation to your clients. All judgments must be their own. If they give one or more yes responses, direct them to their doctor for a review of their medical history before permitting them to complete active test components such as aerobic, strength, or endurance tests. CSEP (2003) has designed the *PARmed-X*, a physical activity-specific checklist to be used by a physician with patients who have had positive responses to the *PAR-Q*. In addition, you can use the Conveyance and Referral Form in the *PARmed-X* to convey clearance for physical activity participation or to make a referral to a medically supervised exercise program.

Personal Observation

The questionnaires discussed here identify most concerns that can make a fitness assessment inappropriate. It is advisable, however, that you make some general observations within the screening process (CSEP 2003). Cancel or postpone the appraisal if clients

- demonstrate difficulty in breathing at rest;
- are ill or have a fever;
- have swelling in their lower extremities;
- are pregnant and do not have the consent of their physicians;
- cough persistently;
- are currently on medication for cardiovascular or metabolic problems;
- have clearly ignored instructions about eating, drinking, and smoking before arrival; or
- exhibit any other trait that you believe may predispose them to unnecessary discomfort or risk.

For some of these observations (e.g., coughing, swelling), direct clients to their physicians; for others (e.g., illness, eating, drinking), instruct them to return once the concern no longer exists.

Informed Consent

Any client who is exposed to possible physical or psychological injury must give informed consent before participation in an assessment or exercise program. The informed consent form should provide clients with an adequate explanation of the tests and program, the potential risks and discomforts that may be involved, and their rights and responsibilities. The client should read, understand, and sign this form before administration of the active appraisal, and you should retain the form as an official record. Filling out the form may prompt questions from your client that provide an

Physical Activity Index (PAI)

Instructions:

Select the appropriate points for each of the following three parts.

Part 1—When you engage in sport, fitness activities, or active leisure, which description is most appropriate?

Intensity descriptions	Points
Very heavy: Continuous intense effort resulting in rapid heart rate or heavy breathing for the length of the activity.	5
Heavy: Bursts of effort that cause rapid heart rate or heavy breathing.	4
Moderate: Requires moderate effort and works up a sweat.	3
Light: Requires light effort and is often intermittent.	2
Minimal: Requires no extra effort.	1

Part 2—When you participate in the activity described in Part 1, how long do you keep at it?

Duration descriptions	Points	Duration descriptions	Points
35 min or more	5	5-14 min	2
25-34 min	4	Less than 5 min	1
15-24 min	3		

Part 3—How often do you participate in the activity described in Part 1?

Duration descriptions	Points	Duration descriptions	Points
Daily	5	1-3 times per month	2
3-6 times per week	4	Less than once per month	1
1-2 times per week	3		

PAI scoring:

Multiply your intensity points times your duration points times your frequency points to obtain your health benefits score.

Physical Activity Index = intensity points ___ × duration points ___ × frequency points. ___

Health benefit rating for PAI scores:

PAI score	Rating	Significance
100 or more	Excellent	This level of physical activity is associated with optimal health benefits.
60-99	Good	This level of physical activity is associated with considerable health benefits.
40-59	Average	This level of physical activity is associated with some health benefits. Increased activity will provide increased health benefits.
20-39	Fair	This level of physical activity is associated with some health benefits and some health risks. Duration or frequency of activity should be increased.
Less than 20	Needs improvement	This level of physical activity is associated with considerable health risks.

From *Client-Centered Exercise Prescription, Second Edition,* by John C. Griffin, 2006, Champaign, IL: Human Kinetics.

PAR-Q & YOU

(A Questionnaire for People Aged 15 to 69)

Regular physical activity is fun and healthy, and increasingly more people are starting to become more active every day. Being more active is very safe for most people. However, some people should check with their doctor before they start becoming much more physically active.

If you are planning to become much more physically active than you are now, start by answering the seven questions in the box below. If you are between the ages of 15 and 69, the PAR-Q will tell you if you should check with your doctor before you start. If you are over 69 years of age, and you are not used to being very active, check with your doctor.

Common sense is your best guide when you answer these questions. Please read the questions carefully and answer each one honestly: check YES or NO.

YES	NO	
❑	❑	**1. Has your doctor ever said that you have a heart condition <u>and</u> that you should only do physical activity recommended by a doctor?**
❑	❑	**2. Do you feel pain in your chest when you do physical activity?**
❑	❑	**3. In the past month, have you had chest pain when you were not doing physical activity?**
❑	❑	**4. Do you lose your balance because of dizziness or do you ever lose consciousness?**
❑	❑	**5. Do you have a bone or joint problem (for example, back, knee or hip) that could be made worse by a change in your physical activity?**
❑	❑	**6. Is your doctor currently prescribing drugs (for example, water pills) for your blood pressure or heart condition?**
❑	❑	**7. Do you know of <u>any other reason</u> why you should not do physical activity?**

If you answered

YES to one or more questions

Talk with your doctor by phone or in person BEFORE you start becoming much more physically active or BEFORE you have a fitness appraisal. Tell your doctor about the PAR-Q and which questions you answered YES.

- You may be able to do any activity you want — as long as you start slowly and build up gradually. Or, you may need to restrict your activities to those which are safe for you. Talk with your doctor about the kinds of activities you wish to participate in and follow his/her advice.
- Find out which community programs are safe and helpful for you.

NO to all questions

If you answered NO honestly to <u>all</u> PAR-Q questions, you can be reasonably sure that you can:

- start becoming much more physically active – begin slowly and build up gradually. This is the safest and easiest way to go.
- take part in a fitness appraisal – this is an excellent way to determine your basic fitness so that you can plan the best way for you to live actively. It is also highly recommended that you have your blood pressure evaluated. If your reading is over 144/94, talk with your doctor before you start becoming much more physically active.

DELAY BECOMING MUCH MORE ACTIVE:
- if you are not feeling well because of a temporary illness such as a cold or a fever – wait until you feel better; or
- if you are or may be pregnant – talk to your doctor before you start becoming more active.

PLEASE NOTE: If your health changes so that you then answer YES to any of the above questions, tell your fitness or health professional. Ask whether you should change your physical activity plan.

<u>Informed Use of the PAR-Q:</u> The Canadian Society for Exercise Physiology, Health Canada, and their agents assume no liability for persons who undertake physical activity, and if in doubt after completing this questionnaire, consult your doctor prior to physical activity.

No changes permitted. You are encouraged to photocopy the PAR-Q but only if you use the entire form.

NOTE: If the PAR-Q is being given to a person before he or she participates in a physical activity program or a fitness appraisal, this section may be used for legal or administrative purposes.

"I have read, understood and completed this questionnaire. Any questions I had were answered to my full satisfaction."

NAME _____

SIGNATURE _____ DATE _____

SIGNATURE OF PARENT _____ WITNESS _____
or GUARDIAN (for participants under the age of majority)

Note: This physical activity clearance is valid for a maximum of 12 months from the date it is completed and becomes invalid if your condition changes so that you would answer YES to any of the seven questions.

 © Canadian Society for Exercise Physiology

Supported by: Health   Santé
Canada   Canada

Source: Physical Activity Readiness Questionnaire (PAR-Q) © 2002. Reprinted with permission from the Canadian Society for Exercise Physiology. http://www.csep.ca/forms.asp

opportunity for dialogue and a chance to gather information and build rapport.

Informed consent does not absolve you from negligence in the administration of an assessment or the prescription of exercise. Although the form should be individualized for each facility or business, the following components should be in every informed consent form (Nieman 1990):

- A general statement of the background and objectives of the program
- An explanation of the procedures to be followed
- A description of any risks or discomfort that may be experienced
- A description of the benefits that can reasonably be expected
- An offer to answer any of the client's questions
- An instruction that the client is free to withdraw consent and to discontinue participation at any time
- An explanation of the procedures to be taken to ensure the confidentiality of the information requested

Fitness Test Item Selection

You do not have to know up front everything there is to know about your client's condition: The client-centered model is flexible, allowing you to loop back at any point and verify needs by assessing your client's current priorities and situation. It's OK to use certain tests, such as standard screening tools, for all first time clients. But when your client has expressed a specific interest or need, be sure to include test items for that component. If your client is intimidated by the idea of exercise, you can gather information from simple field-based tests that may be less threatening to him than more complex assessment tools but that can enable you to design an initial prescription that suits his immediate needs.

Retest sessions need not include all of the initial test items, especially if you used a generic battery of tests. Select only the components that your client has been working on or those in which you anticipate a change. Monitoring throughout the program both shows improvement and indicates when progressions should be made. This may also decrease the need for regular, formal reassessment in areas such as muscular strength. The closer an assessment comes to simulating your client's training activities, the greater the test's sensitivity and validity.

Learn to view assessment in terms of stages of change. Many first-time clients will not be ready to move much beyond an initial counseling and lifestyle appraisal: Pushing on to a full battery of exhaustive tests can destroy what little motivation they have. On the other hand, athletes after preseason training may be very anxious to challenge their limits.

Choosing Laboratory or Field-Based Tests

Before developing a detailed exercise prescription, assess baseline values for selected components of fitness. Sometimes trainers will sample all the components of fitness (i.e., cardiovascular, body composition, flexibility, muscular strength, and endurance). At other times, we may assess only high-priority components. Where appropriate, we may use less expensive and more easily administered field-based tests as supplements to or even as substitutes for laboratory tests.

Chapter 4 discusses a number of assessment tools, and you can readily find details about a variety of assessment protocols (ACSM 2000, CSEP 2003, Heyward 2002, Hoeger and Hoeger 1999). You are encouraged to use these resources when establishing personal assessment batteries. Table 3.1 categorizes a number of assessment tools into laboratory and field-based measures.

The very process of administering a fitness assessment draws attention to the "client-centered" nature of our relationship. The test process and the test results help to educate and motivate clients and stimulate their interest in exercise and other health-related issues. However, the primary function of measurement is to determine status.

Any fitness assessment protocol should meet the following criteria:

- **Validity:** The protocol accurately measures what it is supposed to measure.
- **Reliability:** The protocol gives consistent results when used by different testers or when repeated by the same tester.
- **Economy:** The protocol is relatively inexpensive, efficient, and easy to administer.

Test results are a means to an end. They should not distract you from the purpose of serving your clients. It is better to undertest than to overtest so that you can devote more time to counseling and demonstrating the program. Once your client has begun implementing your initial prescription, careful monitoring under standardized conditions can allow her to continue her workout program while you gain information about her status.

Table 3.1   Laboratory and Field-Based Assessment Tools

	Laboratory	Field-based
Cardiovascular	• Treadmill (e.g., Bruce, Balke) • Bicycle ergometer • Arm ergometer	• Åstrand-Rhyming bicycle test • 1.5/2.0-mile run • Canadian Aerobic Fitness Test • *Physical Activity Index*
Body composition	• Hydrostatic weighing • Bioelectrical impedance • Air displacement plethysmography	• Skinfolds • Circumferences • Height and weight • Body mass index • Bioelectrical impedance

Client-Centered Exercise Prescription

Clients today want more than just aerobic fitness and weight control. We must offer more than just the physiological components of fitness! This includes assisting clients in meeting their fitness and health prescription objectives by explaining and orchestrating their lifestyle factors, environment, genetics, occupation, and personal attributes.

What has recent research told us about the effectiveness of various types and quantities of exercise? How much do the benefits of exercise depend on the type of client? This section discusses these questions, especially as they touch on another question of great importance to our clients: How much exercise is enough? From a health perspective, how does this dose–response relationship influence our exercise prescription?

 ## Traditional and Emerging Exercise Outcomes

We can prescribe exercise programs to produce three potential outcomes:

1. Increased general fitness
2. Performance improvements
3. Health enhancement

For years, guidelines for prescribing exercise were based on improvement in athletic ability or physical performance. As overall fitness grew in popularity, led by a surge of interest in aerobics, the guidelines were modified. Intensity levels were reduced, and workouts were structured to include a balance of all fitness components. Exercises were designed to stress the cardiovascular, metabolic, and musculoskeletal systems, thereby creating physiological and structural changes in the components of fitness.

One of the strongest trends in recent history is the adoption of activity as a health-enhancing strategy. Physical fitness and good health are not synonymous, but they are complementary. **Physical fitness** is the ability to carry out daily tasks with vigor and alertness, without undue fatigue, and with ample energy to enjoy leisure pursuits and to meet unforeseen emergencies. **Good health** is not merely the absence of disease—it is a capacity to enjoy life and withstand challenges. It has social, physical, and psychological dimensions, each characterized on a continuum with positive and negative poles. Health benefits may occur in conjunction with improvements in aerobic power or muscular endurance or with improvements in physical performance capacity. However, some health benefits appear to be achieved by exercise that does not always lead to improved physical fitness (International Federation of Sports Medicine [IFSM] 1990).

General Fitness Components

The essential physiological components of physical fitness are cardiovascular endurance, flexibility, strength, muscular endurance, and body composition.

• **Cardiovascular endurance** is the ability to perform physical work involving large muscle groups continuously for an extended period. This component depends on the efficiency of the oxygen transport system. In the lungs, oxygen moves across a membrane (diffusion) into the red blood cells; it is transported through the arteries to working muscle cells (diffusion and utilization). End products of cellular metabolism (carbon dioxide and at times lactic acid) are transported back through the veins to the heart and lungs. The heart is the key to the oxygen transport system, because it must continuously pump blood to all bodily systems as well as larger quantities to more active tissues.

- **Flexibility** is the capacity of a joint to move freely through a full range of motion without undue stress. For most joints, the limitation of movement is imposed by the soft tissues, including the muscle and its fascial sheaths; the connective tissue, with tendons, ligaments, and joint capsules; and the skin (Wilmore and Costill 2004).

- **Strength** measures the maximum ability of a muscle or muscle group to exert force against a resistance. For example, a person who can maximally curl a barbell weighing 150 lb (68 kg) is twice as strong as the client who can curl only 75 lb (34 kg). Lifting as much as possible in one lift is referred to as one-repetition maximum (1RM).

- **Muscular endurance** is the ability of a muscle or muscle group to exert a force repeatedly or to sustain a contraction for a period of time. A simple measure of muscular endurance involves determining the number of repetitions clients can complete while lifting a fixed percentage of their 1RM.

- **Body composition** refers to the relative amounts of fat and lean body weight in the body. Exercise often decreases total body weight and fat weight and increases fat-free weight (Quinney et al. 1994).

Performance- and Health-Related Fitness Components

Performance-related fitness components are those necessary for sport performance or optimal work performance. The components include motor skills (e.g., speed, agility, balance, and coordination), cardiovascular endurance, muscular power, strength, endurance, size, body composition, skill acquisition, and motivation.

Health-related fitness components include body composition (e.g., subcutaneous fat distribution, abdominal visceral fat, body mass relative to height), muscle balance (strength, endurance, and flexibility—particularly of postural muscles), cardiovascular functions (e.g., submaximal exercise capacity, blood pressure, lung functions), and metabolic components (e.g., blood lipids, glucose tolerance). Very inactive people benefit from even low-intensity exercise, because the detrimental health-related consequences of extreme inactivity are rapidly reversed.

How Do Clients' Needs Affect Their Goals?

The details of each exercise prescription vary with the client's goals, desired outcomes, and risks. Skinner (1987) offered a schematic representation of the goals most common for different populations (figure 3.1).

For the athlete, **performance** is usually the central focus of a physical activity program, and health and fitness are secondary goals. However, sometimes an athlete will want to recover from an injury (health goal) or build a strong off-season base (fitness goal). Skinner (1987) suggested that the average client gets involved in activity for **fitness**, with perhaps an added interest in recreational sport performance. Quality of life and reduction of risk factors (health goals) are still in the minds of these clients. Clients with certain health risk factors or with musculoskeletal injuries obviously are most concerned about improving their **health** and are less oriented toward performance.

Clients may progress through several goals. Consider three hypothetical clients:

- **Active and fit.** This client has progressed with her overall fitness goals to a point where she wants to develop a higher level of performance.

- **Rehabilitation referred.** In the final stages of rehabilitation for a specific injury or health problem, this client will be embarking on a general fitness program to build future resilience.

- **Overuse athlete.** Many athletes train extremely hard and long. To ensure a healthy athlete, you must change the prescription to avoid excessive trauma, regain muscle balance, and reduce inflammation. At the same time, you must help him maintain a competitive level of performance.

Clients are increasingly well informed about fitness. Yet the preceding scenarios show how

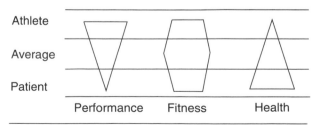

Figure 3.1 Changes in component goals with different clients.

dynamic clients' needs can be and how adaptable you must be to serve them well.

Issues in Prescribing for Physical Activity, Fitness, and Health

You will benefit from understanding the interrelationships among lifestyle, environment, genetics, occupation, personal attributes, fitness, and health. By helping to orchestrate these factors, you can assist your clients in meeting their prescription objectives. How do regular physical activity and fitness contribute to health? Figure 3.2 presents Bouchard's model that defines these interrelationships.

The model demonstrates how physical activity and fitness influence each other. The components of fitness—particularly health-related fitness—are determined by heredity, diet, and patterns of habitual physical activity. Health status also influences both fitness and physical activity. For example, an injury or illness will limit a client's physical activity and eventually will affect her level of fitness. Wellness is a holistic concept of positive health influenced by social and psychological factors, lifestyle habits (e.g., smoking, stress, diet), the environment, and physical well-being. The model also shows that wellness is related to fitness and physical activity.

A purely physiological approach to exercise prescription would ignore many factors in Bouchard's model. To be client-centered, you must first establish whether your client's main concern is activity, fitness (performance), or health. Then consider how the surrounding factors may directly or indirectly affect him. Spend time with your client in these earlier stages so both of you develop a clear vision of what he wants to achieve. The relationships in the model will influence how you reach those objectives and how you package the prescription.

For example, you have a client whose health-related fitness **goal** has already been established. The area of **priority** is appearance and a healthy weight. The specific **objectives** include reduction of body fat (especially in the trunk area) and reduction of blood lipids. These objectives are linked to the health-related fitness components of metabolism and body composition. The purely physiological approach may provide a very sound aerobic exercise prescription, but this would fail to serve all your client's needs. Bouchard's model indicates that your client also will benefit from initiatives in the areas of diet, stress management, social environment, occupational activity, and household chores (that provide continuous moderate activity). You will achieve greater success and a more balanced program if your prescription for one area is made in light of how that area interacts with the other areas. This holistic approach is beneficial for athletes, fitness enthusiasts, and health-conscious clients.

How Much Exercise Is Enough?

"I've been walking, but I hear that to be fit I should be jogging." "Recently I read that living actively, like taking the stairs and walking the dog, will make me fit." "As a distance runner, should I be doing the same weekly mileage even though I am working in intervals?" These are typical client concerns. How much exercise is enough? Enough for whom? Enough for what goal or objective?

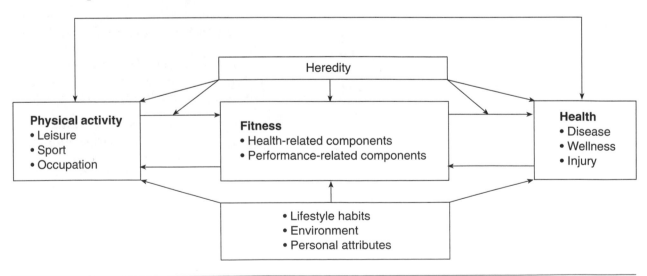

Figure 3.2   Physical activity, fitness, and health model (Bouchard 1994).

Adapted, by permission, from C. Bouchard, 1994, Toward active living, physical activity, fitness, and health: Overview of the Consensus Symposium. (Champaign, IL: Human Kinetics), 8.

The question may not be, "How much is enough?" but rather, "What constitutes an exercise benefit, and how much exercise is required before I see benefits?" Figure 3.3 contrasts two models of the relationship between the acquired benefits of exercise and the amount of exercise performed.

Exercise physiologists traditionally have held that cardiovascular fitness occurs only after a person reaches a threshold of exercise activity. According to this view, there is little or no benefit until the threshold for fitness is exceeded. Benefits continue to accrue as the level of exercise increases beyond this threshold. At an upper limit, the benefits level off (figure 3.3a).

Figure 3.3b shows that some improvements in fitness occur at low levels of exercise, even though the increases are small. At higher exercise levels, benefits accrue at an accelerated rate until an upper limit is reached, beyond which the potential for injury and overuse detracts from the positive effects of training. Proponents of the need for some exercise, even at low levels, believe this gradual increase in benefits is typical of many adaptive responses.

Are the Mechanisms of Change the Same for Health and Fitness?

Improvement in health may be attributable to biological changes different from those responsible for fitness. For example, endurance training will increase endurance capacity and may help prevent coronary artery disease (CAD). The increase in endurance capacity most likely results from an increase in oxygen transport to and utilization by the skeletal muscles. The reduction in CAD risk may result from alterations in lipoprotein metabolism or blood clotting activity (Haskell 1985, La Forge 2001). The accelerated rate of energy production during exercise increases the rate of functioning of other biological systems. With repeated stimulus, these systems will increase their capacity or efficiency, providing many of the health-related benefits of exercise

(Haskell 1985, La Forge 2001). This information can be extremely motivating to a client who sees no immediate changes in other measures.

In some circumstances, the mechanism for health benefits may relate more to physical or mechanical stress placed on the muscles, connective tissue, or skeleton than to increased energy expenditure. For example, retention of postmenopausal muscle tone and bone calcium through exercise probably results from mechanical stress on muscles and bones from weight-bearing activity or resistance exercise (Ross et al. 2000). Joggers may benefit more from the weight-bearing nature of their steps than from elevated heart rates.

Do Health Benefits Build Up or Do They Come and Go?

Although most fitness benefits are somewhat cumulative, this is not always the case with health benefits, which dissipate quickly and require life-long regularity of exercise (Haskell 1985).

Numerous biochemical changes occur during or immediately after a workout. Although these changes may be transient, they can favorably alter the progression of a specific disease if they occur often enough. For example, a single bout of endurance exercise will decrease elevated plasma triglycerides. Exercise on consecutive days further lowers the triglyceride concentration for 48 to 72 hr, but if exercise is not performed for several days, the concentration will return to its elevated level (Haskell 1985). Minimum daily exercise may give rise to discernible health benefits for many clients.

Prescription Guidelines for Health, Fitness, and Performance

There are specific prescription guidelines for each client goal. We will examine these guidelines and

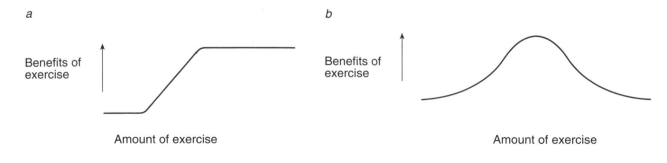

a   b

Benefits of
exercise

Amount of exercise

Benefits of
exercise

Amount of exercise

Figure 3.3   Schematic models of the benefits versus amount of exercise.

follow up from the perspective of three different clients. Client 1 has a number of cardiovascular risk factors and has set a goal of health-related fitness. Client 2 is interested in overall fitness and staying in shape. Client 3 is an athlete interested in performance-related fitness.

Guidelines for Prescription for Health-Related Fitness (Client 1)

Physical fitness and health-related fitness, although not synonymous, are complementary. Although your client may experience the health benefits of exercise along with improvements in fitness and performance (Blair et al. 1989), health benefits also may come from frequent performance of low-intensity exercise that has no fitness training effect.

Research: Benefits of Moderate Exercise

Recent guidelines (ACSM 2000, IFSM 1990, Pate et al. 1995, Wilmore 2003) place less emphasis on vigorous exercise than on moderate-intensity exercise (55-75% maximum heart rate [maxHR] or 40-60% $\dot{V}O_2$max), particularly for sedentary adults. Low-intensity dynamic activity (<50% $\dot{V}O_2$max) may reduce stress, contribute to weight loss, or improve certain biochemical reactions such as the release of endorphines. Performed 30 min or more at least three times per week, low-intensity activity significantly improves blood pressure, lipid metabolism, glucose tolerance, and blood clotting—especially in middle-aged and older persons (Haskell 1995, Malkin 2002). Other metabolic changes, like increases in high-density lipoproteins, appear to respond more to increases in the volume of exercise (amount of time spent) than to intensity. Several studies (De Busk et al. 1990, Ebisu 1985, Kesaniemi et al. 2001) show that multiple periods of moderate-intensity exercise of about 10 min duration spread throughout the day can improve metabolism and body composition. Paffenbarger and colleagues (1986) found that short periods of stair climbing, walking, or light sports proved protection against heart disease.

Factors to Consider for Client 1

One of the most valuable findings of recent research on physical activity is that it produces such health benefits as reduced blood lipids, lowered resting blood pressure, protection from type 2 diabetes, increased metabolic rate (weight loss), and an increased quality of life and independent living in the elderly (Kesaniemi et al. 2001). Exercise is a therapeutic intervention that requires a customized dose (frequency, intensity, time or duration, and type). A dose–response effect exists between exercise and a specific health outcome if there is a consistent relationship between the volume or intensity of the exercise and the health outcome (La Forge 2001). As personal fitness trainers, we must prescribe the appropriate dose of exercise. Like a drug, a prescription that is not client-centered can create adverse effects; these can include overuse strains, fatigue, and immune system dysfunction, resulting in loss in motivation or compliance. The best response will be achieved with a dose-specific health-related exercise prescription based on the information gathered during counseling.

Figure 3.4 (Gledhill and Jamnik 1996) illustrates health gains as related to the volume of physical activity. Lower volumes of physical activity (duration × frequency) show more rapid initial improvement in triglycerides and blood pressure. Improvements in several other health-benefit indicators come at higher volumes of participation. Aerobic fitness depends on the intensity of participation, not just its duration and frequency. The other health-benefit indicators, however, depend primarily on duration and frequency of participation. The authors note that figure 3.4 reflects **general** interpretations of the related scientific literature and is meant to show the **collective** improvement in selected health-benefit indicators. The health benefit zones in figure 3.4 will help your client determine the benefits of his level of activity.

Similar to cardiovascular fitness, there is a dose–response relationship for improvements in health status from better musculoskeletal fitness (Payne et al. 2000). Enhanced musculoskeletal fitness improves bone health, decreases pain in those with chronic low back pain, promotes independent living, and prevents falls and associated injuries (Katzmarzyk and Craig 2002, Warburton et al. 2001). Strength training may preserve bone mineral content and improve psychological well-

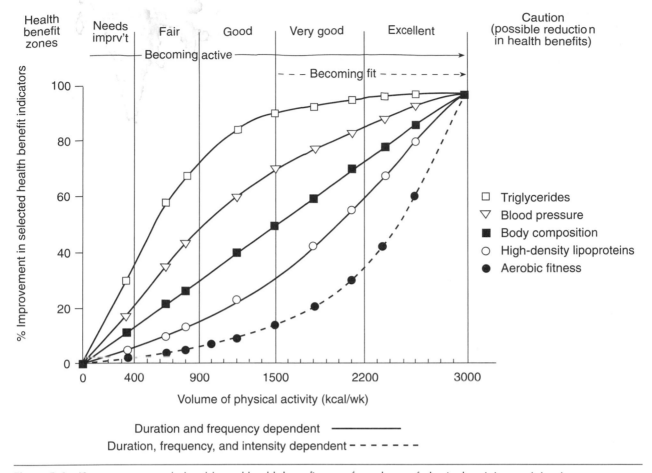

Figure 3.4   Dose–response relationship and health benefit zone for volume of physical activity participation.

The Canadian Physical Activity, Fitness & Lifestyle Approach: CSEP-Health & Fitness Program's Health-Related Appraisal and Counselling Strategy, 3rd Edition © 2003. Reprinted with permission of the Canadian Society for Exercise Physiology.

being. Resistance training may increase high-density lipoproteins, lower diastolic blood pressure, and increase insulin sensitivity (Goldfine et al. 1991, La Forge 2001). Flexibility exercises will improve muscle balance, posture, and musculoskeletal integrity as your client ages. Women and elderly people have the greatest potential for gains in health status and quality of life.

Health-Related Prescription for Client 1

- Recommend moderate-intensity exercise (55-75% maximum HR or 40-60% $\dot{V}O_2$max), a minimum of three sessions per week, 20 min or longer per session.

- Alternatively, have the client perform less intense exercise 5 or 6 days per week or 8 to 10 min bouts of moderate-intensity exercise several times per day, most days of the week.

- For resistance training, have her use large muscle mass exercises, use higher-volume training (i.e., multiple sets, moderate inten-

sity), and avoid exhaustive sets (Feigenbaum and Pollock 1997, Stone, Fleck, et al. 1991).

- Bear in mind that given equal total energy costs, lower-intensity and longer-duration exercise will benefit your older or less fit clients as much as higher-intensity and shorter-duration exercise.

- Also remember that moderate-intensity exercise carries lower cardiovascular risk and lower probability of orthopedic injury, and it enjoys higher compliance.

- If your client is concerned about weight loss, have her exercise at a moderate to low intensity sufficient to burn 300 kcal 3 days/week, or 200 kcal (approximately 30 min) four to five days/week (ACSM 2000). Using frequent short bouts of moderate activity, your client may progress up to a target of 1,500 kcal/week (see table 9.5). To keep abreast of any changes in exercise recommendations, periodically check the ACSM Web site (www.acsm.org).

Guidelines for Prescription for General Fitness (Client 2)

Client 2 wants to be able to perform moderate to vigorous levels of physical activity without undue fatigue and to maintain such ability throughout life. More specifically, he wants to see improvements in cardiovascular condition ($\dot{V}O_2$max), body composition, flexibility, and muscular strength and endurance.

Factors to Consider for Client 2

Intensity is probably the most important variable for improving cardiovascular fitness. Because overall fitness is the primary objective for this client, you must progressively raise the intensity to the recommended level. For instance, if this client is of average capability, the intensity will need to build up to around 70% of his maximum heart rate for substantial cardiovascular improvements.

Wenger and Bell (1986) found intensity and duration of training to be interrelated: Total caloric expenditure (energy cost), which is a direct result of intensity, duration, and frequency, may be the most important factor for cardiovascular and body composition improvements (assuming a minimum intensity of 60% of maximum heart rate). The total energy cost of our client's exercise program, based on a body weight of 70 kg (154 lb), should be approximately 900 to 1,500 kcal per week or 300 to 500 kcal per exercise session (ACSM 2000).

Even if you do not have the resources to measure changes attributable to training, you can be reasonably sure that if the ACSM guidelines are followed, fitness will improve. The proper combination of intensity, duration, and frequency will improve your client's aerobic capacity 15% to 30% over a period of 4 to 6 months (Wilmore and Costill 2004). Programs of lesser intensity, duration, and frequency may produce improvements in the 5% to 10% range (Wenger and Bell 1986); this level of improvement might also result if the client has a high level of initial fitness. If your client stays with the program, he can expect long-term benefits; middle-aged and elderly men who train consistently show less than 5% reduction in aerobic capacity per decade (Wilmore and Costill 2004). Your client may expect slight decreases in his total body weight and in fat weight and increases in fat-free weight (Hagan 1988). The magnitude of these changes will vary directly with the intensity and duration of the activity and the total caloric expenditure (see chapter 9).

Ten-Year Rejuvenation!

Consider an inactive 45-year-old. With his doctor's approval, you design an aerobic program with progressively increased intensity. Over a 6-week period, he works up to exercising at 122 to 125 beats/min (70% maximum HR) and maintains that intensity regularly for another 16 weeks. The increase in his aerobic capacity is 20%. At his age, on average, 0.5% of his capacity is lost per year—so in effect, this client's improvement amounts to a 10-year rejuvenation!

Weight training can increase your client's muscular strength and cause some changes in body composition, but it will yield only a slight improvement in aerobic capacity. Moderate-intensity programs appear superior to high-intensity ones in preventing musculoskeletal injuries and improving adherence to endurance training (Wilmore and Costill 2004).

Exercises for muscle balance (including strength and flexibility) can prevent poor posture, low back complaints, and osteoporosis. Your client's flexibility will increase with static or dynamic stretching or proprioceptive neuromuscular facilitation stretching (chapter 8).

General Fitness Prescription for Client 2

The American College of Sports Medicine (2000) recommends the following for healthy adults:

- **Frequency** of training: 3 to 5 days/week.
- **Intensity** of training: 55% to 90% of maximum heart rate or 40% to 85% of oxygen uptake reserve or heart rate reserve.
- **Duration** of training: 20 to 60 min of continuous aerobic activity. Duration depends on intensity: For example, lower intensity activity should be done for a longer period of time.
- **Mode** of activity: Any activity that uses large muscle groups, can be maintained continuously, and is rhythmic and aerobic in nature—for example, walking–hiking, running–jogging, bicycling, cross-country skiing, dancing, skipping rope, rowing, stair climbing, swimming, skating, and various endurance game activities.
- **Rate of progression:** Proportional to the initial level of fitness and dependent on age

and goals. Clients starting an aerobic training program might achieve a 3% increase per week for the first month, 2% per week the second month, and 1% per week thereafter (Heyward 2002).

- **Resistance** training: Strength training of a moderate intensity, sufficient to develop and maintain fat-free weight (FFW). One set of 8 to 12 repetitions of 8 to 10 exercises that condition the major muscle groups at least 2 days per week is the recommended minimum.
- **Initial level of fitness:** High = higher workload; Low = lower workload.

Guidelines for Prescription for Performance-Related Fitness (Client 3)

For client 3, the serious exerciser or athlete, you will prescribe the upper levels of intensity and volume of exercise. Optimal training for peak performance can be achieved only with a fine balance between intense training and rest. Client-centered prescription for athletes includes training in those components that constitute performance-related fitness: motor skills (e.g., speed, agility, balance, and coordination), cardiovascular endurance, muscular power, strength, endurance, body composition, skill acquisition, and motivation. You can maximize your client's training efficiency only by prudently selecting training methods and appropriately changing the prescription factors of his program as the need arises. Training should be designed with the principles of periodization (Bompa 1999). This training program should

include at least 1 day a week of complete rest to allow for recovery. Monthly schedules should include 1 week that is lighter or used to taper before or recuperate after a competition.

Overtraining

Because most athletes are highly motivated and tend to overstress themselves, they most frequently err on the side of overtraining rather than undertraining. Both you and your athletic clients must be aware of this problem, because overtraining will deny them their full potentials. Hawley and Schoene (2003) referred to the state of persistent muscle soreness, decreased coordination, and frequent upper-respiratory infections as "overreaching" and described it as an expected part of vigorous training. These symptoms usually resolve if followed by a period of lighter training. Your client's performance will increase during this "supercompensation" response. However, if overreaching continues, there will be a decrease in performance and prolonged symptoms characteristic of overtraining (figure 3.5).

But how much exercise is too much? More exercise can be a double-edged sword: It can be helpful or, if poorly directed, harmful. The reinforcement your client receives from his rigorous training regime can easily cross the line to decreased performance and nagging injuries. It is hard to tell such a motivated athlete that he must slow down or change what so far has been a successful prescription. Yet all athletes experience periods when their performance levels off or decreases. This overtraining results from failure to tolerate or adapt to the training load.

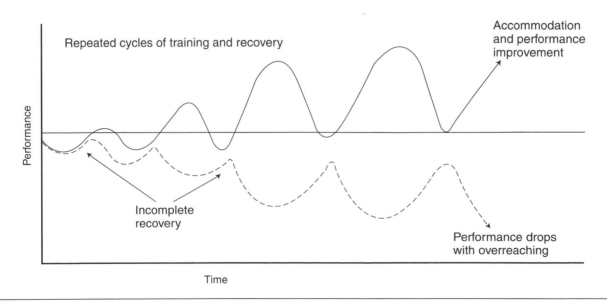

Figure 3.5   Overtraining syndrome.

Stone, Keith, and colleagues (1991) observed two types of overtraining: monotonous program overtraining and chronic overwork overtraining.

• **Monotonous program overtraining** demonstrates a loss or plateauing of performance attributable to the consistent, unvarying use of the same type of exercise. It is not caused by excessive fatigue. It is akin to a batting slump or a goal-scoring void for athletes, a feeling of "the blahs," or a lack of energy in the fitness enthusiast. Stone and colleagues (1991) believe that this type of overtraining may be the central nervous system's adaptation to a lack of appropriate stimulation from different movement patterns.

• **Chronic overwork overtraining** also can result in a plateauing or loss of performance. You need to distinguish the differences between chronic and short-term overwork ("overreaching"). Decreased performance as a result of a few sessions of high-intensity or high-volume training (short-term overtraining) is recovered within a few days. For example, a middle-distance runner may experience slower times after doing cross country training for a few weeks. The recovery period may range from 24 to 72 hr. Likewise, after an intense bout of weight training, the athlete's body generally requires 48 hr to repair the microtrauma to the muscles and connective tissue, to remove waste products (e.g., lactic acid), and to replace energy stores (e.g., muscle glycogen) in the cells (Westcott 1989). Chronic overwork occurs when the overwork is sustained too long or repeated too frequently and the client no longer responds adaptively to training (figure 3.5). This type of overwork can lead to chronic fatigue, exercise burnout, and higher rates of injury. Recovery from chronic overwork may take several weeks or even months (Kuipers and Keizer 1988).

Performance-Related Prescription to Prevent Overtraining for Client 3

Prevent overtraining by insisting on the following:

• **Adequate short-term recovery.** If your client performs a 45 min light aerobic workout with some stretching, he will be able to train harder within 24 hr. If the workout is 90 min and is more vigorous and high impact, he may need to wait 2 or 3 days before a similar workout. Treatment of overtraining may include relative rest that consists of light aerobic exercise using a modality not related to the athlete's sport. Competitive athletes usually prefer a treatment plan based on therapeutic exercise rather than complete rest. Eating well will give the body fuel for healing, and the client might enjoy massage or whirlpool baths.

• **Proper variation.** Varying volume, intensity, and mechanics of training can reduce the likelihood of overtraining. Such variation also encourages "peaking" at the appropriate time and helps maintain a high level of performance (Kuipers and Keizer 1988). Adjust the training according to your client's levels of physical or emotional stress. Adjustments often take the form of decreased training volume with normal intensities. Sudden changes in intensity and volume may create short-term delays in performance gains, but periodic changes in training technique, venue, or stress management techniques can prove rejuvenating.

• **Careful monitoring.** Recognition of overtraining is critically important, yet difficult. Symptoms of monotonous, short-term, and chronic overwork often overlap. By the time they are recognized and differentiated, the client has progressed to a stage where rest is imperative. Keeping a diary or log is essential for the serious performer (see chapter 6). Simple diaries can include quantifying exercise volume and intensity, body weight, diet, sleep patterns, and subjective feelings of general health, fatigue, mood, and ratings of training difficulty. You can provide readings of blood pressure and heart rate, both at rest and postexercise. See that infections are treated, with your client gradually returning to normal training levels. Remember, formal monitoring methods are no substitute for good communication between you and your client.

How to Avoid Runner's Overtraining

The editor of *Runner's World* (Burfoot 1995) provided some practical recommendations:

• Run less when you are tired, more when you find that perfect forest trail.

• Run less when you have a cold, more when you feel strong.

• Run less when your knee hurts, more when you are training for a marathon.

• Run less when you are starting a new job, more when your kids head off to college.

• Run more during some weeks and less during others.

Make running fit into everything else you do. Look at the big picture.

Ensuring Balance and Safety

We are at a point in the prescription journey where a performance, fitness, or health goal has been established. Each specific objective is linked to one or more fitness components. How to reach those objectives and how to package their prescription make up the next stage. If your prescription is to be effective, it must be both balanced and safe.

Creating a Balanced Prescription

Chapters 6, 7, 8, and 9 describe the many tools at our disposal for designing activity programs. They present the physiological bases and advantages of specific methods of training. Effective exercise prescription depends on our ability to achieve selected benefits for specific clients, using popular methods such as weight, flexibility, aerobic, and anaerobic training.

You must integrate the various components of fitness into a balanced workout. To improve or maintain your client's cardiovascular endurance, flexibility, strength, muscular endurance, and body composition, include all the following phases in the prescription:

- Warm-up
- Aerobic conditioning
- Body composition
- Flexibility
- Muscular conditioning
- Cool-down

There are innumerable ways you can tailor each client's prescription to current needs and wants. Here are things you should keep in mind when deciding how to approach the elements of the workout:

- **Order.** There is some room for personal preference in the order of the phases of a workout. Regardless of the order, follow the principle of progressive overload as your client enters the aerobic and the muscular conditioning phases. A gradual increase in intensity will prepare the body for the demands of that phase. The order presented previously allows the tissue temperature to be high when your client works on flexibility. It also stretches muscles tightened during the aerobics, in preparation for the resistance training to follow. However, many clients may feel more comfortable doing their flexibility training before aerobic activity or integrated with their muscular conditioning.

- **Warm-up.** Warming up prepares the muscles that will be used in the workout. When a muscle contracts, not all the individual fibers contract at once. So tension is created among the fibers and the connective tissues between the fibers (Malkin 2004), which can lead to microtears. Warm tissues are less likely to suffer microtears. Three to five minutes of initial warm-up activity often perfuses sufficient warm blood to the active muscles to increase tissue suppleness and allow for more effective stretching in the latter part of the warm-up.

- **Aerobic conditioning.** Both continuous and discontinuous aerobic training can improve cardiovascular fitness (Åstrand and Rodahl 2003). Interval (discontinuous) training consists of a repeated series of exercise bouts with intermittent relief periods. Because interval training permits a variety of activities, it is popular in many sports and has been recommended for symptomatic clients whose primary goal is health (ACSM 1990). Manipulation of the interval prescription factors, such as duration of effort, time of relief, and number of repetitions, can make prescriptions very precise (chapter 6).

- **Body composition.** Body composition changes are achieved through a combination of aerobic and muscular conditioning.

- **Flexibility.** Flexibility through stretching plays a major role in the maintenance of muscle balance. Your client's objectives will determine how, where, and through what technique you integrate flexibility into the prescription (chapter 8).

- **Muscular conditioning.** You can match strength training programs to your clients' objectives. Almost any form of resistance exercise will stimulate some degree of strength gain, especially if your client is unconditioned. Comfort, convenience, and safety therefore become as important for many clients as results. Again, considering the goals of your clients (performance, fitness, or health) will help you select the appropriate resistance training methods.

- **Cool-down.** At the end of aerobic work and to a lesser degree during muscular work, heart rate and blood volume (cardiac output) remain elevated. The return of blood through the venous system requires the rhythmic contraction of muscles to pump blood back to the heart and then to the lungs to oxygenate vital organs and tissues. This can be accomplished by continuing a weight-bearing activity such as walking until the heart rate returns to within about 20 beats/min of the starting rate. An added benefit of an effective cool-down is to help remove metabolites (e.g., lactic acid). With elevated metabolites and fatigue, muscles may feel tight or sore (from earlier eccentric work) and may go into spasm. Stretching while warm will relieve some of these symptoms, promote relaxation, and improve range of motion.

 ## Integrating Safety Into a Balanced Workout

A workout plan, no matter how balanced and client-centered, is appropriate only if it is safe.

What is the safest route through the series of physical stresses presented by each phase of the program? Table 3.2 identifies safety issues prominent during the various phases of a program.

Your clients may wish to improve specific aspects of fitness, optimize sport skills, or develop work hardening tasks. Your prescription must take into consideration the optimal, yet safe, training outcomes and specific benefits provided by weight training, flexibility training, aerobic training, and anaerobic training.

Table 3.2   Safety Issues for Program Segments

Prescription	Safety issues
Preparation (warm-up)	
Range of motion (moving major joints)	Increase joint lubrication and synovial fluid (protect joints) through warm-up. Have client check on how body feels before work. Use warm-up to provide some flexibility gains.
Circulatory warm-up (light aerobic; same mode as cardiovascular work)	Continue warm-up to increase tissue temperature and synovial fluid in preparation for stretching. Use segment to gradually prepare heart and circulatory system. Simulate joint mechanics with low trauma.
Stretching (emphasizing static stretching)	Promote gains in flexibility. Target muscles used, especially if used eccentrically. Use dynamic stretches for sport preparation.
Transition (easing into next segment)	Add a light overload in the activity to follow (start of progressive overload).
Aerobic segment	
Progressive prescription	Build up gradually whether continuous or intervals. Provide adequate relief during intervals. Tear down gradually, avoiding final sprints or sudden stops (better cardiovascular adaptations permitted).
Monitoring	Monitor heart rate, perceived exertion, talk test, and logging. Include stretching for muscular tightness.
Sport-specific segment	
	Try to include the following: • Mini-warm-up and skill practice (especially in intermittent sports such as baseball) • Stretching tight muscles • Tending immediately to minor injuries
Resistance segment	
Progressive prescription	Include progressive overload and adequate relief (depends on training method). Incorporate warm-up sets (e.g., 60% of training). Follow safety rules of the weight room (especially spotting guidelines).
Specific training method (chapter 7)	Follow method guidelines as prescribed.
Muscle balance	Check the balance (agonist and antagonist) of the program (i.e., need for specific muscle stretch or strengthening).

Prescription	Safety issues
Resistance segment	
Monitoring	Have client stretch as needed for muscular tightness.
	Teach client to differentiate between fatigue, soreness, and inflammation.
	Modify the exercise around minor injuries (including avoidance).
	Constantly check for correct breathing, speed of movement, base of support, and alignment such as pelvic stabilization and avoidance of extreme range of motion.
Cool-down	
Stretching (emphasizing static stretching)	Take advantage of warm tissue for greatest flexibility gains.
	Use target muscles, especially if used eccentrically.
	Consider proprioceptive neuromuscular facilitation if flexibility is a priority.
Self-check	Make sure cardiovascular indicators (e.g., heart rate, depth of breathing, blood pressure) are reduced.
	Ensure that muscles feel worked but not sore or tight.
	Ice any "hot spots" or minor injuries.
	Don't underestimate the therapeutic effect of a relaxing shower.

Highlights

1. **Be "client-centered" in your approach to assessment and prescription.**

   In client-centered assessment, we look for things our clients want to do that will satisfy their most important needs in ways that compliment or at least accommodate their lifestyles. Assessment should be viewed in terms of stages of readiness to make lifestyle changes. A client-centered prescription involves decision making that progresses through the issues systematically, making informed selections from a menu of options.

2. **Use lifestyle appraisal tools to change behavior.**

   Inactivity is so common that we have a critical role to play as providers and promoters of health care. A health and lifestyle appraisal may be a client's first step to behavior change. It may be just the extra nudge that a client needs. Its greatest value is as a tool that leads to healthy lifestyle intervention. These lifestyle appraisal tools include *FANTASTIC Lifestyle Checklist*, *RISK-I*, and *Physical Activity Index*.

3. **Screen your clients for risk factors and symptoms.**

   Regardless of the type of preparticipation screening used, information should be interpreted by the appropriate health care professional and results should be documented. Use information from the health and lifestyle appraisals (e.g., *FANTASTIC Lifestyle Checklist* and *RISK-I*) to classify and screen individuals by health status before exercise assessment or prescription. An initial screening of your clients may include *PAR-Q*, personal health history, personal observation, informed consent, and preexercise heart rate and blood pressure.

4. **Select appropriate test items suited to the client.**

   It's OK to use certain tests, such as standard screening tools, for all first-time clients. But when your client has expressed a specific interest or need, include test items for that component. The very process of administering a fitness assessment draws attention to the client-centered nature of the relationship. The test process and the test results help to educate, motivate, and stimulate interest in exercise and other health-related issues. However, the primary function of measurement is to determine status in a valid, reliable, and often economical manner with minimal sources of error.

5. **Describe three potential outcomes of client-centered exercise prescription.**

   We can prescribe exercise programs to produce three potential outcomes: increased general fitness, performance improvements, or health enhancement. For the athlete, performance is the central focus of a physical activity program. Health and fitness are secondary goals. You must be flexible, however—

sometimes an athlete will be recovering from an injury (health goal) or building a strong off-season base (fitness goal). The average client gets involved in activity for fitness, with perhaps an added interest in recreational sport performance. Quality of life and reduction of risk factors (health goals) are still in the minds of these clients. Clients with certain health risk factors or with musculoskeletal injuries obviously are most concerned about improving their health and are less oriented toward performance. We must offer more than just the physiological components of fitness. This includes assisting clients in meeting their objectives by explaining and orchestrating their lifestyle factors, environment, genetics, occupation, and personal attributes.

6. **Identify guidelines for prescription for health-related fitness.**

Although your client may experience health benefits as a result of fitness and performance improvements, health benefits also may come from frequent performance of low-intensity exercise that has no fitness training effect. One of the most valuable findings of recent research is that physical activity of even low intensity reduces blood lipids, lowers resting blood pressure, protects from type 2 diabetes, increases metabolic rate (weight loss), and increases quality of life and independent living in the elderly (Kesani-emi et al. 2001). It is valuable to recognize how exercise prescription can influence the mechanism for health and fitness benefits. Exercise can be a therapeutic intervention that requires a customized dose (frequency, intensity, duration, and type). For health benefits, you should recommend moderate intensity (55-75% maximum HR or 40-60% $\dot{V}O_2max$), a minimum of three sessions per week, 20 min or longer per session. For resistance training, make extensive use of large muscle mass exercises; use higher volume training (i.e., multiple sets, moderate intensity); and avoid exhaustive sets. If your client is concerned about weight loss, have her exercise at a moderate to low intensity sufficient to burn 300 kcal 3 days/week, or 200 kcal (approximately 30 min) 4 to 5 days/week (ACSM 2000).

7. **Identify guidelines for prescription for general fitness.**

Clients interested in general fitness may want to perform appropriate levels of physical activity without undue fatigue and to maintain such ability throughout life. More specifically, they may want to see improvements in cardiovascular conditioning ($\dot{V}O_2max$), body composition, flexibility, and muscular strength and endurance. For healthy adults, ACSM (2000) has recommended the following:

- **Frequency** of training: 3 to 5 days/week.
- **Intensity** of training: 55% to 90% of maximum heart rate or 40% to 85% of oxygen uptake reserve or heart rate reserve.
- **Duration** of training: 20 to 60 min of continuous aerobic activity. Duration depends on intensity.
- **Mode** of activity: Any activity that uses large muscle groups, can be maintained continuously, and is rhythmic and aerobic.
- **Rate of progression:** Proportional to the initial level of fitness and dependent on age and goals.
- **Resistance** training: Strength training of a moderate intensity, sufficient to develop and maintain fat-free weight. One set of 8 to 12 repetitions of 8 to 10 exercises that condition the major muscle groups at least 2 days/week is the recommended minimum.

8. **Identify guidelines for prescription for performance-related fitness.**

For the serious exerciser or athlete, upper levels of intensity and volume of exercise are prescribed. Optimal training for peak performance can be achieved only with a fine balance between intense training and proper rest. Client-centered prescription for athletes requires individualized training in those components that constitute performance-related fitness: motor skills (e.g., speed, agility, balance, and coordination), cardiovascular endurance, muscular power, strength, endurance, body composition, skill acquisition, and motivation. You can maximize your client's training efficiency only through prudent selection of training methods and by appropriately changing the prescription factors of the program as the need arises.

9. **Create a safe, balanced exercise prescription.**

Various components of fitness must be integrated into a balanced workout. To improve or maintain cardiovascular endurance, flexibility, strength, muscular endurance, and body composition, include all the following phases in your client's prescription:

- Warm-up
- Aerobic conditioning
- Body composition
- Flexibility exercises
- Muscular conditioning
- Cool-down

A balanced workout plan is only appropriate if it is matched to the client and identifies safety issues prominent at the various phases of a program (table 3.2).

Client-Centered Assessment

Chapter Competencies

After completing this chapter, you will be able to demonstrate the following competencies:

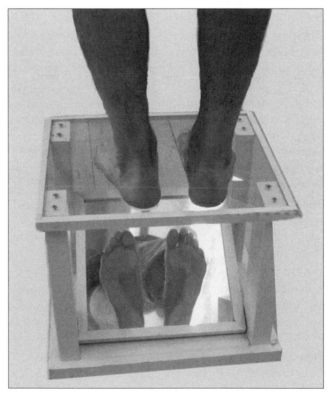

1. Consider client issues in selecting specific field tests.

2. Select a cardiovascular exercise mode and test protocol that are suitable for your client's age, gender, anticipated mode of exercise, and health and fitness status.

3. Identify the advantages of field-based cardiovascular assessment.

4. Identify the strengths, weaknesses, and sources of measurement error of laboratory and field-based body composition assessment tools.

5. Describe the factors to consider in selecting field-based musculoskeletal assessments.

6. Identify the objectives of selected field-based strength and endurance assessments.

7. Identify the objectives of selected field-based flexibility and muscle tightness assessments.

8. Demonstrate competency in administering and interpreting static and dynamic postural analyses.

9. Select and interpret appropriate assessments of your client's muscle balance.

itness testing is not an end in itself but rather is part of the overall exercise program (Nordvall and Sullivan 2002). The client-centered prescription model is flexible, allowing you to verify your client's needs by using selected assessment items that relate to your client's priorities and closely simulate her current training activity. Ultimately, you will validate your client's exercise prescription by using appropriate assessment tools and the baseline values for selected components of fitness.

This chapter introduces laboratory and field-based tests for cardiovascular, body composition, and musculoskeletal components of fitness. The focus is on the selection of field-based assessments and the consideration of maximal effort; normative values; specificity, reliability, and validity; client needs; human error; and equipment availability. We discuss client issues in the selection of test items and describe specific field tests for determining the client's distinct needs. Other laboratory protocols outside of the scope of this text can be found in several texts described in the *Assessment Resources*.

Assessment Resources

The following is a list of assessment resources, including their emphases:

American College of Sports Medicine. 2000. *Guidelines for Exercise Testing and Prescription*. 6th ed. Philadelphia: Lea & Febiger. As an industry standard, this manual provides quick access to the essential details. Chapter 4: Laboratory cardiovascular treadmill and bicycle ergometer protocols and body composition assessments.

Baechle, T.R., and R.W. Earle. 2000. *Essentials of Strength Training and Conditioning*. 2nd ed. Champaign, IL: Human Kinetics. This substantial text is used in conjunction with the National Strength and Conditioning certification. It has some good norms and is somewhat performance oriented. Chapter 15: Musculoskeletal field-based strength and power protocols.

Canadian Society for Exercise Physiology. 2003. *The Canadian Physical Activity, Fitness, and Lifestyle Approach*. 3rd ed. Ottawa: CSEP. This manual is the reference for the Certified Fitness Consultant in Canada. Chapter 7: Field-based body composition, aerobic, musculoskeletal, and back fitness appraisal measures.

Heyward, V.H. 2002. *Advanced Fitness Assessment and Exercise Prescription*. 4th ed. Champaign, IL: Human Kinetics. This is one of the leading references for broad-based assessment protocols for most fitness components. Chapter 4: Cardiorespiratory maximal and submaximal, laboratory and field-based test protocols. Chapter 6: Strength and muscular endurance laboratory and field-based test protocols. Chapter 8: Laboratory and field-based methods for assessing body composition. Chapter 10: Protocols for assessing flexibility.

Hoeger, W., and S. Hoeger. 1999. *Principles & Labs for Fitness & Wellness*. 5th ed. Englewood, CA: Morton. This is a practical text with many easily administered assessments. Field-based testing for body composition (chapter 4), cardiorespiratory endurance (chapter 6), muscular strength (chapter 8), and flexibility (chapter 9).

Kendall, F.P., E.K. McCreary, and P.G. Provance. 1993. *Muscles, Testing and Function: With Posture and Pain*. 4th ed. Baltimore: Williams and Wilkins. Kendall has long been a respected author in the area of physiotherapy with an excellent approach to the assessment of muscle balance. Tests for muscle length and flexibility (chapter 3), tests for posture (chapter 4), and numerous muscle strength tests typically used by physiotherapists.

Nieman, C. 2003. *Exercise Testing and Prescription: A Health-Related Approach*. 5th ed. Mountain View, CA: Mayfield. Nieman uses a health-related approach to test protocol selection. Laboratory and field-based methods for assessing cardiorespiratory fitness (chapter 4), laboratory and field-based methods for assessing body composition (chapter 5), and field-based methods for assessing musculoskeletal fitness (chapter 6).

Norkin, C., and D.J. White. 1995. *Measurement of Joint Motion: A Guide to Goniometry*. 2nd ed. Philadelphia: Davis. This well-illustrated manual covers upper-extremity, lower-extremity, and spinal joint motion testing procedures, most using a goniometer.

Cardiovascular Assessment

Your own experience, training, and educational background will affect the type of test you select. But because you are following the client-centered approach, client factors will be equally important. The following section will help you select laboratory protocols.

Laboratory Tests

You can readily find details for a variety of laboratory-based protocols in the *Assessment Resources*. Table 4.1 compares the four major assessment devices for a number of criteria. You must be able to select an exercise mode and test protocol that are suitable for your client's age, gender, anticipated mode of exercise, and health and fitness status.

Type of Test

The three most common modes used for laboratory cardiovascular assessments are the treadmill, bicycle ergometer, and box step. Here are the advantages and client suitability of each of these protocols:

- **Treadmill protocols** (ACSM 2000, Heyward 2002) are best suited to clients who

    - want a walking, jogging, or running prescription;

    - want to achieve their highest measurable oxygen uptake; or

    - are familiar with running on a treadmill.

Specific protocols (e.g., Balke) use small grade changes each minute with a constant speed and are better suited for sedentary adults who may have trouble jogging. Other protocols (e.g., Bruce) increase grade and speed and may pose limitations to sedentary or older clients due to calf fatigue (Heyward 2002).

- **Bicycle ergometer protocols** (ACSM 2000, Heyward 2002) are best suited to clients who

    - want a cycle or stationary bicycle prescription,

    - already cycle frequently,

    - prefer less joint trauma, or

    - are overweight and unfamiliar with the treadmill.

- **Step test protocols** (CSEP 2003, Heyward 2002, Hoeger and Hoeger 1999) have the following advantages and disadvantages:

    - They predict cardiorespiratory fitness by measuring postexercise recovery heart rates to one or more step rates or step heights.

    - They require little equipment and are both time and cost efficient.

    - They are easy to explain to clients. For example, the modified Canadian Aerobic Fitness Test (CSEP 2003) provides an aerobic fitness score linked to health benefit zones to assist in interpretation and guidance.

    - They may require special precautions for those who have balance problems or are extremely deconditioned.

Table 4.1   Client-Centered Selection of Assessment Method

Performance factor	Treadmill	Bicycle	Step	Arm ergometer
Familiarity and skills required	*	**	***	****
Adjustment of workload	****	** (friction)	*	** (friction)
Instrument calibration	**	*** (friction)	****	*** (friction)
Ability to achieve highest oxygen uptake	****	**	***	*
Ability to obtain blood pressure	***	****	**	*
Ability to obtain $\dot{V}O_2$	***	****	*	**
Ability to obtain ECG	***	****	**	*
Ability to obtain heart rate (stethoscope)	***	****	*	**
Local muscle fatigue	*	***	**	****
Cost and maintenance	*	***	****	**
Client compliance	****	**	***	*

Note. Each mode is rated from * (lowest) to **** (highest) in the various performance factors. ECG = electrocardiogram.

Submaximal or Maximal?

Predictive maximal cycle ergometer tests estimate maximal oxygen uptake from the highest power output completed. These tests are better measures of exercise tolerance than those that simply measure aerobic power, because anaerobic capacity can significantly contribute to performance during the final workload. Submaximal tests are useful tools for tracking training programs and for monitoring blood pressure and heart rate. This added control is suited for older clients. Although the standard error may be about 15%, the measured responses to reproducible workloads provide information for the prescription of cardiovascular intensity (Heyward 2002).

Submaximal tests on the treadmill or bicycle ergometer or with bench stepping are similar to maximal tests but are terminated at a predetermined heart rate. Most submaximal exercise tests determine heart rate at one or more submaximal work rates and use the results to predict $\dot{V}O_2$max or establish a starting intensity. The submaximal test assumes a linear relationship between oxygen uptake, heart rate, and work intensity. In other words, as the workload increases, the oxygen cost of the activity and the heart rate will increase at the same time. Variability in maximal heart rates and mechanical efficiencies usually results in overestimation for highly trained individuals and underestimation for untrained, sedentary clients (Heyward 2002). However, repeated submaximal tests over a period of weeks showing decreased heart rates at a fixed workload can reflect improvements in cardiorespiratory fitness regardless of the accuracy of the prediction of oxygen uptake.

Matching Tests to Client Limitations

It is a challenge to select suitable assessment items for many clients. Conditions such as musculoskeletal problems, overweight, lack of conditioning, advanced age, or high health risks may require that you modify the tests.

Consider the following:

- It is more appropriate to use a bicycle than a treadmill, step, or arm ergometer with clients who need increased monitoring of heart rate or blood pressure.
- Total test time should be less than 15 min for clients who are easily fatigued.
- For clients with poor leg strength, a treadmill is preferable to a bike or step; for those with poor balance, a bike is better than a treadmill or step.

- Clients suspected to have a low oxygen uptake should start at a lower intensity; those who are regularly active can start at a higher intensity.
- Longer warm-ups and smaller increases in workloads are appropriate for those requiring more time to reach steady state.
- Step testing has some technical limitations, such as the client's size and ability to maintain good form.
- Arm ergometry offers a suitable means for testing clients with lower-extremity impairment.

Field-Based Tests

Results from relatively simple field-based tests may be adequate for identifying and quantifying your client's needs. Field-based tests are usually less expensive and more easily administered than lab tests. For the personal trainer or small-facility director, field-based tests may be the only option. They can be very helpful if the regular method of monitoring is similar to that used for the field tests (e.g., minutes per mile, miles per hour, heart rates, or perceived exertion—all easily measured—can be quick indicators of progress).

Walking test protocols can be used for relatively inactive clients who are comfortable with walking but for whom jogging is inappropriate. For participants who are overweight, are older, or have scored less than 40 on the *PAI*, the following walking test (Getchell and Anderson 1982) may be a useful alternative to laboratory assessments.

All you need for this test is a timing device; a track or measured distance of 1, 1.5, and 2 miles; and appropriate weather. Have your client do warm-up stretches and then walk as briskly as she can. If she begins to tire early, encourage her to slow down. If she cannot complete the mile or cannot complete it in less than 20 min, terminate the test. If she reaches the mile in less than 20 min, have her keep going for another half mile. If she reaches the 1.5-mile point in less than 30 min, have her keep going. Her goal now is to reach 2 miles in less than 40 min. Of course, if any signs of intolerance to the exercise start to appear, terminate the test and have your client cool down. Table 4.2 will help you determine a safe and reasonable starting point for exercise prescription, based on the results of the walking test.

Other walk–run field test protocols (Heyward 2002; Hoeger and Hoeger 1999) consist of covering a certain distance in a given period of time (i.e., 12

Table 4.2 Scoring for Walking Test

Test performance	Fitness level (max METs)	Recommended walking program
1.0 mile in more than 25 min	4.0 METs or less	0.5-0.8 miles in 15-20 min
1.0 mile in 20-25 min	4.5 METs	1.1-1.2 miles in 24 min
1.5 miles in 26-30 min	5.0 METs	1.4-1.6 miles in 32 min
1.5 miles in 23-26 min	5.5 METs	1.9-2.0 miles in 40 min
2.0 miles in 35-40 min	6.0 METs	2.3-2.4 miles in 48 min
2.0 miles in 30-35 min	6.5 METs	3.0 miles in 58 min

Note. MET = metabolic equivalent. This measures the energy cost at rest. During a vigorous workout, a fit person may reach 10 to 15 times this resting value (10-15 METs).

Adapted, by permission, from Getchell, B., 1982, *Determining Your Level of Fitness, Being Fit. A Personal Guide.* John Wiley and Sons, Inc. 78.

min run test, Rockport walking test, 1-mile walk test, 1.5-mile run test for time). Because more than one client can be assessed at one time, the run protocols are frequently used with sport teams. Careful visual monitoring is suggested because these tests can be near maximal for some individuals. Maximum oxygen uptake or metabolic equivalent (MET) levels can be estimated from the tests.

Body Composition Assessment

Considering the profound health problems associated with body fat and the public's obsession with body image, the assessment of body composition has become very popular. Most assessment methods assume that the body is made up of fat and fat-free components. Percent body fat (%BF) can be obtained by dividing fat mass by total body weight. The recommended %BF values for adults (18-34 years) are 13% for men and 28% for women, and the standard for obesity is more than 22% BF for men and more than 35% BF for women (Heyward and Wagner 2004). Values vary with age, gender, and activity status. However, comparing clients with norms is often less effective than comparing each client's progress over time with his or her own individual measurements (e.g., girths or individual skinfold sites). Some assessment models have combined skinfold measures, waist girth, and body mass index (BMI) to provide the client with a composite score and health benefit rating (CSEP 2003).

The techniques used for assessing body composition are hydrostatic weighing (densitometry), air displacement plethysmography, bioelectrical impedance, and anthropometry (e.g., skinfold and girth measures). Specific protocols can be found in several of the *Assessment Resources*. These analyses are based on measuring the ratio of fat to fat-free mass. Table 4.3 compares these

Table 4.3 Methods of Body Composition Assessment

Method	Cost	Ease of use	Accuracy
Skinfold	Low	Moderate	Moderate
Hydrostatic weighing	High	Low	High
Electrical impedance	Moderate	High	Moderate

Reprinted, by permission, from T.R. Baechle, R.W. Earle, and D. Wathen, 2002, *Resistance training* (Champaign, IL: Human Kinetics), 407.

three methods for cost, ease of use, and accuracy in measuring body fat.

Client Considerations in the Selection of Tests

Underwater weighing was for many years the gold standard for laboratory assessment of body composition; however, the assumption of a constant density for fat-free mass introduces some error. As well, the time, expense, and expertise needed are often prohibitive. Air displacement plethysmography is based on the same principle but uses air instead of water and has similar practical shortcomings.

Bioelectrical impedance is based on the stature of the body and the resistance to the flow of electrical current (impedance). Because fat-free mass has higher water and electrolyte content, the impedance through fat-free mass is less than it is through fat mass. The variability of the analyzers and the specificity of the equations (age, gender, obesity, activity) are the weaknesses of bioelectrical impedance (Anderson 2003). As better equations are developed and appropriate pretest conditions are followed, bioelectrical impedance should prove to be a most convenient, safe, accurate, and rapid method. It may also have advantages over the skinfold techniques for clients who are overfat or heavily muscled or have thick, tight skin (Kravitz and Heyward 1997).

Body composition determined from skinfold measurement correlates well with underwater weighing (ACSM 2000). Performed by an experienced exercise specialist, the method has several advantages:

- The equipment is inexpensive and portable compared with popular laboratory tests.
- Measures are made quickly and easily.
- Measures correlate highly with body density and provide more accurate estimates of body fat than height-weight ratios (Nieman 2003).

Several studies (e.g., Larsson et al. 1984, Ross et al. 1996) have shown that fat mass located in a centralized area (usually the trunk) versus a generalized pattern of subcutaneous fat distribution is more directly associated with metabolic disorders, overweight, and possibly hypertension. That is, the visceral distribution of adipose tissue, independent of total body fat, is the critical factor in the health risk of obesity. A relationship has been shown between measures of total, abdominal, and visceral obesity and the measures of BMI, sum of five skinfolds, and waist girth (Janssen et al. 2002).

One of the greatest values for clients is the interpretation and education that you provide when explaining body composition measures. These results can be an excellent motivation tool and a useful basis for goal setting and program monitoring.

Simple Field-Based Tests

Field-based tests provide supportive information to estimate body composition and determine a relative health risk. BMI and the waist girth measure are estimates of body composition and, along with skinfold measures, can be effective monitoring measures for individual progress.

Skinfold Measures

Any skinfold protocol's predictive formula is specific to the population with which it was developed. To be more effective and fair to your client, select a protocol suited to her. Many equations have been developed for specific types of people. Heyward and Wagner (2004) discussed the major methods of assessment and ways to apply these methods to different ethnic and age groups as well as clinical populations. The recent trend has been to use generalized rather than population-specific equations. These equations, such as those developed by Jackson and Pollock (1985), apply to a large range of people with some loss in predictive accuracy. The error associated with generalized skinfold equations is only slightly greater (3.7% vs. 2.7%) than that of the hydrostatic weighing technique (Nieman 2003). For example, if the estimated percent body fat is 25%, then a 3.7% error provides a range of accuracy of 21.3 to 28.7% body fat. Another major source of error in skinfold measurements is the variability among technicians. Good training in standardized procedures can reduce this significantly (Heyward 2002).

Body Mass Index (BMI)

The BMI is an indicator of proportional weight or obesity. It is more precise than weight tables, is simple to perform, and allows for comparisons of large groups. Calculate BMI by dividing body weight (in kilograms) by the square of height (in meters).

For example:

Weight = 80 kg; height = 175 cm = 1.75 m

$$BMI = weight/height^2 = 80/1.75^2 = 80/3.06 = 26.1$$

The BMI has the following recommended classifications (NIH, NHLBI 1998):

- <18.5—underweight
- 18.5-24.9—normal (desirable range for adult men and women)
- 25.0-29.9—overweight
- 30.0-34.4—Grade I obesity
- 35.0-39.9—Grade II obesity (medically significant)
- ≥40—Grade III obesity

In the example, the client would be classified as overweight. BMI is most useful when used in conjunction with skinfold measures. A high BMI could be the result of elevated muscle mass, as with a football player, or excessive body fat. If the skinfold measures are high, this is a definite indication of too much body fat and corresponding health risk.

Waist (Abdomen) Girth

Excessive fat in the trunk area is associated with increased morbidity and mortality rates. Some sources (Lean et al. 1998, Ross et al. 1996, NIH, NHLBI 1998) have suggested that waist girth measure provides a valid representation of this pattern of fat distribution.

To measure waist girth, hold the tape horizontally at the level midway between the bottom of the rib cage and the iliac crest and take the measurement at the end of a normal expiration. Maintain tension but do not indent the skin.

Some sources (CSEP 2003) describe waist girth "health-benefit zones" based on age and sex. The National Institutes for Health (NIH, NHLBI 1998) acknowledges that waist girth provides a clinically acceptable measure of a client's abdominal fat content and has identified levels at which relative risk increases:

- Men: >102 cm (>40 in.)
- Women: >88 cm (>35 in.)

Monitoring changes to this measure is simple and can be very encouraging, particularly at the start of an exercise program.

Using BMI, Skinfold Measures, and Waist Girth Measure

If your client has a high BMI, use skinfold measures to determine if it is high because of muscle mass or because of excessive body fat. Next, examine the pattern of fat distribution by measuring waist girth or trunk skinfolds. Even with an acceptable BMI and moderate skinfold measures, there may still be health risks if the waist girth is high and the skinfolds are excessive. These anthropometric measures have been used to establish a health-benefit rating and a method of counseling clients to reduced health risks (CSEP 2003).

Case Histories

For each new client, you must determine what to assess and how to measure it. The following examples trace these decisions about assessments. More details about the individual assessments are described throughout the chapter, and you will find further case histories in chapter 9.

Case History 1

Your first client is a 55-year-old man, moderately overweight. He has been doing some outdoor cycling so he is already in an "action" stage of behavioral change (chapter 1). His doctor has recently encouraged him to get more exercise, and so he has come to your fitness center for guidance.

Is any screening necessary? A number of risk factors become evident in the preliminary counseling, so you select a series of items from the health and lifestyle appraisal (e.g., RISK-I and PAR-Q).

Your client has been cycling outdoors. Considering your preferred mode of assessment, a bicycle ergometer has the advantage of being non-weight-bearing, with no balance concerns. Which method of cycle ergometer assessment is most appropriate? There is no need to push your client to exhaustion. You want to determine his response to various intensities of cycling. Your selection is a three-stage submaximal bike test with the results graphed, allowing you to estimate his heart rate at a large range of workloads.

Because your client's concern about weight comes primarily from a health perspective, your choice for body composition is to use BMI, skinfold measures, and waist girth measure.

Case History 2

Your second client is a previously sedentary 33-year-old woman whose main objective is weight loss. She appears to be moving from a preparation stage to an action stage of behavioral change. She has made it clear that she does not want to be poked and prodded with "those fat pinchers."

How do you proceed with this level of reservation? A health and lifestyle appraisal is a noninvasive way to gain useful information and to continue building rapport. The FANTASTIC Lifestyle Checklist (page 61) takes a holistic approach to weight management; the Inventory of Lifestyle and Activity Preferences (page 18) gives her some choices.

Can you evaluate body composition without skinfold calipers or invasive equipment? BMI (p. 88) uses height and weight measures to provide an indication of relative overweight. You can examine the pattern of fat distribution through the waist girth measure (p. 88), which also provides a barometer for improvement.

If no significant health risks exist and your client does not want a formal cardiovascular assessment, do you even need to do an assessment? You can use a heart rate reserve calculation (p. 172) to determine your client's training zone based on her age, resting heart rate, and desired training level. If you regularly monitor heart rate and compare it with measures of perceived exertion, you can initiate a safe program.

Musculoskeletal Assessment

In this section we examine laboratory and field-based tests for each of the major musculoskeletal components of fitness: strength and muscular endurance, flexibility, and muscle balance. The fitness assessments for strength, muscular endurance, and flexibility, presented in the following pages, can be helpful tools in the assessment of muscle balance. Any misalignments seen in a postural assessment may be attributable to relative tightness or weakness of related muscles.

When selecting field-based assessments, consider the following: joint–muscle relationships; maximal effort; strength level; normative values; specificity, reliability, and validity; body weight test items; client needs; human error; and equipment availability. We discuss client issues in the selection of test items and describe specific field tests for determining the distinct needs of the client. An exercise prescription for a client should be validated using the baseline values for selected components of fitness by using appropriate assessment tools.

Client Considerations in the Selection of Tests

A variety of assessment tools can be used to measure musculoskeletal fitness. Table 4.4 categorizes a number of such tools into laboratory and field-based measures. Because laboratory tests are expensive and more complex to administer, we will deal almost entirely with field-based tests. Field tests are less clinical, more practical, and often performance oriented. Details of the laboratory protocols can be obtained from the *Assessment Resources* (p. 84).

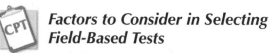

Factors to Consider in Selecting Field-Based Tests

A plethora of field-based assessments are available. When selecting tests, consider several factors:

- **Joint–muscle relationships.** Strength and endurance are specific to the muscle group, the type and speed of contraction, and the joint angle or range of motion. Always consider how your client will be training, the nature of any primary sport participation, the demands of her work environment, or her stated priorities. For example, if your client would like to significantly improve her squash game, you may wish to establish baseline levels of the following:

  - Dynamic strength for shoulder medial rotators through a full range of motion (the power of a forehand shot comes from a rapid contraction of the shoulder medial rotators).

  - Static grip strength (a general indicator of strength and important for racket stability).

  - Dynamic endurance of the knee and hip extensors (extension from a partial crouch position is a movement pattern repeated at high intensities throughout a squash match).

- **Maximal effort.** Most tests require maximum effort. Your client may not be at a stage where this will be accurate or safe. Factors such as time of day, sleep, drug use, and anticipation may also affect a maximum performance. Use caution in pushing clients to their maximum. Flaws in technique usually precede fatigue: Watch clients carefully, and stop the test when they start to struggle.

- **Strength level.** Performance on some endurance tests is highly dependent on strength. Use tests that are proportional to a percentage of the client's maximum strength or proportional to her body weight such as with the five-level sit-up (p. 94).

Table 4.4 Laboratory and Field-Based Musculoskeletal Assessment Tools

	Laboratory	Field-based
Muscular strength and endurance	Isokinetic dynamometer (e.g., Cybex, Kin-Com) Cable tensiometer Load cell	Grip dynamometer Free weights and exercise machines (repetition maximum percent 1RM) Calisthenics (e.g., sit-ups, push-ups)
Flexibility	Leighton flexometer	Goniometer (e.g., ankle, hip) Sit-and-reach Indirect measures (e.g., back hyperextension, shoulder flexion)
Muscle balance		Postural assessment Muscle tightness tests Back fitness test

- **Normative values.** Although some age- and gender-based norms exist (see *Assessment Resources*), many tests lack up-to-date norms against which you can compare your client's results—especially for adults over 25 years. However, test results may serve other functions: Use them to establish baseline levels for measuring improvement (especially if the test resembles the training) or to determine starting points for exercise prescriptions.

- **Specificity, reliability, and validity.** Some very reliable laboratory methods have limited usefulness because they are too specific. For example, the sophisticated isokinetic dynamometers normally measure only one joint action. Yet compound movements involving two joints, such as a leg press action, are common in sports. Another example is the cable tensiometer, which is a good measure of isometric strength but is specific to the angle of contraction and may not reflect dynamic strength.

- **Body weight test items.** Calisthenic tests produce highly variable results. People with high body fat have relatively less muscle and therefore a lower strength level for their body weight. Because the resistance is the client's weight or a portion of that weight, these clients are lifting a relatively higher load (expressed as a percent of their maximum strength). Distribution of body weight affects the results of sit-up tests, because those with relatively more weight in their lower bodies have less resistance with their lighter upper body. On a positive note, calisthenics are cheap, they usually require no equipment, and they can be modified to vary the resistance by changing body and limb positions.

- **Client needs.** Strength testing can be used to effectively monitor rehabilitation after injury and provide objective criteria for the resumption of activity. Many nonathletes use strength training for aesthetic as well as functional reasons. Postural misalignment or compensatory movement patterns may indicate a need for muscle balance assessment. Testing can also provide a guideline for prescription and provide a means of monitoring progress.

- **Human error.** A source of error in muscular fitness testing is the human factor. Our clients must be familiar with the testing procedures and the equipment. They may need time to practice to control for the effects of learning on performance. We need to motivate our clients during and after their trials to encourage maximal performance (using caution, as noted previously). To obtain accurate results, follow the standardized starting positions and testing procedures. Clients may inadvertently modify a position or technique particularly as they fatigue. Observe and spot your clients accordingly.

- **Equipment availability.** Many personal fitness trainers are mobile and travel light or for other reasons do not have assessment equipment readily available to them. Large or expensive equipment is often not necessary. In fact, more than 20 assessments are described in this chapter, and all but one can be performed with only a tape measure, watch, goniometer, aerobic step, and plumb line.

Limitations of Specific Musculoskeletal Fitness Tests

Many traditional physical fitness tests have long been accepted as measures of muscular strength, endurance, or flexibility. Unfortunately, these tests have become evaluations of performance rather than measures of physical fitness. Emphasis is on speed of performance, number of repetitions, or extent of stretching rather than on quality and specificity of movement. Following are examples:

- **Push-ups.** Properly executed push-ups involve scapular abduction during the up phase. When the serratus anterior is weak, the scapulae do not move—and yet the push-up may still be performed. Because other muscles can compensate for this weakness, you may fail to note small changes in body mechanics, such as incomplete flexion of the elbow or an unacceptably wide hand position. The purpose of push-ups is to test the strength or endurance of arm muscles. Winging and lack of abduction of the scapula reveal a weak serratus anterior. If such weakness is not noticed, the test's validity is reduced, and push-ups are not a good index of muscular endurance of the arms.

- **Bent-knee sit-ups.** Exercise specialists often measure endurance of abdominal muscles by having clients perform as many bent-knee sit-ups as possible in 60 s. The curled trunk requires a strong contraction of the abdominals to hold this position. Many people start the test with the trunk curled, but their backs begin to arch because their abdominals are not strong enough to maintain the position. Because the speed and length of the test magnify the problem, the low back is strained. The result is that clients with weak abdominals may pass this test using poor mechanics of the low back and possibly assistance from the hip flexors.

Recent evidence (Chen et al. 2003) shows that curl-ups recruit high abdominal muscle activity, whereas sit-ups do not challenge the obliques, they have a higher psoas activity, and they are ill-advised for an unstable back.

• **Trunk flexion.** One of the most common tests for flexibility is forward trunk flexion, or **sit-and-reach.** Sitting with knees extended, the participant reaches forward toward or beyond the toes. Designed to measure flexibility of the low back and hamstrings, the test focuses on how far the person can reach. The test fails to consider variables that can affect the results:

- There may be limitations attributable to imbalances between length of back and hamstring muscles.
- Poor flexibility in the low back may go undetected if hamstrings have excessive flexibility.

Clients with such imbalances may do well on the test, whereas people with normal flexibility may not do well. Moreover, some trainers would wrongly prescribe therapeutic exercise to increase spinal flexibility or stretch hamstrings when it is unnecessary or contraindicated.

Field-Based Strength and Muscular Endurance Assessment

The term **muscular fitness** has been used to describe the integrated status of muscular strength (maximal force of a muscle) and muscular endurance (ability of a muscle to make repeated contractions or resist muscular fatigue) (ACSM 2000). Assessing muscular fitness involves a continuum of tests that allow few repetitions to measure strength and a greater number of repetitions or longer time held to measure endurance.

Unlike laboratory-based tests for muscular strength and endurance, field-based tests often closely simulate the training activity of your clients, thereby increasing the validity and sensitivity of the assessments. The tests are usually inexpensive and easy to administer and often can be modified to suit desired resistance levels (see *Strength and Endurance Testing,* p. 93). They can help you establish starting prescription levels if the tests closely resemble the exercise.

Strength Test 1: Relative Muscular Endurance in RM Weightlifting

When measuring strength with weights, increase the load to find a weight the client can lift only once (1RM). To test for relative muscular endur-

ance, assign a submaximal load—that is, a percentage of a repetition maximum (1RM). The load should be specific to the objective of the client: a particular sport, a work task, a rehabilitative goal. The exercise used for the test should also reflect the client's objective and reflect a muscular balance between agonist and antagonist. More easily standardized exercises include bench press, latissimus dorsi pull-down, leg curl, leg extension, leg press, arm curl, and triceps extension.

A modification of the 1RM test involves lifts to fatigue between 2RM and 10RM. Estimates of 1RM can be made from the results without having to reach an exact number of repetitions. Figure 4.1 illustrates the average number of repetitions possible when compared with 1RM (Sale and MacDougall 1981). This graph may be used to evaluate results of relative load tests. It shows the percentages of the 1RM that you can try with your client when prescribing at an 8-10RM level or a 1-3RM level. Baechle and Earle (2000) combined similar data to provide a relationship between percentage 1RM and repetitions (table 4.5). To estimate 1RM from results obtained between a 2RM and 10RM, divide the weight lifted by the corresponding %1RM.

For example:

Weight lifted = 140 lb (63.6 kg)

Number of repetitions = 8

1RM: 140 lb/0.80 = 175 lb (79.5 kg)

These estimates are helpful guidelines when prescribing training loads but may vary depending on age and gender, size of muscle group (smaller muscle groups may not produce as many repetitions as predicted), number of sets performed, and type of machine or free weights (Baechle and Earle 2000).

Strength Test 2: Biering–Sorenson Back Endurance

Following screening for back pain, the client lies prone, with legs on a table or portable steps and trunk hanging at a right angle. The iliac crest is positioned at the edge of the table and the appraiser secures the lower thighs. The client raises her trunk to a horizontal position, crosses her arms on the chest, and then maintains that position as long as possible to a maximum of 180 s (figure 4.2). Details of the procedure and interpretation of the Biering–Sorenson back endurance test are in the *Canadian Physical Activity, Fitness and Lifestyle Approach* manual (CSEP 2003).

Strength and Endurance Testing

Client: _____ Date: _____

Assessor: _____

Muscle	Test	Rating system (circle one)	Comments
1) _____ 2) _____ 3) _____ 4) _____	Weightlifting	Exercise: _____ 5-10RM ___; 1RM ___ Exercise: _____ 5-10RM ___; 1RM ___ Exercise: _____ 5-10RM ___; 1RM ___ Exercise: _____ 5-10RM ___; 1RM ___	
Erector spinae	Biering–Sorenson	E.g., Age 20-29 male (M) and female (F) (s) Needs improvement / Fair / Good / Very good / Excellent M ≤85 86-98 99-132 133-175 176-180 F ≤65 66-101 102-135 136-179 179-180	
Rectus abdominis	Five-level sit-ups	1) _____ 2) _____ 3) _____ 4) _____ 5) _____ Number of reps _____	
Lower abdominals	Leg lowers	75° = poor; 60° = fair; 30° = good; 5° = excellent ° = Degrees when back arches while lowering legs	
Quadratus lumborum	Lateral lift	**Right shoulder** Grade 1: Shoulder 12 in. off floor without difficulty Grade 2: Shoulder 12 in. off floor with difficulty Grade 3: Shoulder 2-6 in. off floor Grade 4: Unable to raise shoulder off floor **Left shoulder** Grade 1: Shoulder 12 in. off floor without difficulty Grade 2: Shoulder 12 in. off floor with difficulty Grade 3: Shoulder 2-6 in. off floor Grade 4: Unable to raise shoulder off floor	
Serratus anterior	Push-up	*Strong* = Scapulae flat in down phase *Weak* = Scapular "winging" in down phase	

Complete norms and health benefit zones are available for Biering-Sorenson test in CSEP (2003).

From *Client-Centered Exercise Prescription, Second Edition*, by John C. Griffin, 2006, Champaign, IL: Human Kinetics.

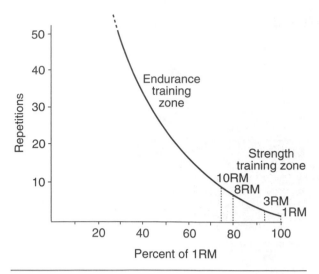

Figure 4.1   Percent of 1RM and number of repetitions.

Reprinted from: *The Canadian Journal of Applied Sports Sciences,* Vol. 6. Published by the Canadian Society for Exercise Physiology, 1981, pp. 87-92.

Table 4.5   Percent of the 1RM and Repetitions Allowed (%1RM–Repetition Relationship)

% 1RM	Number of repetitions allowed
100	1
95	2
93	3
90	4
87	5
85	6
83	7
80	8
77	9
75	10
70	11
67	12
65	15

Reprinted, by permission, from T.R. Baechle and R.W. Earle, 2002, *Essentials of Strength Training and Conditioning,* 2nd ed. (Champaign, IL: Human Kinetics), 407.

Back extensor endurance has been positively related to back health. When coupled with other test results that indicate low abdominal endurance and hip flexor and low back tightness, a Biering–Sorenson finding of poor back extensor endurance has a very strong association with the development of low back pain (Albert et al. 2001).

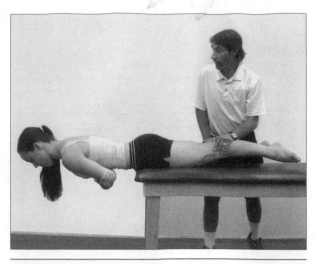

Figure 4.2   Back extensor endurance is associated with back health.

Strength Test 3: Five-Level Sit-Up

With calisthenics, you can use simple biomechanics to change the position of certain body segments and create changes in loading. The five-level sit-up test uses a modified arm position to change the resistance. The knee is at 90° to minimize the involvement of the hip flexors. Figure 4.3 illustrates the procedures for the five levels from least difficult (Level 1) to most difficult (Level 5). The client executes each level one at a time starting with Level 1. If the execution is appropriate, allow a brief rest and then attempt Level 2, and so on (Griffin 1998).

Scoring: If your client visibly strains on the attempt but does manage to perform it correctly, this is considered her "strength level." If she has to modify her technique to complete the sit-up (such as extending her legs or using momentum), the previous level is considered her strength level. To assess her "endurance level," select the sit-up one level below her strength level. To test for muscular endurance, have your client complete as many correct repetitions as possible for 1 min or to the point of fatigue. The test may also be terminated when she performs a second technical flaw (any flawed repetitions are not counted).

Before using the results of the tests to prescribe an exercise program, determine your client's objectives: strength, strength–endurance, or endurance. From the results of the strength and endurance tests, you can prescribe the level of sit-ups and the number of repetitions to suit her objective (also see chapter 7). By having her move her heels 2 to 4 in. closer to the buttocks, you can make the level slightly more difficult and fine-tune her prescription.

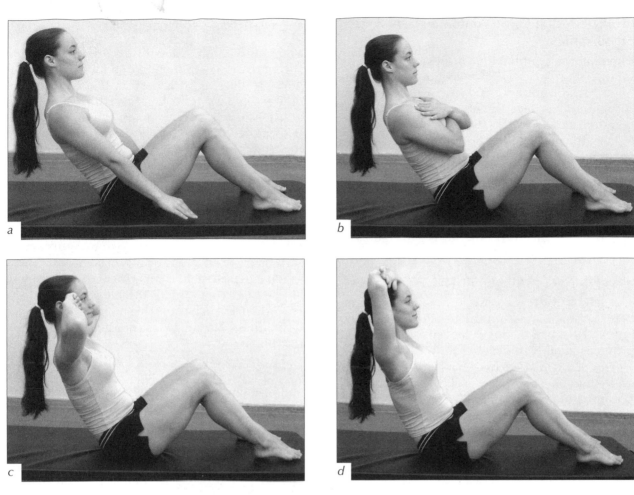

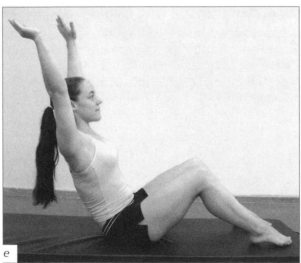

Figure 4.3 Five-level sit-ups provide a starting point for the prescription.

Strength Test 4: Lower Abdominal and Pelvic Stabilization

The client lies supine on a hard surface with her knees bent (figure 4.4). The examiner places one hand, palm up, under the low back. The client straightens her legs directly up in the air (90°) and then slowly lowers her extended legs, trying to keep the pressure on the appraiser's hand. The test is terminated when the spine begins to rise off the appraiser's fingers. The angle between the legs and the floor at this point represents the stabilizing strength of the abdominals as they counter the eccentric pull of the hip flexors. An angle of 75° is poor strength, 60° is fair, 30° is good, and 5° is excellent (Ellison 1995).

Strength Test 5: Lateral Lift Test

The lateral lift test assesses the quadratus lumborum, which is part of the back extensor group but is also a prime mover for lateral flexion and provides lateral support to the spine and pelvis.

The client lies on his side with arms folded across the chest and feet stabilized (figure 4.5). While maintaining the body straight with no twisting, the client raises his shoulder off the floor as high as possible and holds it briefly. He should avoid jerking movements or pushing off with the elbow. The scoring is seen in *Strength and Endurance Testing* (p. 93) (Imrie and Barbuto 1988).

Strength Test 6: Serratus Anterior (Push-Up)

Push-ups are commonly performed as part of a musculoskeletal test battery (figure 4.6). An indication of a weak serratus anterior is a winging of the scapulae when your client executes the down phase of a push-up (Michaelson and Gagne 2002).

Flexibility Assessment

You can determine flexibility directly by measuring the range of motion of a joint or series of joints in degrees with devices like goniometers or flexometers. The Leighton flexometer has a test–retest reliability ranging from .90 to .99 (Heyward 2002). With goniometers, locating the true joint center is critical to obtaining true readings. Goniometer test–retest results with the same appraiser are stronger than between different appraisers (Norkin and White 1995). Indirect assessment methods, using measuring tapes, are often criticized as crude and lacking normative data. As well, because the length or width of body segments can affect the results of some tests, such as the sit-and-reach, comparing individuals may not be highly valid with these tests. These tests nevertheless can be effective monitoring tools for individuals. No single test predicts overall body flexibility.

The range of motion of a joint may be limited by a number of factors including skeletal contact and ligaments as well as tight muscles. There are a number of excellent field tests for muscle tightness that do not involve putting the joint through a full range of motion.

Flexibility and Muscle Tightness Field-Based Assessments

For this component of flexibility, it is particularly important to be client-centered. Each joint and range of motion are unique. Careful questioning can help you focus on the areas of potential concern. Test joint range of motion to determine if it is limited, excessive, or within normal limits.

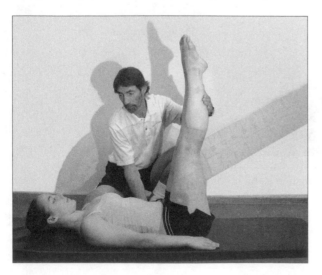 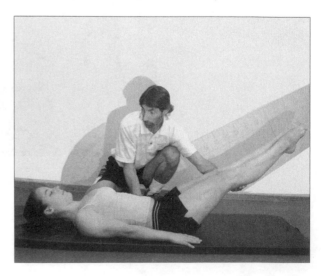

Figure 4.4   Lower abdominal strength is important for core stability.

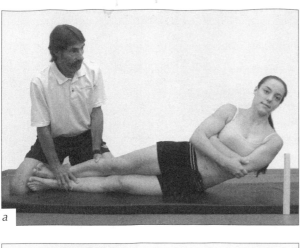

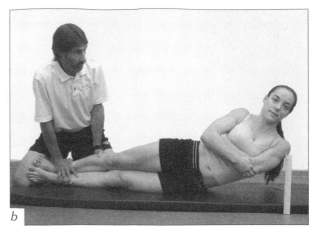

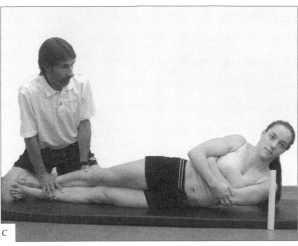

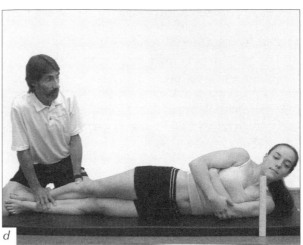

Figure 4.5 Lateral lift test: *(a)* grade 1: excellent, *(b)* grade 2: average, *(c)* grade 3: fair, and *(d)* grade 4: poor.

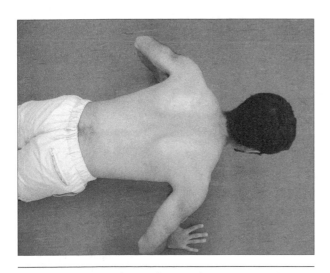

Figure 4.6   Winged scapulae: weak serratus anterior.

A summary of the results of these assessments can be recorded in *Field-Based Assessments of Flexibility and Muscle Tightness* (see p. 98).

Flexibility Test 1: Sit-and-Reach

The client sits, legs extended, with soles of feet (bare) vertical against the flexometer, 6 inches (15 cm) apart and at the 10 inch (26 cm) mark of the ruler (figure 4.7). Instruct her to bend and reach forward gradually with arms even, palms down, and knees straight. She lowers her head and holds at a comfortable distance near maximum for 2 s. Complete details of the test procedure and scoring are in the *Canadian Physical Activity, Fitness, and Lifestyle Approach* manual (CSEP 2003).

Field-Based Assessments of Flexibility and Muscle Tightness

Client: _____ Date: _____

Assessor: _____

Shoulder, chest assessment	Results (observations)	Normal ROM	Pain Y/N
Shoulder internal (medial) rotation: (tightness of infraspinatus, teres minor)	L: _____ R: _____	70°	
Shoulder external (lateral) rotation: (tightness of subscapularis)	L: _____ R: _____	90°	
Pectoralis major (sternal) length		Table level	
Pectoralis minor length	L: _____ R: _____		
Shoulder joint abduction (see dynamic shoulder alignment)		180°	

Interpretation and comments:

_____

_____

_____

Back assessment	Results (observations)	Normal ROM	Pain Y/N
Spinal rotation: Lumbar Cervical	L: _____ R: _____ L: _____ R: _____	45° 65-70°	
Sit-and-reach test: (actual) (visual)		Good: 11-13 in (28-33 cm) (males) 13-15 in. (32-37 cm) (females)	

Interpretation and comments:

_____

_____

_____

(continued)

Hip, knee assessment	Results (observations)	Normal ROM	Pain Y/N
Hamstring length	L: _____ R: _____	80° (males) 90° (females)	
Hip flexors: 1 joint (tightness of iliopsoas)	L: _____ R: _____	Thigh table level	
Hip flexors: 2 joints (tightness of rectus femoris)	L: _____ R: _____	Knee: 80°	
Tensor fascia latae tightness	L: _____ R: _____		
Hip internal (medial) rotation (tightness of gluteus maximus, piriformis)	L: _____ R: _____	35°	
Hip external (lateral) rotation (tightness of gluteus minimus, anterior gluteus medius)	L: _____ R: _____	45°	

Interpretation and comments:

_____

_____

_____

Ankle assessment	Results (observations)	Normal ROM	Pain Y/N
Ankle plantar flexion: (tightness of tibialis anterior)	L: _____ R: _____	45-50°	
Ankle dorsiflexion: 1 joint (tightness of soleus)	L: _____ R: _____	20°	
Ankle dorsiflexion: 2 joints (tightness of gastrocnemius)	L: _____ R: _____	10°	

Interpretation and comments:

_____

_____

_____

Note. ROM = range of movement.

From *Client-Centered Exercise Prescription, Second Edition,* by John C. Griffin, 2006, Champaign, IL: Human Kinetics.

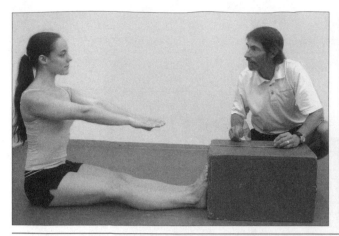 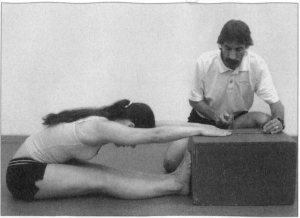

Figure 4.7 Sit-and-reach test may indicate back or hamstring tightness.

Normal: "Good" scores range from 11 to 13 in. (28 to 33 cm) (males) and 13 to 15 in. (32 to 37 cm) (females) for those up to 40 years of age (CSEP 2003). However, this test does not indicate where limitation or excessive motion has taken place (Alter 2004). Various combinations of short hamstrings, back muscles, shoulder muscles, or gastrocnemius may be the cause of poor performance. Watch your clients carefully while they execute this test to identify where movement is restricted (e.g., flat back).

Flexibility Test 2: Ankle Range of Motion

The full range of motion for the ankle is conservatively 65 to 70°. These field-based tests are more sensitive to where the muscle tightness may be restrictive. Armed with the information, you can be more client-centered with your prescription (figure 4.8).

- **Plantar flexion (length of dorsiflexor muscles).** Have the client sit on the edge of a table with knees at 90° and legs dangling. Align the center of the goniometer with the center of the lateral malleolus. Next, align one arm of the goniometer with the head of the fibula, and set the other arm at 90°. The neutral position of the ankle has the lateral sole of the foot parallel to the lower arm of the goniometer. Ask your client to actively plantar flex the ankle. An average range of motion should be 45-50° (Kendall et al. 1993). A range of motion much less than 40° may affect your client's ability to buffer the trauma of bearing weight—particularly when running or engaging in other locomotor activities.

- **Dorsiflexion (length of one-joint plantar flexor muscles).** Client and instrument are set up as previously described. Ask the client to actively dorsiflex the ankle. An average range of motion

should be 20° (Kendall et al. 1993). Clients with a range of motion less than this have tight soleus or tibialis posterior muscles and possibly weak dorsiflexors. Runners and other aerobic exercisers may experience lower-leg rotation or overstretching of the Achilles tendon if these plantar flexor muscles are tight.

- **Dorsiflexion (length of two-joint plantar flexor muscles).** Have client sit on a table or floor with knees straight. Align the goniometer as described previously. Ask client to actively dorsiflex the ankle. An average range of motion should be 10° (Kendall et al. 1993). Clients with a range of motion less than this have a tight gastrocnemius muscle. This muscle crosses over the back of the knee; when the knee is extended, the gastrocnemius pulls tight and further restricts the ankle in dorsiflexion. With practice, the angle from the neutral position can be estimated quite accurately without a goniometer.

Flexibility Test 3: Shoulder Internal and External Rotation Range of Motion

Have the client supine on a table, with knees bent and the spine in a neutral curve (figure 4.9). Arm is abducted to 90°, elbow is at 90° and off the table, and forearm is perpendicular to the floor. The goniometer axis is aligned with the humerus, the stable arm is perpendicular to the floor, and the moving arm is aligned with the styloid process. Internal (medial) rotation movement should be 70° (measuring infraspinatus and teres minor tightness). The external (lateral) rotation should be 90° (measuring subscapularis tightness). Instruct your client to avoid protracting shoulder girdle, rotating trunk, lifting shoulder, and changing angle at shoulder or elbow (DeLisa 1998).

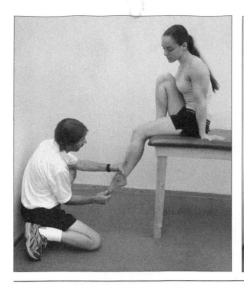 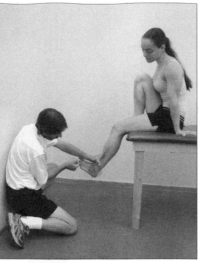 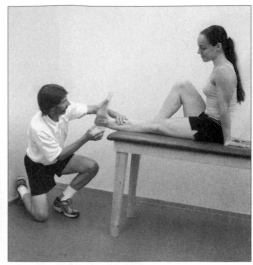

Figure 4.8   Ankle range of motion is important for clients involved in running activities.

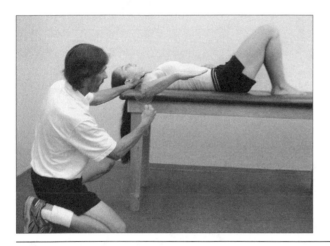 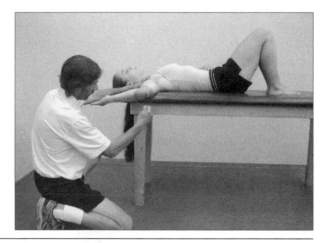

Figure 4.9   Shoulder rotation is important for clients involved in throwing activities.

Flexibility Test 4: Hip Internal and External Rotation Range of Motion

Have your client sit with knee flexed at 90° and leg dangling (figure 4.10). The center of the goniometer is on the patella, aligned with the femur. The stable arm is perpendicular to the table, and the moving arm is aligned with the middle of the anterior ankle. Internal (medial) rotation movement should be 35° and external (lateral) rotation should be 45°. Avoid rotating trunk or lifting thigh from the table (DeLisa 1998).

Flexibility Test 5: Spinal Rotation Range of Motion (Cervical and Lumbar/Thoracic)

Have the client sit with arms folded across her chest or with hands on anterior thighs. The goniometer is horizontal with the axis over the center

cranial head with the examiner standing behind and looking down (figure 4.11).

- **Cervical rotation.** The stable arm is aligned parallel to an imaginary line between the two acromial processes. Align the moving arm with the nose. Rotation to the right and left should be 65 to 70° each. Have the client stabilize his shoulder girdle on the back support of the chair to prevent rotation of the thoracic and lumbar spine.

- **Lumbar and thoracic rotation.** The stable arm is aligned parallel to an imaginary line between the two anterior iliac spines. Align the moving arm with the nose. It must remain aligned with the sternum (i.e., the cervical spine does not rotate). Rotation to the right and left should be 45° each. Check that the client stabilizes his pelvis to prevent any other spinal movement (Norkin and White 1995).

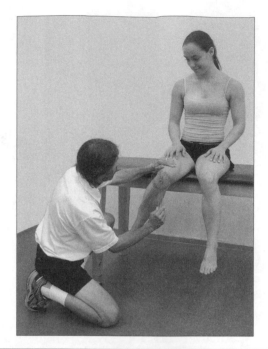

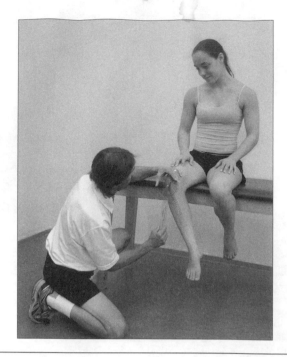

Figure 4.10 Lack of hip rotation can increase strain on knees and low back.

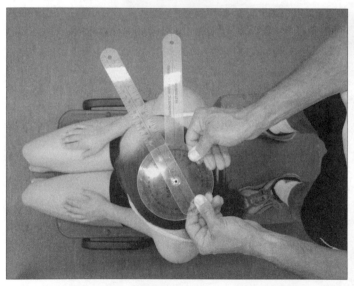

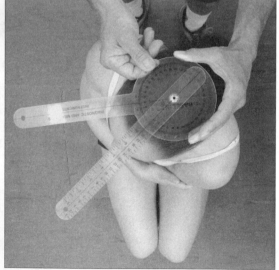

Figure 4.11 Many functional activities are dependent on good spinal rotation.

Muscle Tightness Tests

Examine the needs and demands of your client. Has a joint area been overworked, possibly causing muscle tightness? For example, clients who play a weight-bearing sport or who regularly perform a weight-bearing locomotor activity should have ankle flexibility assessed. Clients who sit for long periods of time should be checked for tightness of the hip flexors and in some cases the trunk extensors. Many manual workers tend to have tight anterior chest muscles such as the pectoralis major and minor. Overuse or underuse of back muscles may leave them tight and the joints inflexible.

A horizontal bench or one of the longer portable aerobic steps may substitute for an examination table for the following assessments.

Tightness Test 1: Length of Pectoralis Minor (Kendall et al. 1993)

1. Have the client lie supine, knees bent and low back neutral, palms up (figure 4.12).

2. Look from above the head; determine whether the shoulders are significantly off the table and are equal.

3. Gently push the shoulders to judge the resistance and to see if muscle tightness is slight, moderate, or marked.

Tightness Test 2: Length of Pectoralis Major (Sternal) (Kendall et al. 1993)

1. Have client lie supine, knees bent, and low back neutral.

2. Assist client to slowly lower arm at 135° abduction.

3. Be sure shoulder is laterally rotated and elbow is straight.

Normal: arm should rest, relaxed on the table.

Tightness Test 3: Length of Hip Flexors (Kendall et al. 1993)

1. With the client seated at the very edge of the table, help her roll back to a tucked supine position. Appraiser has one hand behind client's back and the other under her knee.

2. Have the client pull one thigh toward the chest only enough to flatten the low back and sacrum to the table.

3. The opposite thigh is allowed to slowly lower over the edge of the table with the knee freely relaxed.

4. Note the angle of thigh and knee.

Normal one-joint hip flexor (e.g., iliopsoas): thigh remains on the table (any lift is measured in degrees).

Normal two-joint hip flexor (e.g., rectus femoris): knee flexion of 80°.

Note: If the hip abducts and internally rotates with some knee extension, the tensor fascia latae are probably tight.

Tightness Test 4: Length of Hamstrings (Kendall et al. 1993)

1. Have client lie supine on the table or floor.

2. See that client's legs are extended, with low back and sacrum pushed flat on table.

   If low back is not flat (short hip flexors), use a rolled towel under the knees just enough to flatten the back.

3. Hold one thigh down and assist client to gently raise the test leg.

4. Be sure the knee is straight and the foot is relaxed.

5. Have the client raise her leg until restraint is felt.

Normal: 80 to 90°.

Muscle Balance Assessment

Muscle balance does not mean equal strength between agonists and antagonists (e.g., hamstrings and quadriceps). And it means more than a proper

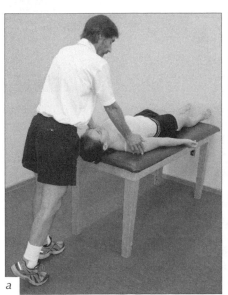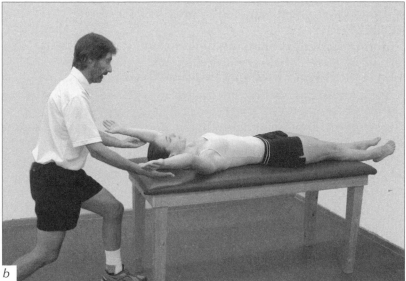

Figure 4.12   Muscle length assessments of the shoulder: *(a)* pectoralis minor and *(b)* pectoralis major (sternal).

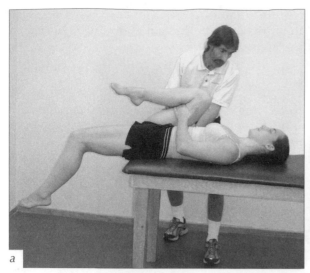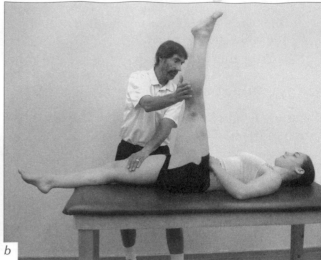

Figure 4.13   Muscle length assessments of the lower body: *(a)* hip flexors and *(b)* hamstrings.

ratio of strength or muscular endurance of one muscle group relative to another muscle group. Muscle balance exists when there is a proper relationship between the strength, length, and neural excitation of related muscles. This relationship should exist between agonists and antagonists, between synergistic muscles that work together, and between prime movers and stabilizers. When certain muscles become stronger or tighter than their counterparts, muscle imbalance occurs. Muscle imbalance is also a major cause of faulty movement patterns.

A battery of fitness assessments for strength, muscular endurance, and flexibility, similar to what we have just discussed, can be helpful tools in assessing muscle balance. However, a more focused client-centered approach is most effective.

First, you will probably notice some indication of muscle imbalance: For example, a past injury, a complaint of localized tightness or aching, or an occupation or sport that requires repetitive movement patterns may come up during the preassessment counseling. A closer examination may be afforded with a postural assessment. Any misalignments may be attributable to relative tightness or weakness of related muscles. Further probing with respect to symptoms, history, or lifestyle may shed new light at this point. To verify relative tightness or weakness, select relevant tests outlined in this chapter. With this data in hand, specific to the symmetry of your client, you are much better prepared to set clear objectives and design effective prescriptions.

Postural Assessment

Good posture involves all body parts in a state of balance and the muscles holding the body erect against gravity without fatigue. A misaligned human body does not collapse—rather it twists out of shape to compensate for imbalances and requires extra muscular energy and tension to hold itself up.

Postural assessment is a very effective screening tool (figure 4.14). By carefully observing alignment, we can detect strain produced by faulty relationships of various body parts. By keeping the postural assessment simple, we increase the speed of assessment and can go directly to the next stage of muscle balance assessment: muscle tightness and weakness testing.

Alignment While Standing

Have your clients remove shoes and socks. Women should wear a two-piece bathing suit, and men should wear trunks, to allow a clear view of landmarks. You will find a plumb line and a horizontal line grid very helpful but not necessary for screening purposes. A brick or cement block wall also is helpful. Assess your client in a standing position from three positions—side, back, and front. Ask your client to stand in an upright, relaxed position, looking forward. Figure 4.14 shows the anatomical structures that coincide with the line of reference. Your observations should be referenced to the *Segmental Postural Assessment* forms on pp. 107-109.

Figure 4.15 illustrates ideal alignment and figure 4.16 illustrates common postural faults.

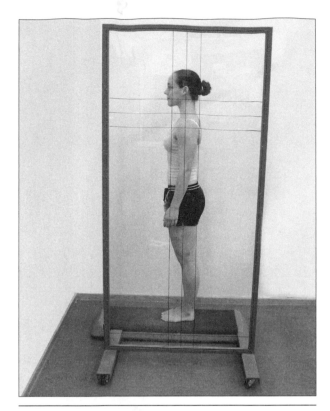

Figure 4.14   Portable postural grid.

Practice in judging good and faulty posture will quickly improve your skill levels.

The "standard posture" (Kendall et al. 1993) represents an ideal skeletal alignment that minimizes stress and maximizes efficiency. No one will match the standard in every respect.

- **Side view.** The following points coincide with a vertical line of reference in a lateral view:

    - Slightly anterior to lateral malleolus
    - Slightly anterior to axis of knee
    - Slightly posterior to axis of hip
    - Bodies of lumber vertebrae
    - Shoulder joint
    - Bodies of most of cervical vertebrae
    - Mastoid process (Kendall et al. 1993)

Check alignment of knees, position of pelvis, curves of the spine, head position, and chest position. If the spinal curves appear excessive, have the client stand with heels 3 in. from the wall with the buttocks, scapulae, and head touching the wall. Slide your cupped hand, fingertips against the wall, behind his neck to approximate normal cervical lordosis. Place your cupped hand behind his low back to check for excessive lumbar lordosis. If the cupped hand fits easily between the spine and the wall, the lordosis is pronounced.

- **Back view.** Start by observing alignment of the Achilles tendon, angle of the femurs, height of the posterior iliac spines, lateral pelvic tilt, spinal deviations, position of shoulders and scapulae, and angle of the head.

- **Front view.** Observe the following: position of the feet, knees, and legs; height of the longitudinal arch; pronation or supination of the foot; rotation of the femur as revealed by the patella; knock-knees or bowlegs; rotation of the head; or prominence of the ribs.

Segmental Postural Assessment Charts

The body is a series of kinetic chains where misalignment in one area can set off a number of compensatory adjustments that may be seen, and felt, a far distance from the original problem. For this reason, a complete static postural assessment from at least three views should be done. However, because of time or prior knowledge of the problem area, the examiner may elect to do a "segmental" postural analysis. Separate assessments (see forms on pp. 107-109) may be done for the lower body, upper body, and spine. These forms overlap slightly to reflect muscles that extend into adjacent areas that may exert imbalanced forces. Therefore, the scores for each segment cannot be summed and are merely helpful benchmarks for reassessment.

The left column of each segmental postural assessment form (pp. 107-109) lists key body areas to be examined. As an ideal standard, there is a column describing "good alignment." The best vantage point for viewing this alignment (A = anterior; P = posterior; L = lateral) is suggested in the preceding column. A description of faulty alignment is included to contrast the good alignment and to cue the examiner toward specific observations. A clear indication of the faulty posture would score a 3. The table allows the recording of left or right sides and any other comments or observations (e.g., "chin forward") or relevant client remarks.

Static and Dynamic Foot Alignment

For any client who will be running or walking, carefully observe the longitudinal arch as part of a static and dynamic postural assessment.

- **Longitudinal arch.** While the client is standing, feet shoulder-width apart, have him lift one foot off the floor so you can observe his arch. This assessment may also be done in a sitting position if it is more comfortable. The idea is to

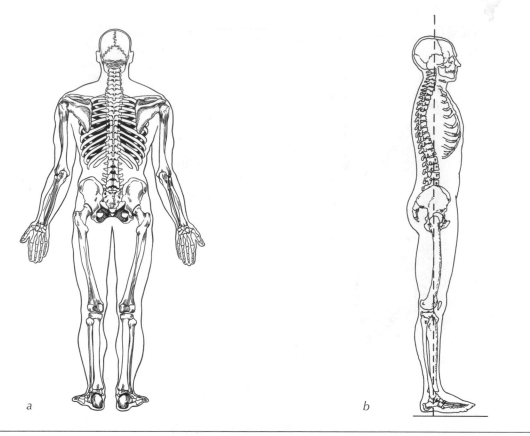

Figure 4.15   Ideal alignment: *(a)* back view and *(b)* side view.

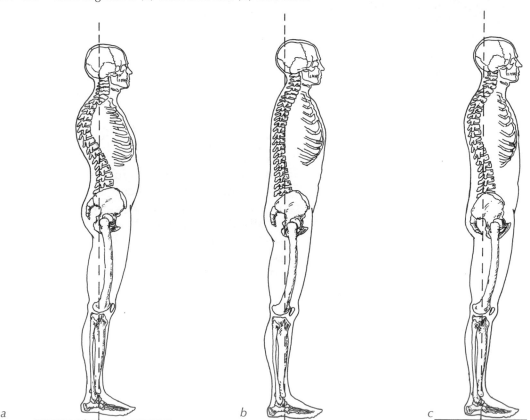

Figure 4.16   Common postural faults: *(a)* kyphosis–lordosis posture, *(b)* flat-back posture, and *(c)* posterior pelvic tilt.

Segmental Postural Assessment: Lower Body

Alignment scale:

5 (good)	4	3 (faulty)	2	1 (very faulty)

Joint	View	Good alignment	Faulty alignment	Score	Left/right	Comments
Foot	A	Half dome arch	Low arch, flat foot			
	A/P	Feet toe out slightly	Significant toeing out or in Pronation or supination			
Knees and legs	A/P	Vertically aligned	Bowlegs (genu varum) or knock-knees (genu valgum)			
	A	Kneecaps face ahead	Kneecaps inward or outward (rotated femur)			
	L	Knees straight, not locked (lateral view)	Flexed or hyperextended knee			
Spine and pelvis	A/P	Hips level, weight even on both feet	One hip higher (lateral tilt), hips rotated (forward one side)			
			Score	___/30		

Note: A = anterior; P = posterior; L = lateral.

Recommendations:

_____

_____

_____

From *Client-Centered Exercise Prescription, Second Edition,* by John C. Griffin, 2006, Champaign, IL: Human Kinetics.

Segmental Postural Assessment: Upper Body

Alignment scale: 5   4   3   2   1
                   (good)   (faulty)   (very faulty)

Emotional stress may cause any combination of these misalignments.

Joint	View	Good alignment	Faulty alignment	Score	Left/right	Comments
Head	L P	Erect and balanced	Protruding, chin forward Tilted or rotated			
Arms and shoulders	A	Arms relaxed, palms facing body	Arms stiff, away from body Palms facing backward			
	L	Shoulders back	Shoulders rounded or forward			
	A/P	Shoulders level	One or both shoulders up, down, or rotated			
	P	Scapulae: flat on ribcage, 4-6 in. (10-15 cm) apart	Scapulae: prominent winged, far apart			
			Score	___/25		

Note: A = anterior; P = posterior; L = lateral.

Recommendations:

_____

_____

_____

From *Client-Centered Exercise Prescription, Second Edition,* by John C. Griffin, 2006, Champaign, IL: Human Kinetics.

Segmental Postural Assessment: Spine

Alignment scale: 5 (good) 4 3 (faulty) 2 1 (very faulty)

Joint	View	Good alignment	Faulty alignment	Score	Left/right	Comments
Spine and pelvis	A/P	Hips level, weight even on both feet	One hip higher (lateral tilt), hips rotated (forward one side)			
	P	No lateral curve to spine (posterior view)	C- or S-curve scoliosis Ribs prominent one side			
	L	Natural lumbar curve	Lordosis: forward tilt of pelvis Flat back: pelvis tilts backward			
	L	Natural thoracic curve	Kyphosis: thoracic rounding			
	L	Natural cervical curve	Cervical lordosis: forward head			
Trunk	L	Flat or slightly rounded abdomen	Lower or entire abdomen protrudes			
	L	Chest slightly raised	Hollow chest or rounded back			
Head	L P	Erect and balanced	Protruding, chin forward Tilted or rotated			
		Score	__/40			

Note: A = anterior; P = posterior; L = lateral.

Recommendations:

_____

_____

_____

From *Client-Centered Exercise Prescription, Second Edition,* by John C. Griffin, 2006, Champaign, IL: Human Kinetics.

assess the arch in a non-weight-bearing position (Griffin 1989). Another alternative is to have your client remove his shoes and immediately stand on a noncarpeted surface. When he steps off, an imprint of his foot showing his arch should be visible (figure 4.17).

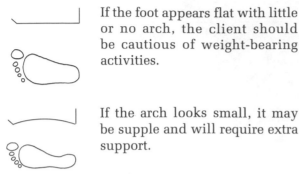

If the foot appears flat with little or no arch, the client should be cautious of weight-bearing activities.

If the arch looks small, it may be supple and will require extra support.

If the arch looks full it is probably healthy, mechanically sound, and able to support trauma.

Figure 4.17 Poor arch support can lead to lower leg overuse injuries.

• **Dynamic foot alignment.** Whether pronation or a flattened arch was present during the static postural assessment, you should observe the back and front of the foot for the degree of rolling inward while the client walks or jogs. This assessment is best performed with the client wearing no shoes (Griffin 1989) (figure 4.18).

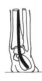

If the heel or forefoot rolls inward, "flattening the arch" while the client is walking or jogging lightly, the client pronates.

If the heel rolls inward somewhat while the client is walking or jogging lightly, the client should avoid overuse.

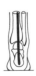

If the heel remains stable and the Achilles tendon is vertical while client is walking or jogging lightly, then the ankle is aligned.

Figure 4.18 Foot pronation should be assessed with all clients involved in running activities.

Dynamic Shoulder Alignment

During the static posture assessment, you may have recognized rounded shoulders, forward head, abducted or winged scapula, protracted head with a cervical lordosis, or backward-facing palms (see *Segmental Postural Assessment: Upper Body,* on p. 108). Repetitive movements that overemphasize one muscle group, movement compensations perhaps caused by injury, lack of range of motion, or even emotional stress may cause any combination of these misalignments.

A more functional approach examining dynamic shoulder alignment may give us a better idea of muscular or neural imbalances. The Shoulder Clock Test (figure 4.19) will help you observe the dynamic relationship between the shoulder girdle and the shoulder joint. The client is positioned with her head, back, and arms pressed against the wall with her feet approximately 1 ft (30 cm) away from the wall. Ask her to slide her extended arms up the wall, palms forward, in a slow and deliberate manner, as high as she can without her back, head, or arms leaving the wall (Michaelson and Gagne 2002). This may also be repeated with the client facing the wall so you can better observe the scapular movement and trapezius contraction.

Watch for a number of things:

• Excessive elevation (shrugging) of the scapula may indicate dominant or neurally facilitated upper trapezius. It may also reflect a weakness in the lower trapezius and serratus anterior if normal upward (lateral) rotation of the scapula is not seen. (*Note:* Weakness of the serratus anterior and possible tightness of the pectoralis minor may be present if your client's scapulae "wing" during the down phase of a push-up.)

• If the arms leave contact with the wall, the pectoralis major or the latissimus dorsi may be tight (Michaelson and Gagne 2002).

• If the client cannot keep his low back in a neutral position and you observe excessive lumbar lordosis while he raises his arms, he may have tight anterior chest or medial shoulder rotators, and his arched back is allowing his arms to remain against the wall.

• The client should demonstrate symmetry: Do his arms rise at the same speed; does one lose contact with the wall; does the head lean to one side; does one scapula rise before or higher than the other?

• Shoulder joint abduction range of motion should approach 180°.

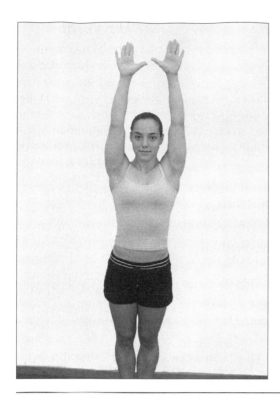 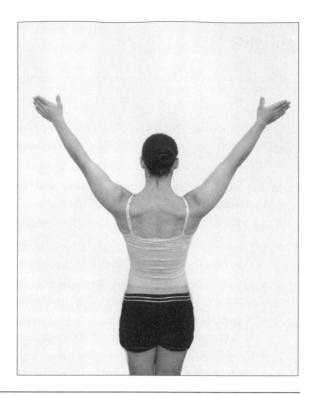

Figure 4.19   Shoulder girdle and shoulder joint should work synchronously.

- If pain occurs, perhaps resulting from impingement, note the angle at the onset of the symptom—beyond this range should be avoided.

Tightness and Weakness Assessment

When postural screening reveals faulty alignment or body mechanics, consider the possibility that your client has a muscular imbalance. Confirm those results by applying specific flexibility (p. 96) or muscle tightness (p. 102) tests and strength and muscular endurance tests (pp. 92) to the joint areas. The postural analysis will help you determine which musculoskeletal tests you should perform.

Although flexibility is often defined as a range of motion of a joint, it is not a simple matter: It involves both the length and strength of muscles. A short muscle restricts the normal range of motion. A shortened muscle may not be a strong muscle because there are fewer cross-bridge sites available with the overlap of the actin and myosin filaments. Muscles that are too short hold the opposite muscle in a lengthened position. Excessively long muscles are usually weak and allow adaptive shortening of antagonists. It is the old argument: "Did the chicken or the egg come first?"

When prescribing to improve muscle balance, use exercise movements that

- **lengthen** short muscles by increasing the distance between the muscles' origin and insertion opposite to the direction of the muscle action, and

- **strengthen** weak muscles that have been elongated by tight antagonist muscles.

You will encounter a large number of clients, particularly middle-aged people, with musculoskeletal injuries or low back problems. Most low back problems are attributable to postural misalignment and a lack of muscle balance. The highest incidence of aerobic and running injuries involve the lower leg precipitated by muscle tightness and poor range of motion around the ankle. Careful questioning can help you focus on the areas of potential concern.

A preoccupation with instrumentation has left many personal trainers feeling inadequate when faced with the measurement of flexibility and strength. Yet physiotherapists, athletic trainers, and physicians rely successfully on their skills of manual assessment. Although, as a personal fitness trainer, you are not qualified to diagnose, treat, or directly prescribe treatment for any injuries, you must develop the knowledge and skill base to recognize what exercises will help strengthen weak muscles, stretch tight muscles, or correct negative muscular imbalances, thus aiding prevention or rehabilitation of an injury.

Highlights

1. **Consider client issues in selecting specific field tests.**

    The client-centered prescription model is flexible, allowing you to verify your client's needs by using selected assessment items that relate to your client's priorities and closely simulate her current training activity. This text focuses on the selection of field-based assessments and the consideration of maximal effort; normative values; specificity, reliability, and validity; client needs; human error; and equipment availability.

2. **Select a cardiovascular exercise mode and test protocol that is suitable for your client's age, gender, anticipated mode of exercise, and health and fitness status.**

    It is a challenge to select suitable assessment items for many clients. Consider the following:

    *   It is more appropriate to use a bicycle than a treadmill, step, or arm ergometer with clients who need increased monitoring of heart rate or blood pressure.
    *   For clients with poor leg strength, a treadmill is preferable to a bike or step; for those with poor balance, a bike is better than a treadmill or step.
    *   A lower intensity is appropriate for clients suspected to have a low oxygen uptake; high intensity is appropriate for those who are regularly active.
    *   Longer warm-ups and smaller increases in workloads are appropriate for those requiring more time to reach steady state.

3. **Identify the advantages of field-based cardiovascular assessment.**

    Results from relatively simple field-based tests may be adequate to identify and quantify your client's needs. Field-based tests are usually less expensive and more easily administered than lab tests. For the personal trainer or small facility director, they may be the only option. They can be very helpful if the regular method of monitoring is similar to that used for the field tests (e.g., minutes per mile, miles per hour, heart rates, or perceived exertion—all easily measured—can be quick indicators of progress). Walking test protocols can be used for relatively inactive clients who are comfortable with walking but for whom jogging is inappropriate. Because more than one client can be assessed at one time, the running protocols are frequently used with sport teams.

4. **Identify the strengths, weaknesses, and sources of measurement error of laboratory and field-based body composition assessment tools.**

    The techniques used to assess body composition are hydrostatic weighing (densitometry), air displacement plethysmography, bioelectrical impedance, and anthropometry (e.g., skinfold and girth measures). These analyses are based on measuring the ratio of fat to fat-free mass. Underwater weighing and air displacement plethysmography were for years the gold standard for laboratory assessment of body composition; however, the assumption of a constant density for fat-free mass introduces some error. As well, the time, expense, and expertise needed are often prohibitive. With bioelectrical impedance, the variability of the analyzers and the specificity of the equations (age, gender, obesity, activity) are their current weaknesses. Bioelectrical impedence may have advantages over the skinfold techniques for clients who are overfat, are heavily muscled, or have thick, tight skin. Body composition determined from skinfold measurement correlates well with underwater weighing when performed by an experienced exercise specialist. Body mass index (BMI) and the waist girth measure are estimates of body composition and, along with skinfold measures, can be effective monitoring measures for individual progress. Waist girth measure provides a valid representation of trunk fat distribution, which is associated with health risk. Comparing clients with norms is often less effective than comparing each client's progress over time with his or her own individual measurements.

5. **Describe the factors to consider in selecting field-based musculoskeletal assessments.**

    The selection of field-based assessments should consider the following:

    *   Joint–muscle relationships: Strength and endurance are specific to the muscle group, the type and speed of contraction, and the joint angle or range of motion.

- Maximal effort: Your client may not be at a stage where this will be accurate or safe.
- Normative values: Many tests lack up-to-date norms; use them to establish baseline levels for measuring improvement or to determine starting points for exercise prescriptions.
- Specificity, reliability, and validity: Some very reliable laboratory methods have limited usefulness because they are too specific.
- Body weight test items: Calisthenic tests produce highly variable results but they can be modified to vary the resistance by changing body and limb positions.
- Client needs: Testing can also provide a guideline for prescription and a means of monitoring progress.
- Human error: To obtain accurate results, follow the standardized starting positions and testing procedures.
- Equipment availability: Many personal fitness trainers are mobile and do not have assessment equipment readily available to them.

6. **Identify the objectives of selected field-based strength and endurance assessments.**

Strength and Endurance Assessments

Muscle	Test	
1) 2) 3) 4)	Weightlifting	The load should be specific to the objective of the client: a particular sport, work task, or rehabilitative goal. The exercise used for the test should also reflect the client's objective and reflect a muscular balance between agonist and antagonist.
Erector spinae	Biering–Sorenson	When coupled with other test results that indicate low abdominal endurance and hip flexor and low back tightness, a Biering–Sorenson finding of poor back extensor endurance has a very strong association with the development of low back pain.
Rectus abdominis	Five-level sit-ups	With calisthenics, you can use simple biomechanics to change the position of certain body segments and create changes in loading.
Lower abdominals	Leg lowers	The angle between the legs and the floor represents the stabilizing strength of the abdominals as they counter the eccentric pull of the hip flexors and stabilize the pelvis.
Quadratus lumborum	Lateral lift	The lateral lift test assesses the quadratus lumborum, which is part of the back extensor group and provides lateral support to the spine and pelvis.
Serratus anterior	Push-up	Winging of the scapula in the down phase indicates a weakness within the shoulder girdle stabilizers.

7. **Identify the objectives of selected field-based flexibility and muscle tightness assessments.**

Shoulder and Chest

Shoulder internal (medial) rotation: tightness of infraspinatus, teres minor

Shoulder external (lateral) rotation: tightness of subscapularis

Pectoralis major (sternal) length

Pectoralis minor length

Shoulder joint abduction (dynamic shoulder alignment)

Back

Spinal rotation: lumbar and cervical

Sit-and-reach test: actual measure: erector spinae and hamstrings; visual: pelvis and back curvature

Hip and Knee

Hamstring length

Hip flexors: one joint (tightness of iliopsoas)

Hip flexors: two joints (tightness of rectus femoris)

Tensor fascia latae tightness

Hip internal (medial) rotation: tightness of gluteus maximus and piriformis

Hip external (lateral) rotation: tightness of gluteus minimus and anterior gluteus medius

Ankle

Ankle plantar flexion: tightness of tibialis anterior

Ankle dorsiflexion: one joint (tightness of soleus)

Ankle dorsiflexion: two joints (tightness of gastrocnemius)

8. **Demonstrate competency in administering and interpreting static and dynamic postural analyses.**

   The body is a series of kinetic chains where misalignment in one area can set off a number of compensatory adjustments that may be seen and felt. By carefully observing alignment, we can detect strain produced by faulty relationships of various body parts. For this reason, a complete static postural assessment from at least three views should be done involving "segmental" postural analysis (see forms on pages 107-109).

9. **Select and interpret appropriate assessments that indicate your client's muscle balance.**

   Muscle balance exists when there is a proper relationship between the strength, length, and neural excitation of related muscles. When certain muscles become stronger or tighter than their counterparts, muscle imbalance occurs. When postural screening reveals faulty alignment or body mechanics, consider the possibility that your client has a muscular imbalance. Confirm those results by applying specific flexibility or muscle tightness tests and strength and muscular endurance tests to the joint areas. The postural analysis will help you determine which musculoskeletal tests you should perform.

Exercise Analysis, Design, and Demonstration

Chapter Competencies

After completing this chapter, you will be able to demonstrate the following competencies:

1. Anatomically analyze the joint movements, muscles used, and types of contraction for exercises and activities common to fitness programming.

2. Apply biomechanical principles to optimize exercise benefits for your clients and at the same time attend to their limitations through biomechanical alterations of the exercise.

3. Describe and use the five-step exercise design model.

4. Use the client-centered exercise demonstration model to provide personal exercise demonstrations involving preexercise explanations, trainer demonstration, client trial, performance feedback, and follow-up.

5. Apply technical knowledge and people skills in exercise demonstration.

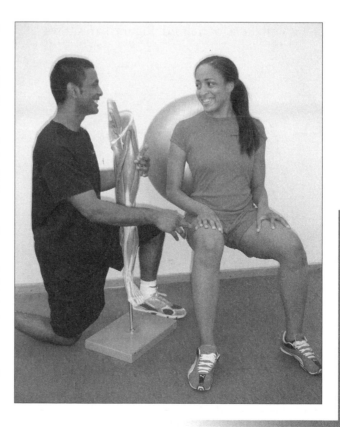

This chapter outlines two types of exercise analysis: anatomical and biomechanical. Numerous examples of popular exercises are used, and their suitability to client needs is determined. A progressive model for exercise analysis and a five-step approach to client-centered exercise design are provided as pivotal points in the prescription model. Finally, one of the most frequent tasks of a personal fitness trainer—exercise demonstration—is presented as both a science and an art using a four-step model.

Exercise design is optimized when each exercise is client-centered. There are three broad criteria for client-centered exercise:

1. Meeting the client's needs

2. Achieving the purpose for which the exercise was designed effectively and safely

3. Being accepted by the client as something he wants to do

Only if an exercise meets these criteria will it be included in the prescription.

Client personalization comes a step closer with the "selection + modification" approach. Modification molds an exercise to meet exact specifications—for example, to simulate a movement pattern used in a work task or sport skill. Figure 5.1*a* shows a resisted horizontal adduction of the shoulder joint that strengthens the pectoralis major and anterior deltoid. Figure 5.1*b* shows a modification suitable for an athlete whose sport includes throwing. The modified exercise involves the same muscles but works them at a slightly different angle and includes a medial rotation (subscapularis) and some trunk rotation.

We must meet the needs of our clients with appropriate modifications. Most often we recognize the need to modify an exercise during the **demonstration.** At this time, our counseling skills (chapter 1) play a critical role as we observe body language, question the client effectively, provide clarifications, and encourage two-way feedback. We change designs based on answers to a number of questions: Does it work the targeted muscle? Does the joint action suit the purpose? Is the difficulty level appropriate? Does this exercise maintain a balance with the rest of the prescription? Does the client need unique modifications? Are the starting position and range of motion safe and effective? Is the equipment appropriate; is it needed at all? Will the client enjoy or value the exercise? What is the effectiveness versus risk ratio? Do monitoring techniques need to be integrated? How does the client feel about the comfort, difficulty, and effectiveness of the exercise? Our system of exercise design must be simple to use but sensitive enough to deal with these issues.

The skills in this chapter involve **breaking down** exercises to determine their purpose (i.e., **analysis**) and **building** exercises based on need (i.e., **design**). These skills are invaluable for

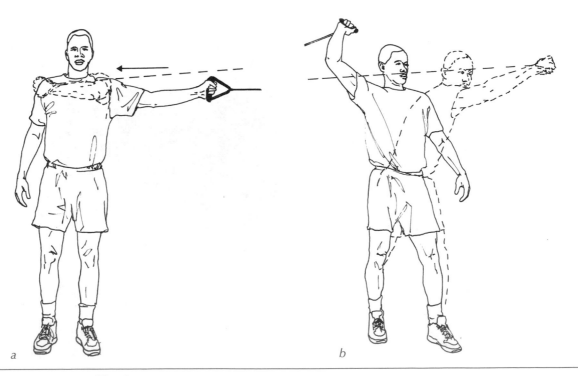

a   b

Figure 5.1   Design modifications.

- **exercise analysis** to aid in selection or modification of an exercise;

- **sport skill analysis** to aid in selection of exercises that simulate the movements and muscular patterns of a skill; and

- **work task analysis** to aid in design of exercises that build the required muscular strength and endurance or to balance the overuse effects of repetitive or prolonged tasks.

You should be able to anatomically analyze the joint movements, muscles used, and types of contraction for exercises and activities common to fitness programming. To analyze, design, and demonstrate exercises, you need to understand the anatomy of the targeted area, recognize the degree of risk, know how to deal with alignment or compensation issues, and be able to provide modifications and alternatives.

Anatomical Analysis of Exercise

You must understand the muscular focus of an exercise and know if that focus is appropriate for your client. To the untrained eye, identifying the muscles responsible for various exercises can be confusing. The following should help you judge your current skills of anatomical analysis.

Imagine you are with a client at the local fitness center and he asks what the difference is between exercises being done by the people in figure 5.2.

Because the movements of the arm look very similar, one might assume that the same muscles are responsible for each exercise. In each case, rubber tubing is providing the resistance in a muscular conditioning exercise for the upper body. However, this is where the similarities end.

In figure 5.2, the muscles working are as follows:

- **Exercise *a*:** Middle and posterior deltoid, middle and upper trapezius, and rhomboids

- **Exercise *b*:** Pectoralis major, anterior deltoid, serratus anterior, and pectoralis minor

- **Exercise *c*:** Infraspinatus and teres minor

Even the seasoned exercise specialist must scrutinize an exercise carefully. Watch the exercise several times and perhaps repeat it yourself slowly. Notice which body parts are moving and which are stabilizing without movement. Are joints bending or straightening through a full range of motion or to the end of their range of motion? Are the muscles being stretched or are they contracting, and if so, how? The following anatomical analysis section shows how to determine the targeted muscle group for each exercise.

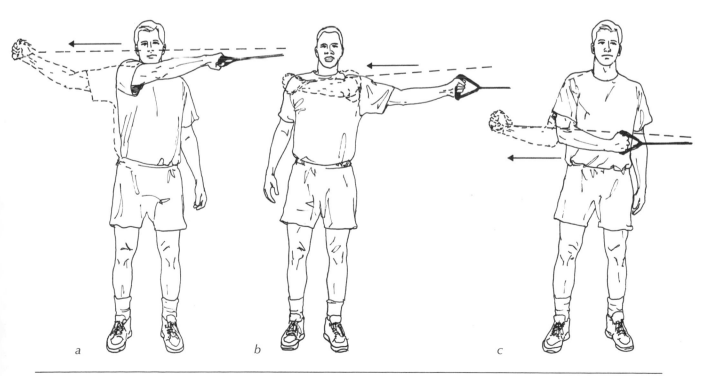

Figure 5.2 Determining exercise differences.

You should analyze every exercise you prescribe. You should also apply the following steps when critiquing an existing program (written or demonstrated), observing a class or workshop, reading a fitness journal or book, receiving a program from a rehabilitation referral, seeing exercise equipment promotions, or trying new things yourself. With practice, the following simple five-step approach to anatomical analysis will become second nature to you:

1. Analyze phases.
2. Analyze joints and movements.
3. Analyze types of contractions.
4. Analyze which muscles are being used.
5. Evaluate purpose, effectiveness, and risk.

Step 1: Analyze Phases

Break the exercise into phases. Most exercises have two discernible phases: up and down, in and out, push and pull, or left and right. For example, exercise *a* in figure 5.2 has "out" and "back" phases. The phases are not technical terms but are chosen as brief and descriptive. New phases generally are determined by the point when a joint movement stops and a new movement begins. In muscular conditioning exercises such as with free weights or calisthenics, the phases are usually "up" and "down" to take advantage of gravity's opposition on the up phase. In figure 5.3, the side-lying position optimizes the force of gravity in the up and down phases of the exercise.

Some complex sports skills have several phases. The **power phase** is illustrated in the batter example (figure 5.4). The power phase is the time of the greatest force generation and is often the part of the movement that ends with contact (e.g., in batting) or release (e.g., in throwing). The **preparatory phase**, or wind-up, precedes the power phase—usually in the opposite direction—and serves two functions: to increase the range of motion through which the force can be applied in the power phase and, if done quickly, to prestretch the muscles responsible for the power phase and thereby increase their force.

After the power phase is the **follow-through phase.** By watching the follow-through, you can get a good idea about the direction of force application. This phase has no effect on the amount of force transferred from the body (or bat). These three phases are typical of many sport skills. You will focus your analysis on the power phase—for this is where the client will need the greatest strength or power.

Step 2: Analyze Joints and Movements

Within specific segments of exercise phases, determine which joints are involved and what movements they are performing. Joints move when muscles crossing those joints contract. During concentric (shortening) contractions, the insertion of the muscle moves toward the origin. To be more effective in exercise analysis, review your knowledge of anatomy so that you can accurately describe major joint movements (see figure 5.5).

Movements Performed at Several Joints

The following are definitions of the major movements at joints throughout the body (Batman and Van Capelle 1992). All movements are from the anatomical position. The **anatomical position** involves the body standing at an erect position, arms and legs straight, head facing forward, with palms and toes also facing forward.

- **Flexion:** Bending; bringing the bones together; reducing the angle at a joint. The exception is flexion at the shoulder joint, which occurs when the humerus is moved forward.

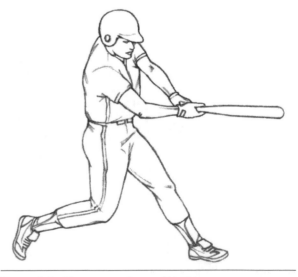

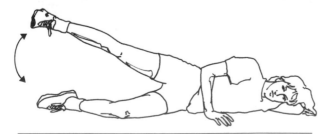

Figure 5.3   Side leg raise with up and down phases.

Reprinted, by permission, from B.B. Cook and G.W. Stewart, 1996, *Strength basics* (Champaign, IL: Human Kinetics), 72.

Figure 5.4   The power phase of batting.

Reprinted, by permission, from G. Carr, 1997, *Mechanics of sport* (Champaign, IL: Human Kinetics), 177.

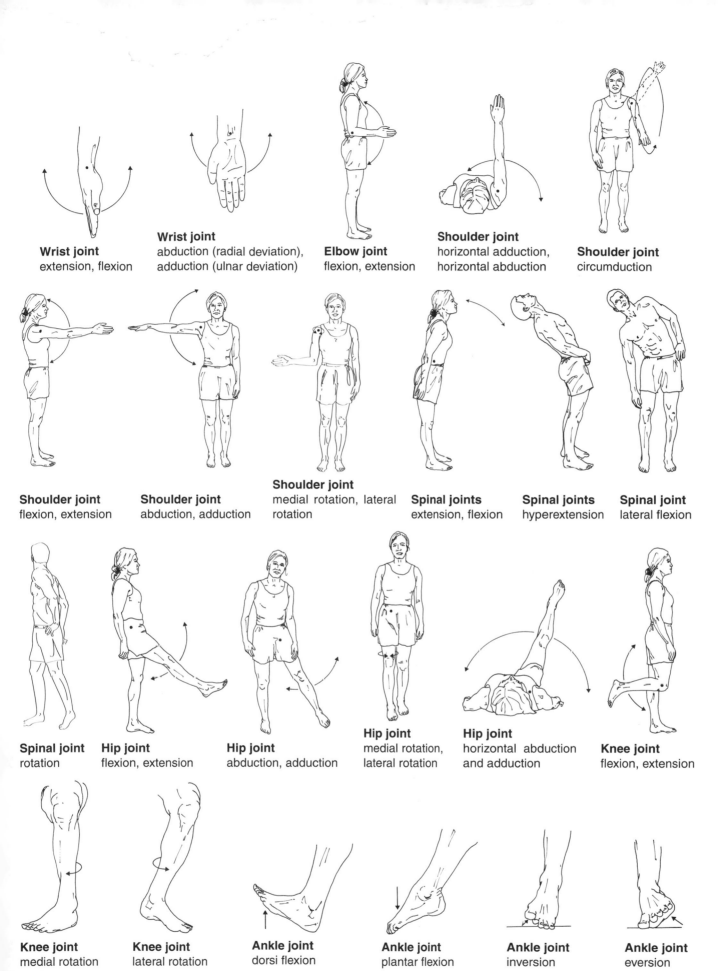

Wrist joint
extension, flexion

Wrist joint
abduction (radial deviation),
adduction (ulnar deviation)

Elbow joint
flexion, extension

Shoulder joint
horizontal adduction,
horizontal abduction

Shoulder joint
circumduction

Shoulder joint
flexion, extension

Shoulder joint
abduction, adduction

Shoulder joint
medial rotation, lateral
rotation

Spinal joints
extension, flexion

Spinal joints
hyperextension

Spinal joint
lateral flexion

Spinal joint
rotation

Hip joint
flexion, extension

Hip joint
abduction, adduction

Hip joint
medial rotation,
lateral rotation

Hip joint
horizontal abduction
and adduction

Knee joint
flexion, extension

Knee joint
medial rotation

Knee joint
lateral rotation

Ankle joint
dorsi flexion

Ankle joint
plantar flexion

Ankle joint
inversion

Ankle joint
eversion

Figure 5.5 Action at specific joints.

119

- **Extension:** Straightening; moving bones apart; increasing the angle at a joint. The exception is extension at the shoulder joint, where the humerus is brought back toward the body.
- **Abduction:** Movement away from the midline of the body—for example, moving the arms and legs away from the trunk in a sideways motion.
- **Adduction:** Movement toward the midline of the body—for example, moving the arms or legs toward the trunk in sideways motion.
- **Medial rotation:** Rotation of a limb toward the midline of the body—for example, rotating the arms or legs toward the trunk.
- **Lateral rotation:** Rotation of a limb away from the midline of the body—for example, rotating the arms or legs away from the trunk.
- **Supination:** Lateral rotation movement at the radioulnar joint (below elbow) or a roll to the outside of the heel at the subtalar joint (below the ankle).
- **Pronation:** Medial rotation movement at the radioulnar joint (below elbow) or a roll to the inside of the heel at the subtalar joint (below the ankle).
- **Horizontal abduction:** Movement of a limb away from the midline of the body in a horizontal plane—for example, moving the arm from a front horizontal position to a side horizontal position.
- **Horizontal adduction:** Movement of a limb toward the midline of the body in a horizontal plane—for example, moving the arm from a side horizontal position to a front horizontal position.
- **Circumduction:** Circular movements at a joint; combines many other movements—for example, occurs at shoulder joint, hip joint, and spinal joint.

Movements Unique to Specific Joints

Some movements occur only at one pair of joints.

Shoulder Girdle

This joint is a combination of three joints that work together. The movements are often difficult to see. The following actions describe movements of the shoulder girdle, which comprises the scapula and clavicle.

- **Elevation:** Movement of the scapula upward.
- **Depression:** Movement of the scapula downward.

- **Abduction:** Movement of the scapula away from the spinal column.
- **Adduction:** Movement of the scapula toward the spinal column.
- **Upward rotation:** Rotation of the scapula upward. The inferior angle (bottom) moves outward and upward.
- **Downward rotation:** Rotation of the scapula downward. Inferior angle moves down and in.

Although its joints can move independently, the shoulder girdle mainly supports and assists movements of the shoulder joint. The shoulder girdle actions allow the arm (humerus) to move through a wide range of motion. When you analyze shoulder joint and shoulder girdle movements, it might be helpful to use table 5.1 to identify the action at the shoulder joint and then look across to the corresponding action of the shoulder girdle.

Pelvic Girdle

The following actions are specifically related to the pelvic girdle.

- **Forward tilt:** Movement of the pelvic girdle forward.
- **Backward tilt:** Movement of the pelvic girdle backward.
- **Lateral tilt:** Movement of the pelvic girdle such that one side drops.

Table 5.1   Combined Actions of the Shoulder Girdle and Shoulder Joint

Shoulder joint action	Shoulder girdle action
Abduction	Upward rotation Abduction
Adduction	Downward rotation Adduction
Flexion	Upward rotation Abduction
Extension	Downward rotation Adduction
Medial rotation	Abduction
Lateral rotation	Adduction
Horizontal abduction	Adduction
Horizontal adduction	Abduction

Foot

The following actions are uniquely related to the ankle and foot.

- **Dorsiflexion:** Same as flexion only at the ankle joint.
- **Plantar flexion:** Same as extension only at the ankle joint; pointing the foot.
- **Eversion:** Turning the sole of the foot outward, where the weight is taken on the inside of the foot. Occurs at the subtalar joint.
- **Inversion:** Turning the sole of the foot inward, where the weight is taken on the outside of the foot. Occurs at the subtalar joint.

Figure 5.5 shows actions performed by specific joints. Some of those listed here as unique to certain joints are not listed.

Practicing Steps 1 and 2

At this point, you are able to divide the exercise into phases, identify all joints that are involved for each phase, and determine the movement or movements for each joint.

You should practice these skills. In the following exercises, determine the phases, the joints involved, and the movements taking place at those joints:

- Curl-ups
- Resisted toe points
- Prone scapular retraction

To make your analysis easier, sketch three "analysis charts" with columns labeled "phase," "joint," and "movement." Leave at least five rows between each chart for your analysis. After you have analyzed these three exercises, compare your conclusions with tables 5.2, 5.3, and 5.4. Using a grid such as these tables will make your analyses easier.

Table 5.2
Exercise: Curl-Up

Phase	Joint	Movement
Up	Spine (lumbar)	Flexion
Down	Spine (lumbar)	Extension

Illustrations: Reprinted, by permission, from B.B. Cook and G.W. Stewart, 1996, *Strength basics: Your guide to resistance training for health and optimal performance* (Champaign, IL: Human Kinetics), 121.

Table 5.3 Exercise: Resisted Toe Points

(With tubing around foot, press foot down.)

Phase	Joint	Movement
Out	Ankle	Plantar flexion
In	Ankle	Dorsiflexion

Illustrations: Reprinted, by permission, from B.B. Cook and G.W. Stewart, 1996, *Strength basics: Your guide to resistance training for health and optimal performance* (Champaign, IL: Human Kinetics), 91.

Table 5.4 Exercise: Prone Scapular Retraction

(Pinch shoulder blades together with arms out from sides and elbows bent.)

Phase	Joint	Movement
Up	Shoulder joint	Horizontal abduction
Up	Shoulder girdle	Adduction
Down	Shoulder joint	Horizontal adduction
Down	Shoulder girdle	Abduction

Step 3: Analyze Types of Contractions

To cause a movement, a muscle must produce tension and contract. While under tension, the muscle may shorten during the contraction, lengthen, or stay the same length.

With a **concentric contraction**, the muscle develops tension great enough to overcome a resistance and produces an action by shortening. The "up" phase of calisthenics, free weights, sports skills, and many resistance machines involves concentric contraction of the muscles producing joint movements in that direction. For example, in the up phase of a biceps curl, the biceps shorten under tension (concentric contraction) to produce flexion at the elbow. The biceps are creating enough tension to overcome the resistance of gravity, the weight of the arm, and the external weight.

With an **eccentric contraction,** the tension generated by the muscle is less than the resistance and the muscle will lengthen. Eccentric contractions occur when

- muscles attempt to counter the force of gravity, such as when the body or a limb is lowered, or

- muscles attempt to counter the force of momentum by slowing down the action (e.g., the ballistic action of the follow-through of a batter).

Eccentric contractions do not increase flexibility, because the muscle is producing tension while it is lengthening. In fact, eccentric contraction can generate more tension than a shortening contraction (Wilmore and Costill 2004). The down phase of calisthenics, free weights, sports skills, and many resistance machines involves eccentric contraction of the muscles that produce joint movements in that direction. Remember, the force of gravity produces significant acceleration if an object or limb is allowed to fall freely. In most exercises, the down phase involves eccentric contractions of the muscles that initiated the up movement. We control the speed of the descent with eccentric contractions. For example, the biceps lower the weight in the biceps curl at a rate slower than gravity, thus controlling the free fall.

It is sometimes difficult to understand that the same muscle groups are responsible for both the up and down phases of an exercise. These muscles shorten on the way up with a concentric contraction and lengthen on the way down with an eccentric contraction. Eccentric contractions are a big part of everyday life—for example, the landing phase of each step of a jog, or lowering yourself to sit, walking down the stairs, lowering a fork from your mouth, and bending down.

Eccentric contractions also occur when we slow down something that is moving quickly or that has significant momentum. We are still attempting to control a movement. When a person throws a ball, for example, the anterior shoulder muscles contract concentrically to produce the movement (power phase), but after the ball has been released (follow-through phase), the arm must be slowed down to prevent injury. This control comes from tension in the muscles on the posterior shoulder. The momentum of the arm keeps it moving forward, but the lengthening contraction slows the movement. Many high-power sports and ballistic exercises (such as arm actions with hand weights) involve rapid eccentric contractions. The greatest muscular forces are generated with rapid eccentric contractions, and more strain is placed on connective tissue when it is elongated under tension.

Proper execution of an exercise or skill may involve the stabilization of a joint. If a muscle develops tension but there is no visible movement of the joint, it is called an **isometric contraction.** Although the information is not included on our analysis chart, you should identify the major muscles involved in any isometric contraction where stabilization is a critical part of your client's activity. For example, upper-body exercises involving barbells or dumbbells such as the lateral arm raises in table 5.5 require the shoulder girdle to be stabilized. An isometric contraction of the shoulder girdle elevators and adductors will form a strong base for shoulder joint movements. Also note the following:

- There is no movement in the elbows and wrists, which are stabilized (isometric contractions) during both phases of the exercise.
- In the first 60° of shoulder joint abduction, there is little or no movement of the shoulder girdle. Shoulder girdle adductor muscles contract isometrically to stabilize.

It is useful, then, to expand the analysis chart to include the type of contraction.

Synergists

Synergists are muscles that act together to create a combined force. They can be separate parts of the same muscle, as when the anterior and posterior parts of the gluteus medius work together for hip abduction or the upper and lower trapezius muscles complement one another in shoulder girdle adduction. Synergists may also be opposing muscle parts that work together for one action but neutralize each other because of opposing roles: for example, wrist muscles that flex and abduct work in synergy with others that flex and adduct. The result

Table 5.5 Exercise: Lateral Arm Raises

(Raise arms out from the body.)

Phase	Joint	Movement	Contraction type
Up	Shoulder joint	Abduction	Concentric
Up	Shoulder girdle	Upward rotation Abduction	Concentric
Down	Shoulder joint	Adduction	Eccentric
Down	Shoulder girdle	Downward rotation Adduction	Eccentric

Illustrations: Reprinted, by permission, from B.B. Cook and G.W. Stewart, 1996, *Strength basics: Your guide to resistance training for health and optimal performance* (Champaign, IL: Human Kinetics), 135.

is stronger wrist flexion with neither abduction nor adduction. In the foot, both invertors and evertors combine to plantar flex without rotation. A common effect of this synergistic muscle action is greater joint stabilization.

Step 4: Analyze Which Muscles Are Being Used

Here are two helpful visualizations for exercise analysis:

- Muscles affect movement of the joints that they cross. An obvious example is the biceps at the elbow. Flexion of the elbow is the primary movement, but the biceps also crosses the radioulnar joint and the shoulder joint and can be recruited to cause movements at these joints.

- If alignment of the muscle–tendon unit is in the direction of the movement, the influence of that muscle will be optimal (see the section on biomechanical analysis of exercise, p. 125).

Once you have determined the joint action and type of contraction, your final and most important step is to identify the active muscles. Determining individual muscles responsible for a movement can be simplified by following this principle: **The muscle group causing the action is named by that**

joint and action (if the contraction is concentric). For example, in the up phase of a biceps curl, the elbow flexes—and the muscle group used is the elbow flexors. In lateral arm raises, the shoulder joint abducts in the up phase; therefore, the shoulder joint abductors are responsible.

For a more detailed analysis, we will look at a bench press (see table 5.6).

Table 5.6 concisely presents the active joints, their movements, the primary muscles, and how they are contracting during the phases of the bench press. The most challenging part of the anatomical analysis is recalling the specific muscles responsible for the joint actions (Tortora and Grabowski 2003). To facilitate this step, the end of the chapter presents **JAM** charts (tables 5.14-5.20): these are quick references indicating joint, actions, and muscles (pp. 145-147).

Let's apply the JAM charts for anatomical analysis of a partial squat designed to strengthen the lower body—particularly the quadriceps. The exercise is effective in producing gains but does carry some risk. The patellar–femoral pressure increases dramatically as the angle of the knee approaches 90°. Use a light weight and restricted range of motion to begin.

Remember the principle: The muscle group causing the action is named by that joint and action (if the contraction is concentric). This directs us to the JAM chart columns for hip extensors (table 5.17), knee extensors (table 5.18), and

Table 5.6   Exercise: Bench Press

(Press bar up; lower bar near chest.)

Phase	Joint	Movement	Contraction type	Muscles
Up	Shoulder joint	Horizontal adduction	Concentric	Pectoralis major Anterior deltoid (Shoulder joint horizontal adductors)
Up	Shoulder girdle	Abduction	Concentric	Serratus anterior Pectoralis minor (Shoulder girdle abductors)
Up	Elbow	Extension	Concentric	Triceps (Elbow extensors)
Down	Shoulder joint	Horizontal abduction	Eccentric	Pectoralis major Anterior deltoid
Down	Shoulder girdle	Adduction	Eccentric	Serratus anterior Pectoralis minor
Down	Elbow	Flexion	Eccentric	Triceps

Illustration: Reprinted, by permission, from E.T. Howley and B.D. Franks, *Health fitness instructors handbook*, 3rd ed. (Champaign, IL: Human Kinetics), 310.

ankle plantar flexors (table 5.19). Reading down each column of the JAM chart, select the prime movers (PM) and insert them in the analysis chart (table 5.7). Remember, the down phase is the opposite movement but the same muscles are contracting eccentrically. Notice the advantage in always analyzing the up phase first.

Step 5: Evaluate Purpose, Effectiveness, and Risk

Evaluate each exercise, using the information gained during steps 1 through 4. Having completed the anatomical analysis of an exercise, you know what muscles it will work. Is this what you want for your client? With the client-centered counseling approach, you have established her priorities by considering her needs, wants, and lifestyle. It is time now to evaluate how well the exercise fills its purpose, its effectiveness, and the degree of personal risk it carries.

• **Purpose.** Establish the general purpose of the exercise, that is, which primary fitness component is being challenged. The purpose of the exercise must coincide with the component and body area that the client identifies as an area of priority. Discussion in this chapter will focus primarily on the components of flexibility and muscular conditioning. It is sometimes difficult to differentiate between a flexibility and a strengthening exercise. To assist, try the three simple checks in *Checking for Purpose*. The checks should verify that a stretch will pull the muscle, extend its length without creating much tension, and leave the muscle more relaxed after the stretch, whereas a strengthening exercise will shorten the muscle, create significant tension, and result in fatigue.

Define the purpose more specifically by referring to the areas of the body targeted by the exercise. For example, the purpose of an exercise may be to stretch the calves, to strengthen the abdominal area, or to develop power needed for a vertical jump.

Table 5.7   Exercise: Partial Squat

(Keeping back straight and head up, lower the bar by flexing the knees to 90°. Return.)

Phase	Joint	Movement	Contraction type	Muscles
Up	Hip	Extension	Concentric	Gluteus maximus Semitendinosus Semimembranosus Biceps femoris
Up	Knee	Extension	Concentric	Rectus femoris Vastus lateralis Vastus intermedius Vastus medialis
Up	Ankle	Plantar flexion	Concentric	Gastrocnemius Soleus
Down	Hip	Flexion	Eccentric	Gluteus maximus Semitendinosus Semimembranosus Biceps femoris
Down	Knee	Flexion	Eccentric	Rectus femoris Vastus lateralis Vastus intermedius Vastus medialis
Down	Ankle	Dorsiflexion	Eccentric	Gastrocnemius Soleus

Illustrations: Reprinted, by permission, from V. Heyward, 1998, *Advanced assessment and exercise prescription*, 3rd ed. (Champaign, IL: Human Kinetics), 272.

Checking for Purpose

Checks	Stretch	Strength
Attachment points (i.e., origin and insertion)	Pulled farther apart	Moved closer together (concentric contraction)
Muscle tension	Slight	Moderate to high
Gradual feeling	Relief and relaxation	Hardness; fatigue

• **Effectiveness.** Effectiveness refers to how well an exercise fulfills its purpose. No two clients will take exactly the same route to reach an objective. Effectiveness is not just what researchers have said about an exercise or training method—effectiveness varies considerably among clients. The bottom line to effectiveness is, "Will the exercise do what I want it to do for my client?" Ask the following questions:

- What is the appropriate overload to challenge the desired fitness component?

- Does the stretch avoid excessive tension, and is the alignment such that the stretch is in the direction of the fibers and elongation of the muscle?

- For a strengthening exercise, is fatigue felt in the targeted muscles, and are they directly resisted by an external resistance such as free weights, equipment, elastic bands, or gravity?

- Is the exercise effective from the physiological point of view?

- What monitoring can be built into the design to track its effectiveness?

• **Risk.** Careful risk analysis is inherent in any client-centered prescription. Exercise execution and other training errors are called extrinsic risks. Biomechanical risks or structural weaknesses that clients bring with them are referred to as intrinsic risks. Details of how to control these risk factors are discussed in chapter 10.

Biomechanical Analysis of Exercise

Biomechanical analysis examines the method of execution of an exercise. We can apply biomechanical principles to optimize exercise benefits for our clients and at the same time attend to their limitations through biomechanical alterations of the exercise. Such analyses enable us to advise our clients concerning

- choosing the best starting position for an exercise,
- finding the optimal speed for their objectives,
- determining the position of joints to isolate specific muscles,
- aligning the movement to the muscle,
- combining muscles for optimal results, and
- modifying the leverage to gain a greater strength output.

The next section is guided by a number of biomechanical principles. The purpose, effectiveness, and risk of an exercise or sport skill may be affected by any of the following:

- Muscle length and force
- Biarticular (two-joint) muscle action
- Composition of forces
- Leverage and strength
- Direction of force application/alignment
- Alignment of external resistance

Muscle Length and Force

The amount of force produced by a muscle is related to the physical length at which the muscle is held. You can use this information to direct your prescription and optimize the results when you understand the answers to the following questions.

What Causes the "Sticking Point" in Weightlifting?

A person working with weights will begin to feel weak at some point during the exercise. Getting the weight started and completing the last few degrees are the two usual sticking points. The maximum tension that can be generated in the muscle will occur when the muscle is activated at a length slightly greater than its resting length—up to about 120% of the resting length. When a muscle is shortened to about 50% to 60% of its resting length, its force is minimal because actin and myosin filaments are doubled over and few cross-bridges are formed (first sticking point). The second sticking point occurs as the muscle is elongated beyond 120% of the resting length and there is slippage of the cross-bridges (fewer are formed) and less force is generated (Edman 1992). In addition, the angle of pull of the muscle on the bone changes as the joint moves through its motion. Maximal force occurs when the angle of pull of the muscle is at 90° to the long axis of the bone. As a result of both factors, your clients will feel weak at the ends of the range of motion. Select weights that he can lift through a full range of motion for the prescribed repetitions or assist him through the sticking points.

How Can Your Client Tap an Energy Reserve?

If your client is working with weights, a slight increase in the stretch of the muscle before the contraction will summon an energy reserve for increased performance. The reason is that the total tension or force generated in a shortening muscle receives a contribution from the passive (stretch) tension of the tendon and the connective tissue in the muscle (figure 5.6). This stored elastic energy or passive tension plus the voluntary muscular tension provides the total tension or force output. Your clients can apply this principle in training or in athletic activities by placing the joint in a preparatory phase (prestretched) before the power phase (e.g., the back swing of a batter or the squat of a volleyball spiker). This stored energy can be used only if the shortening contraction occurs within 0.0 to 0.9 s after the stretch and if the muscle is not lengthened too much (Komi 1992). With eccentric

training, the force increases as the velocity of the lengthening contraction increases, up to a point where control is lost. These principles are the basis for plyometric training (chapter 7).

Biarticular (Two-Joint) Muscle Action

Biarticular muscles are those that cross two joints and affect movement at both joints. You can apply this understanding to help clients stretch muscles from both ends, isolate muscles for conditioning, and perform aerobics more efficiently.

How Can a Biarticular Muscle Stretch From Both Ends?

Biarticular muscles are not long enough to allow a full range of motion simultaneously at both joints. If one of the two joints is moved to the end of its range of motion, the attempt to move the second joint to the end of its range will stretch the biarticular muscle nearer the second joint. For example, the hamstrings attach above the hip and below the knee. Once the knee is pulled tight to the chest, it is not possible to fully extend the knee because the hamstrings are too short. Attempting to extend the knee, however, will stretch the lower hamstrings. To stretch the upper hamstrings, extend the knee and rotate the pelvis forward as the trunk flexes. Hamstring strains are more common in the upper area of the hamstrings, suggesting that stretching this area may be of greater value for prevention or rehabilitation. "Feeling" where the stretch is centered provides feedback that the biarticular principle is being used effectively.

Other biarticular muscles (and the joints they cross) that can be effectively stretched in this manner include these:

- Gastrocnemius (ankle and knee)
- Rectus femoris (knee and hip)
- Iliopsoas (hip and pelvis)
- Erector spinae (pelvis and spine)
- Levator scapulae (shoulder girdle and cervical spine)
- Triceps (shoulder joint and elbow)

Check the JAM charts at the end of the chapter for joint movements (pp. 145-147).

How Can We Isolate a One-Joint Muscle for Conditioning or Stretching?

If both ends of a biarticular muscle are brought closer together, the muscle is too short to exert a

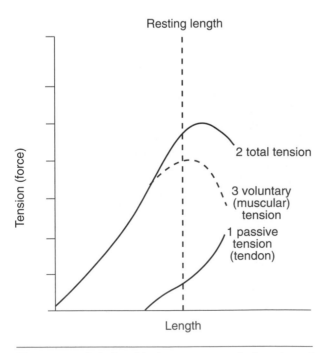

Figure 5.6   Relationship between muscle length and tension.

maximum force output, and therefore single-joint muscles can be isolated. This principle is used to isolate the abdominals in a curl-up. When the knees and hips are bent, the biarticular hip flexors (rectus femoris) are short and slack and do not contribute appreciably to the action. The work feels more difficult because the abdominals are being isolated. Adjustment of even one joint can shorten a muscle and decrease its involvement. For example, as the knee flexes during a resisted leg flexion exercise (figure 5.7), the hamstrings lose their force as their origin and insertion come closer together. The individual therefore seeks help from the assistant movers for knee flexion. The JAM charts (pp. 145-147) indicate that these include the sartorius, gracilis, and gastrocnemius muscles.

In another example, the biarticular gastrocnemius (which attaches above the knee) is more heavily activated during a standing calf raise than when it is shortened during a seated calf raise, thereby isolating the soleus (figure 5.8).

This method of isolation will also help you to analyze flexibility exercises. With the previous example of the gastrocnemius (two-joint) and soleus (one-joint), both muscles are stretched when the ankle is dorsiflexed. When the knee is straight, the gastrocnemius is maximally stretched; when the knee is flexed, the two-joint gastrocnemius is slack and the soleus stretch is optimized.

How Do You Get More Force From a Biarticular Muscle?

Prestretching a biarticular muscle can significantly improve its force output. For example,

the flexor muscles of the wrist act as assistant movers for elbow flexion. When the wrist is slightly hyperextended during elbow flexion, the increased tension in these muscles contributes to the force of the movement. This is also seen in the leg flexion exercise (figure 5.7), in which the force of the hamstrings is improved when the pelvis is rotated forward and the muscle is elongated. Because greater resistance can be applied, the training results are increased. Caution your clients about excessive pelvic rotation in this exercise, which can increase the lumbar curve and force the low back muscles into contracture.

How Do Biarticular Muscles Increase Efficiency?

Two-joint muscles, particularly in the lower extremity, save energy by allowing concentric work at one joint and eccentric work at the adjacent joint. This mechanical coupling of joints allows for a rapid release of stored elastic energy (passive tension; Hamill and Knutzen 1995). For example, in a vertical jump, the gastrocnemius concentrically plantar flexes the ankle. At the knee, which is extending, the gastrocnemius is eccentrically storing elastic energy. These joint couplings occur frequently in walking and jogging and reduce the work required from the single-joint muscles. **Closed kinetic chain exercises** (see chapter 8) that involve direct weight bearing use this mechanical coupling. They are quite useful, and clients wanting to strengthen their knees would benefit from closed kinetic chain leg exercises.

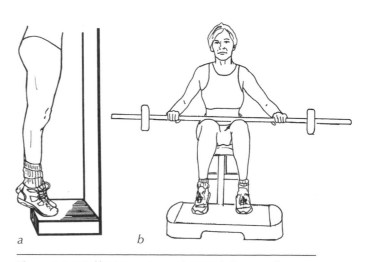

Figure 5.7 Leg flexion.

Figure 5.8 Calf raises: (a) standing and (b) seated.

(a): Reprinted, by permission, from T. O'Brien, 1997, *The personal trainer's handbook* (Champaign, IL: Human Kinetics), 103.

Composition of Forces

Try to visualize the combination of muscles involved in a particular joint movement. Teach your clients to use this visualization to direct their focus to the right muscles and provide helpful sensory feedback.

It is often possible to modify a movement to isolate a targeted muscle or muscle part. Joints do not always follow traditional movements. For instance, they may move halfway between flexion and abduction. Many sport skills or work tasks involve similar oblique movements. Think of a muscle as a string on a mannequin causing joint movement in the direction of the pull of the string. Each muscle acting on that joint is like a string pulling at a different angle. When more than one force is acting on the joint, you can apply the technique of **composition of forces** to help visualize the relative contribution of those muscles to the final movement. For example, the pectoralis major has two parts, combining the sternal (S) and clavicular (C) forces to produce a resultant force (R) that produces movement in a different direction from that caused by either part of the muscle by itself. This resultant force causes shoulder joint horizontal adduction (figure 5.9).

To use this technique, try the following:

1. Draw (or visualize) the movement as an arrow. This is called the resultant force.

2. Select, from the anatomical analysis, the two primary muscles causing the movement.

3. Represent these muscle forces with arrows, where the arrowheads indicate the direction of pull of the muscles and the length of the arrow depicts the relative strength of that muscle's involvement.

4. Place the base of the two forces (S and C in this example) together on or near the point of attachment of the two muscles.

5. Draw a parallelogram from the arrows.

The diagonal of the parallelogram represents the composition of the forces—that is, the **resultant force.**

The final stage of this technique involves identifying which muscle you want to isolate. Alter the direction of the resultant force closer to the direction of that muscle. You can see in figure 5.9b that as the movement (R₂) is angled more upward, the clavicular arrow becomes larger (C₂). This means that the clavicular part of the pectoralis major is generating more force, effectively isolating it.

Here are more examples of the composition of forces:

- Acting alone, the anterior (A) and posterior (P) parts of the deltoid flex and extend the shoulder joint, respectively (figure 5.10). Their combined action (resultant-R) is shoulder joint abduction. When someone lifts an object by abducting the shoulder joint, she calls into play the anterior deltoid more heavily because the object is in front of the body. If she has a rounded shoulder posture, how would you modify the shoulder joint abduction to emphasize the posterior deltoid? Recall

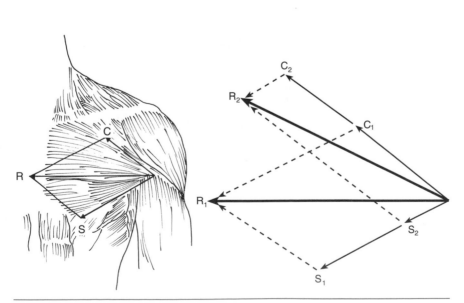

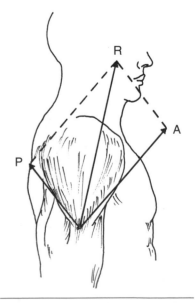

Figure 5.9   Resultant force: pectoralis major. S = sternal; C = clavicular; R = resultant force.

Figure 5.10   Resultant force (R): deltoid.

that the posterior deltoid is a prime mover for shoulder joint extension and horizontal abduction (table 5.14).

• The two heads of the gastrocnemius, pulling in lateral (L) and medial (M) directions, together exert an upward force (R) on the Achilles tendon and cause plantar flexion of the ankle (figure 5.11). Toeing in will slightly prestretch the lateral head of the gastrocnemius, allowing a small increase in the force output of that head during plantar flexion. Only the most avid bodybuilders would want this advantage during an exercise such as a calf raise (figure 5.8).

• The pull of the quadriceps on the patella guides the patella through the path of motion (figure 5.12a). Sometimes (figure 5.12b) the patella is directed laterally (R) by the quadriceps (Q) and patellar tendon (P)—particularly if the vastus medialis (M) is weak. This muscle imbalance can lead to inflammation on the posterior side of the patella.

• A resultant force acting on the knee in a different direction (figure 5.13) is the pressure exerted on the back side of the patella from the quadriceps muscles (Q) and patellar tendon (P). As the knee flexes (as in a squat or a lunge), the resultant force increases (R_1 vs. R_2). Have your clients take precautions with the depths and applied loads during these types of exercises.

Leverage and Strength

Lever systems can help you modify exercises to optimize your clients' efforts. If a client is having difficulty with an exercise or wants to make it more challenging, you can adjust the intensity by changing the lever system.

How Do You View the Body As a Series of Lever Systems?

To view the body as a series of lever systems, consider the joint as the fulcrum and the bones as lever arms that move around the fulcrum. Muscle contraction is the force applied to the lever (at the point where the tendon attaches to the bone), whereas the weight of the body parts plus any external weight being lifted is resistance to the force (figure 5.14).

The majority of levers in the body are third class, which means that the force is applied between the resistance and the fulcrum. The biceps acting around the elbow joint is an example of a third-class lever. In figure 5.14, the elbow is the fulcrum, the radius is the lever arm, the biceps exerts the force, and the weight of the box and the forearm is the resistance.

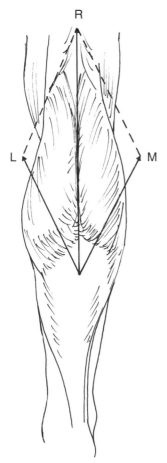

Figure 5.11 Resultant force (R): gastrocnemius.

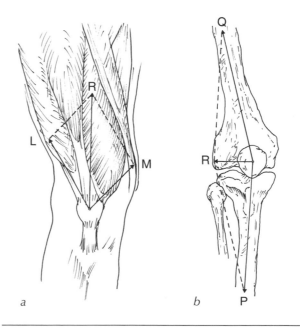

Figure 5.12 Resultant force: quadriceps. R = resultant force; Q = quadriceps; P = patellar tendon; M = vastus medialis.

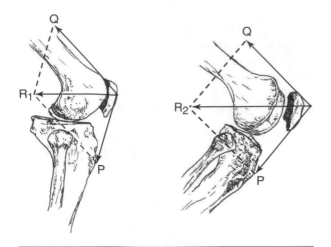

Figure 5.13   Resultant force: patellar pressure.

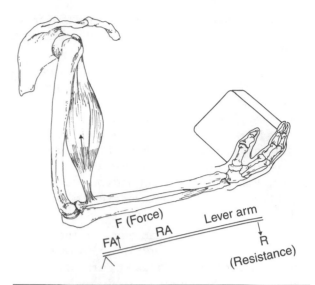

Figure 5.14   The arm as a lever system (e.g., third-class lever). FA = force arm; RA = resistance arm.

The tendon of the biceps inserts to the radius just below the elbow. The distance from the fulcrum (elbow) to the force (biceps insertion) is called the force arm (FA). The distance from the fulcrum (elbow) to the resistance is called the resistance arm (RA) (figure 5.14).

 ### How Can You Adjust a Lever System to Modify the Difficulty of an Exercise?

You can modify the intensity or difficulty of an exercise by changing aspects of the lever system. Depending on your client's situation, you can adjust the resistance, force, force arm, or resistance arm.

Resistance

If your clients are lifting weights or have load adjustments on their machines, it is easy to change the resistance. You can introduce (or change the thickness of) tubing or elastic bands. Water offers increased resistance and an added safety element for joints. Increased resistance is the overload of choice when your client's goal is strength.

Force

Force is the strength or the speed of the muscular contractions that cause a movement. Sometimes performing an exercise slowly demands more control and is more difficult than doing it more quickly. As your clients' muscular condition improves, they can generate greater forces in a more coordinated manner. Increased speed of movement is the overload of choice when your client's goal is muscular power. The speed adjustments on isokinetic and hydraulic machines (chapter 7) change the potential force outputs. Even aerobic machines like stair

climbers have similar setting options (i.e., slower speed settings generate greater force). With certain flexibility training methods, the isometric contraction phase of a proprioceptive neuromuscular facilitation (PNF) stretch (chapter 8) can modify the force of contraction, changing that element of the lever system and ultimately the effectiveness of the stretch.

Force Arm

The distance between the joint and the insertion of the muscle (FA) cannot be changed, but it partially explains differences in performance among clients whose muscular conditioning (force) appears to be equal.

Resistance Arm

Changing the distance between the joint and the resistance arm (RA) is the easiest way to adjust the body's lever systems. As the resistance moves closer to the joint, the muscle will need less force to move the resistance. The challenge is to recognize the parts of the lever system in question: Which joint is the acting fulcrum? What represents the resistance? What is the best way to shift the resistance arm? There are often multiple lever systems working at once, and you must identify the one most appropriate to adjust. The examples in table 5.8 illustrate the answers to these questions.

Direction of Force Application and Alignment

Tension or force from a muscle is transferred through the tendon to the bone. The angle of

Table 5.8   Adjusting the Resistance Arm (RA)

Exercise	Fulcrum	Resistance (R)	RA adjustment
Curl-up	Low back	Upper-body weight	Arms above the head move R away from the fulcrum—harder
Push-up	Shoulder joint	Weight of entire body	Done from the knees moves a reduced R closer to the fulcrum—easier
Dumbbell flys	Shoulder joint	Dumbbell and arm	Changing the angle of the elbow moves the R
Leg (knee) flexion and extension (machine)	Knee	Assigned weight and lower leg	Adjusting the position of the pad lower—harder
Standing knee lifts	Hip	Weight of leg (could use ankle weight or tubing)	Lifting leg with an extended knee; R farther from hip—harder
Bent-over rowing	Low back (not shoulder joint)	Weight of upper body and barbell	Upright rowing brings R closer to lower back—less load on back structures

attachment of the muscle dictates the direction of force application, which produces the movement (figure 5.15). Near the middle of the range of motion, the angle of insertion of the tendon usually directs more of the force perpendicular to the bone, resulting in its strongest position.

Force application is optimized when the muscle–tendon unit is directly aligned with the plane of movement. This can be seen with the prime movers for specific joint actions. In fact, careful alignment of the movement can emphasize the contribution from particular parts of a given muscle. With this information, you can personalize exercises for your clients. The external obliques are a good visual example. The muscle fibers run diagonally and therefore are most effective when pulling the trunk in the diagonal direction (such as in a curl-up with a rotation). In a straight curl-up, the external oblique muscle is not as effective—with spinal flexion, the pull of the muscle is at an angle to the action and the entire force is not used for the movement. Here are some other examples:

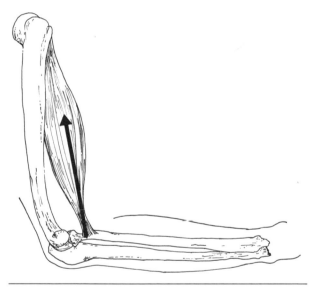

Figure 5.15   Direction of force application. Force increases as the angle between the tendon and the bone approaches 90°.

- **Crossovers** (figure 5.16) using pulleys, tubing, or elastic bands are versatile exercises because the angle of the pull is easily changed to suit the targeted muscle or the sport skill.

- The **pull-down** exercise uses the latissimus dorsi. Different secondary muscles are pulled into play, however, if the bar is pulled down in front of or behind the head. In front, the pectoralis major is used because of the slight flexion. Pulling behind the head forces the shoulder joint backward and activates the posterior deltoid.

- The **bench press** uses a horizontal movement of the shoulder joint and uses the sternal or horizontal fibers of the pectoralis major. With the incline bench press, the shoulder joint is angled upward and activates the upper clavicular part of the pectoralis major.

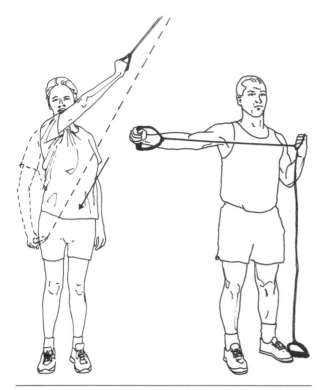

Figure 5.16 Crossovers with different directions.

- **Rowing** action with any device may be done with elbows in or out. With elbows in, the shoulder joints extend to involve the latissimus dorsi and pectoralis major as prime movers. With the elbows up, the shoulder joints horizontally abduct through contraction of the posterior deltoid, infraspinatus, and teres minor. A small change in alignment can significantly change the purpose of the exercise.

Alignment of Muscle Action

Question: Which muscles are working in a side leg raise? What changes take place if the toe is pointing upward? (Remember, the line of pull of a muscle across a joint will determine the functions of that muscle.)

Answer: The hip abductors lift the leg in a side leg raise. When the toe is pointed upward, the task of lifting the leg has shifted to the hip flexors, which are directly in the line of pull.

 ## Alignment of External Resistance

Do not leave the interface between your client and his equipment to chance. It is not the machine's job to know the proper alignment, stabilization, range of motion, and application of resistance—it is yours. Ask yourself the following questions:

- Is the path of motion defined by the machine the same as your client's path of motion?
- Is the direction of the force application safe and optimal?
- Does the equipment allow proper alignment between the machine's fulcrum and the center of the moving joint?

Path of Motion

Many machines have a guided range of motion that may cause problems for smaller or larger clients. If seats and lever arms cannot be adjusted and your client looks or feels unnatural throughout the movement, the machine path is probably unsuitable. Always ascertain the following:

- A correct position of the joint before the exercise begins
- A safe end point to the range of motion (the machine may have a range-limiting device)
- A smooth arc of motion of the joint

Monitor your client carefully for these three checks, especially during spinal movements and shoulder rotations. New technology is addressing this issue. Some pec decks (e.g., Cybex) now use a dual-axis technology that allows clients to determine their own optimal arc of movement and range of motion. You should monitor the path of motion even when using low-tech body weight resistance. For example, take care that your client does not go too low during dips and excessively hyperextend her shoulder.

The ankle, knee, and hip joints form a kinetic chain. When the foot is stabilized or fixed, this kinetic chain is closed. An open kinetic chain exists when the foot is not in contact with the ground or some other surface. Knee flexion and extension using a machine are examples of open kinetic chain exercises. In a closed kinetic chain, the foot is weight bearing: The forces begin at the ground and work their way up through each joint. There is an advantage in having forces absorbed by various anatomical structures rather than simply dissipated as in an open chain.

Direction of Force Application

There is a direction of movement that generates maximal muscular force. Always determine if the force angle allows for the maximum resistance to be lifted.

With pulley systems, tubing, or water, your role involves establishing the correct body position for your client. The purpose of the exercise will significantly affect the line of pull and the position of the joints. The example in figure 5.2 (p. 117) shows the line of pull and the position of the shoulder considerably different in three similar exercises.

Similarly, various angles on an incline bench can be used to isolate targeted muscles when using free weights. For example, a 10° decline on the bench when a bodybuilder is doing flys can help him focus on the lower fibers of the sternal section of the pectoralis major. A 45° incline will swing the emphasis to the clavicular section of the pectoralis major.

Proper Alignment

If the fulcrum of the machine does not align with the center of the moving joint, that joint will experience additional shearing force (making it slide apart) that increases more rapidly than the resistance on the machine (Hamill and Knutzen 1995). Clients with previous injuries to that joint are at significant risk. The following examples illustrate this problem on various pieces of equipment.

- Many pec decks have their pivot points in front of the shoulder, forcing the shoulder girdle to abduct significantly and decreasing the effectiveness of the exercise.

- The knee is particularly vulnerable to shearing forces. Joint alignment on leg extension machines is critical. Correct placement of shin pads (not too low) and a resistance varied by a cam reduces knee stress and optimizes strength gains.

- The leg curl machine involves similar issues. An angled bench that elevates the pelvis will help maintain alignment of the low back as the knee flexes.

- Hack squat machines keep the pelvis and back quite stationary (unlike a regular squat), so that the knees are placed under greater shearing stress.

- Abdominal machines are particularly difficult because multiple pivot points change throughout the range of motion. Actions that have the trunk flexed well forward creating an L position increase low back stresses (Hamill and Knutzen 1995). Crunching downward or bringing a tucked lower body upward is a preferred movement if no pain is present. Some say that this movement focuses the intensity of contraction to the lower abdominals. More important for people with low back problems, this movement appears to present less compression on the discs of the lower back.

Anatomical and Biomechanical Analysis of a Weight-Training Exercise

A full and effective exercise analysis combines anatomical and biomechanical analyses. You must achieve the desired purpose of the exercise, meet your client's needs, account for any limitations, and validate the exercise design. You should always alter exercises—anatomically and biomechanically—to take your client's limitations into account and reduce the risk of injury.

The Situation

Maria worked as a sorter in the post office. She was interested in adding weights to her fitness program. Sometimes her shoulders tired at work, and she wanted to improve her shoulder endurance and prevent the injuries she had seen in some of her coworkers. Their injuries resulted from impingement (chapter 11), where the soft tissue between the head of the humerus and the acromion process of the scapula can be jammed.

One of the core exercises I designed for her was a lateral arm raise.

Anatomical Analysis

The purpose of the lateral arm raise is to develop the shoulders and upper back. The exercise effectively targets the deltoids and upper shoulder girdle muscles (table 5.9). Heavier weights and arms lifted above the horizontal can magnify the risk of impingement. Keeping the thumbs up provides the largest space for the tissues and a reduced risk (see Rotator Cuff Tendinitis [Impingement Syndrome]—chapter 11, p. 314). Because Maria had no shoulder problems, I expected that application of a progressive overload would bring the desired results with no complications. I advised Maria to avoid rapid movements, especially much beyond the horizontal. If she began to feel any discomfort, she was to stop and ice her shoulder after the workout.

Table 5.9   Anatomical Analysis of Lateral Arm Raises

Phase	Joint	Movement	Contraction type	Muscles
Up	Shoulder joint	Abduction Lateral rotation (thumbs up)	Concentric Isometric	Middle deltoid Supraspinatus Infraspinatus Teres minor
Up	Shoulder girdle	Upward rotation Abduction Elevation	Concentric	Serratus anterior Trapezius I and II Levator scapulae[a]
Down	Shoulder joint	Adduction Lateral rotation (thumbs up)	Eccentric Isometric	Middle deltoid Supraspinatus Infraspinatus Teres minor
Down	Shoulder girdle	Downward rotation Adduction Depression	Eccentric	Serratus anterior Trapezius I and II Levator scapulae[a]

[a]Pectoralis minor and trapezius IV are depressors and less effective in this exercise.

Biomechanical Analysis

The middle deltoid and supraspinatus have a direct line of pull for shoulder joint abduction. As the deltoid lifts the arm near the horizontal, the deltoid is shorter and not as strong. At this point, the shoulder girdle muscles play a more significant role.

The anterior deltoid assists with shoulder joint abduction. As Maria began to be fatigued, I noticed that she was lifting the weights a little more in front of her body to recruit more of the anterior deltoid. This change in alignment alters the composition of forces. Similarly, the thumbs-up position rotates the starting position of the shoulder, involving two more of the rotator cuff muscles (infraspinatus and teres minor). This change in alignment is not only a safety feature—it makes the lateral arm raise into a conditioning exercise for the rotator cuff. Because Maria's work required that she raise her arms over her head, I encouraged her to use the thumbs-up position.

A lateral raise is a third-class lever where the fulcrum is the shoulder joint, the lever arm is the humerus, the primary force is the deltoid, and the resistance is the weight of the arm and the dumbbell. Increasing the bend of the elbow brings the resistance closer to the fulcrum, reducing the resistance arm and making the exercise easier. I encouraged Maria to use this position at the beginning. As she progressed, I began to have her straighten her elbows somewhat before changing the weight.

Effective exercise analysis allowed me to achieve the desired purpose of the exercise and to meet Maria's needs. You should always alter exercises—anatomically and biomechanically—to account for your client's limitations.

Client-Centered Exercise Design Model

Just as a patient approaches the physician or pharmacist with the request, "Give me something for my . . . ," clients approach personal fitness trainers requesting specific exercises. The proliferation of strength training technique seminars and exercise design workshops for aerobic leaders and personal trainers is a testament to the interest in exercise design (Griffin 1986b). Yet many people in the industry are on the verge of "design template syndrome" where every program they design starts to look the same. In contrast, we should be able to draw on a variety of exercises to personalize our prescriptions—particularly in the component areas of flexibility, muscular balance, and conditioning.

After we analyze possible exercises, we select those that most closely match the needs of our client. We usually need to make modifications to improve the client "fit." And if the fit is still not right, we can build the ideal exercise for our client from scratch.

Training methods and exercise equipment are the setting for the real actors—the individual exercises. The script for these actors starts with the design of the exercise and continues with adjustment of the prescription factors (FITT—Frequency, Intensity, Time, and Type of exercise) to suit the client.

Steps in the Exercise Design Model

The following method, which puts together the techniques learned in this chapter, is a simple five-step approach to guide you through this process of exercise design:

1. **Identify the component and training method.**
2. **Target the muscles.**
3. **Determine the appropriate joint movements or position.**
4. **Design and modify.**
5. **Finish with a safety check.**

Step 1: Identify the Component and Training Method

Sometimes you will have to take your client's vision and translate it into a physiological component. For example, your client may want to make it through his work day without low back pain. This may require exercises for stretching the hip flexors, low back, and hamstrings; muscular endurance for the abdominals and gluteals; and some aerobic work. Your client's objectives may also involve multiple components. For example, someone who wants aerobic work but has a lower-leg problem must deal with modifications of the aerobic task while rehabilitating the leg. As the client makes gains, the importance of some of the components may decrease (e.g., lower-leg strength) while others may increase (e.g., cardiovascular endurance).

Careful selection of a training method (chapters 6-9) can assist in balancing several components. For your client with a lower-leg problem, you might consider rowing, swimming, or circuit training with aerobic activities involving the upper body. For muscular conditioning, consider simple sets, closed kinetic chain exercises, or a calisthenic circuit using surgical tubing. Even PNF stretching will develop isometric strength while improving joint flexibility.

Step 2: Target the Muscles

Step 2 identifies the goal area of the body and then targets the primary muscle groups (figure 5.17).

In this step you must consider muscular balance and postural stabilizers . For example, someone who spends many hours at a computer has asked for exercises to help his baseball throwing ability. The exercise illustrated in figure 5.1b will strengthen the anterior chest and shoulder muscles used in throwing. However, these muscles are tight because of the client's constant computer posture. Targeted muscles must strike a muscular balance with their antagonists. Therefore, your prescription should include stretches for the active chest muscles and strengthening of the upper back and posterior shoulder muscles (i.e., posterior deltoid, latissimus dorsi, and trapezius). Chapter 8 will show you how to analyze and work with muscle balance and posture.

Please note: Narrow targeting with muscle "isolations" is sometimes appropriate, but it may leave gaps in your client's program. Some machines can prevent muscles from working together naturally with other muscles as synergists or co-contractors. For example, there is little correlation between performance on isokinetic knee extension machines and functional performance in a weight-bearing sport or activity that uses the quadriceps (Ellison 1993).

Step 3: Determine the Appropriate Joint Movements or Position

You can read the JAM charts in reverse to determine the movement needed for an exercise design (see pp. 145-147). Here is an example:

- Use the tri-set system of training (chapter 7) to target the gluteus maximus. Table 5.17 (p. 146) indicates that the gluteus maximus is a prime mover for hip extension and lateral rotation and an assistant mover for hip abduction. In Step 4 you will see how to design three muscular endurance calisthenics that use these hip movements, or a single exercise modified in three ways. The JAM charts are a reminder that multiple movements are required to fully challenge all fibers of a muscle.

- A second example involves a client who has tension in the upper back. Step 2 targeted the upper trapezius muscles, levator scapulae, and the erector spinae of the cervical spine. Step 4 will explain how to design some static stretches for these muscles—but in what positions should the shoulder girdle and cervical spine be placed to stretch all of these muscles? Table 5.15 of the JAM charts (p. 145) shows that the levator scapulae and trapezius I and II are responsible for shoulder girdle elevation, upward rotation, and some assisted adduction. Taking the opposite position

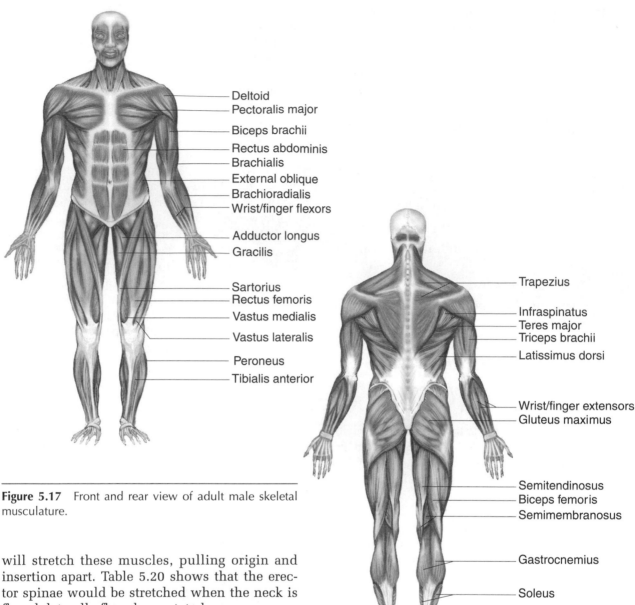

Figure 5.17 Front and rear view of adult male skeletal musculature.

will stretch these muscles, pulling origin and insertion apart. Table 5.20 shows that the erector spinae would be stretched when the neck is flexed, laterally flexed, or rotated.

Step 4: Design and Modify

This system establishes the requirements before an exercise is selected. Your guidelines are the muscle actions or movements. You are not restricted to a menu of exercises. Let the creative juices flow!

In the first example, figure 5.18 suggests three calisthenics that work the gluteus maximus in *(a)* lateral rotation with extension tubing (dynamic), *(b)* extension (isometric), and *(c)* abduction (dynamic). Dynabands could be used in all three exercises; ankle weights could be used from a standing position in exercises 1 and 3; or the range of motion could be increased in all three movements.

In the second example (figure 5.19), the first

exercise *(a)* stretches both sides of the erector spinae, trapezius I, and levator scapulae. The second exercise *(b)* focuses on one side at a time and stretches all four muscles. If your client has tension at his computer work station, you could modify the second exercise to be done in a chair. Grasping the bottom of the chair seat, she would lean to one side with a lateral flex to the neck.

Part II will provide sample program cards to record the exercises for your client. Consider the quality and format of the way you present the exercise on the program card. A diagram or photograph will be of immeasurable help at the early stages of the program when you are not around. Provide an

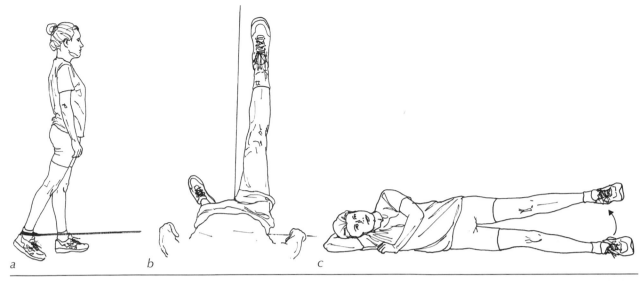

Figure 5.18   Strengthening exercises for the gluteus maximus.

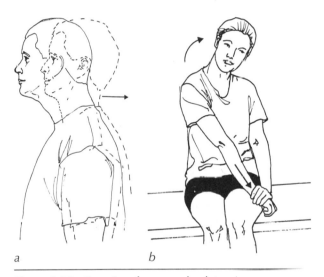

Figure 5.19   Exercises for upper back tension.

exercise name and the primary muscles involved. Select your wording carefully as you describe the exercise, from the initial body position through all sequenced movements. Give helpful cueing such as what to stabilize and include all relevant safety precautions.

Step 4 may also involve refinement and modification of exercises. To generate creative ideas, consider changes in body position, joint angle, or range of motion; the addition of other body segments, stages of the exercise, or combining movements; or simulation of a work task or sporting skill. Let's work with lateral arm raises (table 5.5) and consider a variety of modifications suited to specific scenarios. You are training at a home and only have 10 lb (3.7 kg) dumbbells, and your client is having some difficulties. Modify the exercise by having your client slightly bend his elbows to bring

the resistance closer to the joint. Another client is a water polo player and needs core stability while using the shoulders. Have this athlete perform the exercise while sitting on a stability ball with varying degrees of leg support. Or you may have a recreational tennis player who feels weak on her backhand topspin. Have this client start the lateral lifts from a bent elbow position and, as the arm is raised, lift the weight to point straight up (lateral rotation of the shoulder joint). This compound movement simulates a backhand topspin.

Step 5: Finish With a Safety Check

After creating your design, scrutinize it for safety. Check for risk in the design and later in the execution. Look for repetitive forces contributing to overuse, excessive force in the development of momentum, or forces applied when joints are not aligned. Modify the design further if the exercise has high injury risk (see table 5.10). During an exercise program demonstration, you present a lot of information for your client to retain. One of the real values of a personal fitness trainer is that you provide ongoing safety checks.

Your client may already have some areas of weakness to which you need to be sensitive, such as muscle imbalances, joint instability, muscle tightness, or previous injuries. I recall demonstrating a program to a strong, very fit client who followed my instructions and demonstration with good safe form. After a few sessions, I left him on his own for a few weeks and when I returned, he was doing one exercise with a form that was contraindicated. I had given him wall squats with a

Table 5.10 Program Segment Safety

Prescription	Safety issue
Preparation (warm-up) segment	
ROM (major joints are moved through their ROM)	• Use warm-up to increase joint lubrication and synovial fluid (protect). • Allow client to assess how body feels before work. • Use warm-up to provide some flexibility gains.
Circulatory warm-up (light aerobic; same mode as CV work)	• Continue warm-up to increase tissue temperature and synovial fluid in preparation for stretching. • Use segment to gradually prepare heart and circulatory system. • Simulate joint mechanics with low trauma.
Stretch (emphasis on static stretching)	• Promote flexibility gains. • Target muscles, especially those to be used eccentrically. • Provide dynamic stretches for sport preparation.
Transition (ease into next segment)	• Continue warm-up with a light overload in the activity to follow (start of progressive overload).
Aerobic segment	
Progressive prescription	• Build up gradually whether continuous or intervals. • Provide adequate relief during intervals. • Tear down gradually; avoid final sprints or sudden stops (better CV adaptations permitted).
Monitoring	• Monitor heart rate, perceived exertion, talk test, logging. • Have client stretch as needed for muscular tightness.
Sport (sport-specific)	Look for opportunities to • Do mini-warm-ups and skill practice (especially in intermittent sports such as baseball) • Stretch tight muscles • Tend immediately to minor injuries
Resistance segment	
Progressive prescription	• Provide progressive overload and adequate relief (depends on training method). • Incorporate warm-up sets (e.g., 60% of training weight). • Follow weight room safety rules (especially spotting guidelines).
Specific training method (chapter 6)	• Follow method guidelines as prescribed.
Muscle balance	• Check the balance (agonist and antagonist) of the program (i.e., need for specific muscle stretch or strengthening).
Monitor	• Have client stretch as needed for muscular tightness. • Differentiate between fatigue, soreness, and inflammation. • Modify the exercise around minor injuries (including avoidance). • Conduct ongoing check for correct breathing, speed of movement, base of support, and alignment such as pelvic stabilization and avoidance of extreme ROM.
Cool-down segment	
Stretch (emphasis on static stretching)	• Take advantage of warm tissue for greatest flexibility gains. • Target muscles used, especially if used eccentrically. • Consider PNF if flexibility is a priority.
Self-check	• Ensure that CV indicators (e.g., heart rate, depth of breathing, blood pressure) are well down. • Ensure that muscles feel worked but not sore or tight. • Ice any "hot spots" or minor injuries. • Don't underestimate the therapeutic effect of a relaxing shower.

Note. ROM = range of motion; CV = cardiovascular; PNF = proprioceptive neuromuscular facilitation.

stability ball behind his back, but he had adjusted his feet well back toward the wall with his toes pointing outward. He said he made the changes because he developed some shin splints from running and this position gave him some relief. I knew at a glance that the shear and torque on the knee were not safe and eliminated that exercise until he could perform the squat correctly without shin pain.

Weekend Warrior

A word of caution about the "weekend warrior," the impetuous client who charges from his week of sedentary living directly to the competitive playing field. He is a prime candidate for muscle or connective tissue injury caused by a rapid or forceful eccentric contraction. Avoidance is not the message he wants to hear, and a few cold stretches do little to prepare his body for the trauma. A longer warm-up integrating progressive eccentric actions similar to those in the sport will help. Also add a supplemental program to strengthen (eccentrically) the muscles used in the sport, particularly in preseason. Always critically evaluate eccentric contraction patterns within your client's activity prescription.

What other counseling would be appropriate for this type of client? Why?

Common Design Faults . . . and Why

When you assign "cookbook" exercises to your clients, the chances of missing important individual differences in the mechanics of the movement are high. Another significant source of design faults is the failure to watch for execution errors during the demonstration. A client's errors may not simply be a learning issue; it may be that an area of instability is causing the altered mechanics. Table 5.11 identifies a number of common faults in the design or execution of popular resistance exercises.

Client-Centered Exercise Demonstration Model

First impressions about the prescription begin in the demonstration stage and continue to be reinforced through subsequent workouts and all the stages of monitoring. There is a relative paucity of articles concerning the teaching and demonstra-tion of new exercise skills despite the fact that this often constitutes a vast majority of time for a personal fitness trainer. Teaching behaviors such as exercise explanations, demonstrations, positive reinforcement, and performance feedback increase the level of exercise focus.

Clients need to understand how an exercise will help them. They need to see it demonstrated and then try it with some expert feedback. Finally, the exercise may need to be modified or integrated into a full prescription. These are the steps involved in the *Exercise Demonstration Model Checklist*. Adapt this model to suit your client and situation.

Exercise Demonstration Model Checklist

The one-on-one exercise demonstration is a core element of your client-centered services. *The Exercise Demonstration Model Checklist* identifies more than two dozen critical behaviors that make up a single demonstration.

There are four distinct steps.

1. The **predemonstration** sets the scene, in which you ensure that the client is comfortable, find out about the client's previous experience, and provide an idea of what is to come and why.

2. The actual **demonstration** stage teaches the client how to perform the exercise correctly and safely. Effective use of verbal and physical techniques adds clarity to the teaching.

3. The third stage is the **client trial,** in which you observe carefully and provide specific feedback.

4. The **follow-up** allows you to gather feedback from the client and provide client-centered prescription guidelines.

The items on the checklist guide you through this process. For many of the items, the checklist provides examples of behaviors or methods of showing that item. They are merely suggestions that may guide your actions or dialogue with your client.

Encouraging an Experiential Approach

You can encourage an experiential approach to the program demonstration and follow-up by designing situations that offer all the ways adults like to

Table 5.11 Common Design and Execution Faults for Selected Resistance Exercises

Exercise	What's wrong?	Why? Key points
Lat pull-down	Pulling down behind the head	Muscle imbalances such as rounded shoulders can compromise the position of the scapula and shoulder joint at the start of the movement. At times a restricted lateral rotation of the shoulder can force the lumbar spine into increased lordosis.[a] Wide grip with bar and a pull to anterior chest require more work from lats.[b]
Seated row	Leaning forward to start and backward to finish	Rounded low back may create compression in a flexed position. Rounded shoulders create a loosely packed, unstable position. Leaning back activates the erector spinae, not the desired lats, posterior deltoids, and mid-traps. More weight may be lifted but not by the intended muscles.
Dumbbell press	Lowering the weights too far	The problem can be caused by excessive microtrauma of the chest musculature. The client may be in a position of lumbar lordosis as the chest rises. Also, subacromial space diminishes (potential impingement) when the elbows are brought down.[c]
Fly cable crossover	Failing to lock elbows throughout range of motion	Bringing elbows from a bent to a straightened position will use the triceps. Keeping elbows stable in a slight flex will focus horizontal movements on the pectoralis.
Squat	Squatting to a depth where the thighs are parallel to the ground	Most lifters will bend forward excessively at the hips, which rotates the pelvis forward and increases lumbar lordosis in an attempt to stay upright. Some may round the back (flex at the spine) creating a shear force with the compression on the intervertebral disc. Spine should be stable in a neutral position.
Leg press or hack squat	Bringing the weight too low Turning the feet inward or outward to isolate parts of the quads	When the knee tracks beyond the toes, excessive forces are placed on the posterior cruciate ligament.[d] There is no consensus that foot position can alter quad muscle recruitment.[e] Select the most comfortable foot position that poses the least stress.
Hamstring curl	Allowing buttocks to rise from the bench and the hips to flex	This may be one of three things: (1) the weight is too high; (2) the rectus femoris is too tight, pulling to rotate the pelvis; or (3) the abdominals are too weak to hold a neutral spine position.
Triceps kickback	Positioning elbow below the body	The ROM in which the triceps have to lift against gravity is reduced. However, a raised elbow puts the long head of the triceps in a shortened position, so this head has less involvement. A modification of a triceps exercise in which the upper arm is raised (shoulder flexion) will involve the long head as well as the medial and lateral heads.
Barbell curl	Moving the torso or shoulder joint	Extending the torso in the up phase creates momentum. Flexing the shoulder joint draws assistance from the anterior deltoid and upper pectoralis major. These actions do not allow the elbows to move through a full ROM and decrease the muscle fiber recruitment of the biceps.
Theraball crunch	Using a position on the ball that does not allow for a ROM suited to the client's strength	A position of support in the middle and upper back will decrease the ROM and reduce the lever arm length, creating an easier modification. A lower starting position allowing the spine to slightly hyperextend will prestretch the abdominals, change the fulcrum, and increase the lever arm, therefore increasing the contractile ROM.

Note. ROM = range of motion.

[a]Hagan 2000; [b]Signorile et al. 2002; [c]Lyons and Orwin 1998; [d]Escamilla et al. 1998; [e]Lockwood 1999.

Exercise Demonstration Model Checklist

1. Predemonstration

____ Set climate by making client feel comfortable and being receptive and responsive.

____ Provide overview by explaining the purpose of this session and what is to happen in this session.

____ Determine client's background and experience by asking, Have you done this exercise before? Have you used this type of equipment before? What was your experience?

____ Clarify purpose of exercises by explaining the specific muscles used (major prime movers) and relevance to stated needs and wants.

____ Encourage the client to ask questions and provide input.

2. Demonstration

____ Provide precise and appropriate verbal instructions.

____ Provide clear physical demonstration (before client trial).

____ Ensure overall technical execution was smooth and confident.

____ Ensure beginning position alignment.

____ Isolate the movement (i.e., no compensation or inappropriate movements).

____ Stabilize the pelvis and key joints.

____ Ensure terminal points of range of motion appropriate.

____ Demonstrate safety, including controlled breathing and no Valsalva maneuver.

____ Demonstrate safety, including controlled speed and no momentum at the end of the range of motion.

____ Ensure efficient use of time with descriptions and explanations.

3. Client trials

____ Set client up by positioning and alignment.

____ Select appropriate weight (moderately difficult).

____ Ensure trial safety by controlling breathing, momentum, and plane of movement and ensuring no joint locking.

____ Ensure effective spotting by being in position to observe and assist with starting and finishing positions.

____ Have client execute a full set.

____ Provide feedback to the client, which may include providing specific information and monitoring, focusing on behavior and not the person, correcting one aspect at a time, and being positive and helpful (providing success).

____ Demonstrate verbal skills such as cueing during execution paraphrasing, summarizing, and questioning.

____ Demonstrate nonverbal skills such as using correct body position, being engaged, providing eye contact, and ignoring distractions.

4. Follow-up

____ Obtain feedback from client by asking how it felt (i.e., awkward, comfortable, difficult) and encouraging the client to ask questions and provide input.

____ Demonstrate active listening skills by responding to feedback.

____ Provide prescription guidelines (including weight, reps, and sets, or frequency, intensity, time, and type) that integrate and interpret information from client trial.

____ Suggest a method of progression or encourage self-monitoring and assessment.

From *Client-Centered Exercise Prescription, Second Edition*, by John C. Griffin, 2006, Champaign, IL: Human Kinetics.

learn. Here are four different learning styles, each followed by an example of how you would use that learning style with a client:

- **Learning by doing:** Have the client perform a series of abdominal exercises at a very slow and controlled pace, rather than the faster pace to which she is accustomed.

- **Learning by observation:** Ask your client to comment on specific items she observed or felt—for example, "How did the slow exercises feel? Was there more energy required to perform the series slow or fast?"

- **Learning by knowing the theory:** This is a combination of your client's experience and observations; ask, for example, "What does this mean about the next time you will do sit-ups?"

- **Learning by applying the information to individual situations:** Have your client consider how this information will apply to other exercises he executes. "What would be the best way to perform muscle endurance exercises? Where else can this information apply?"

Base the amount of information you share with your client on his current stage of learning as well as on his preferred learning style. In the beginning stages, focus on giving only the important points. As your client becomes more experienced, offer more alternative exercises, allowing your client to make his own selection.

Exercise Demonstration

Demonstrating an exercise is both an art and a science. It requires a balance between your technical knowledge and your people skills. With practice, you will learn to alter the technical aspects to suit each client's personality and learning style.

Science of Exercise Demonstration

You should always observe, analyze, and modify technique. You must have a sound knowledge of the biomechanics of the exercises and an ability to design multiple variations in technique to suit the abilities of your clients. In addition to designing appropriate exercises, you must reinforce good technique both by demonstrating new exercises and by observing your client as she attempts to duplicate your demonstrations.

There are four technical issues on which you must focus to provide effective exercise demonstration:

- **Initial body position.** Focus on overall body posture. Instruct your client to "set" herself into a good body position before any exercise. Focus on exactly where you want your client to begin. For example, when beginning a bench press, your client should press her low back into the bench, with feet on the bench (if possible) and hands slightly wider than shoulder-width apart. Establish what will be stabilized and how that will feel (e.g., shoulder girdle or pelvic stabilization).

- **Movement pattern.** From the starting position, describe the sequence of movements and the body or joint position at the end of the exercise.

- **Cueing.** Give alignment and "feeling" cues to assist in the execution phase of the exercise. For example, when your client is doing side-lying lateral leg raises, show how the hips are aligned one on top of the other, raising to approximately 45°, with knees facing forward.

- **Safety and quality.** Using your knowledge of the demands and biomechanics of the exercise, provide appropriate safety guidelines. Focus on quality versus quantity. This refers to the number of repetitions your client performs correctly and the speed at which they occur. When resistance equipment is being used, remember the issues we raised in *Direction of Force Application and Alignment* (p. 130):

  - Is the path of motion defined by the machine the same as your client's path of motion?

  - Is the direction of force application safe and optimal?

  - Does the equipment allow proper alignment between the machine's fulcrum and the center of the moving joint?

Other Issues

Spotting and positioning are also technical in nature but relate directly to client execution. Poor spotting or positioning could result in serious injury to the client or trainer; good spotting provides a trust-building experience that rivals any counseling technique.

- **Spotting.** Spotting is an important component of exercise demonstration. Spotting refers to the visual and physical aspects of monitoring clients as they execute exercises. Visual spotting is done for all exercises, whereas physical spotting is used primarily in weight training. Watch for correct body alignment, signs and symptoms of fatigue, signs of discomfort, control of movements, and the direction of the exercise energy.

Assist the client to make technique corrections, attempt more repetitions, or complete the range of motion. For clients who are more advanced, verbal reinforcement cues are effective to correct their technique. Once the neural pattern (motor schema) has been cemented, the cues can prompt fluid modification during the repetition (Baker 2001). The simple use of one or two key words such as *head up, pelvis stable,* or *pinch* provides sufficient feedback based on the client's current knowledge of performance. Spotting the client provides an excellent opportunity to monitor good form. Table 5.12 lists the major spotting guidelines for monitoring technically sound mechanics.

• **Positioning.** While you are training or demonstrating to your client, your positioning can help you and affect your rapport with your client. Position yourself for the best view of the client's technique if you are not spotting. From the side you should also be able to view her face and most of her body. Match your client's upper body level, and avoid talking down to her. Like an athlete, be in a ready position to assist your client. Being casual by leaning or sitting can make you appear unprofessional.

• **Touching or not touching.** Many personal fitness trainers touch their clients to adjust their position. We must always respect individual boundaries. If you have not received permission to touch your client or are hesitant to ask, you can use a few strategies to help position your client without touching her. Demonstrate the exercise and then point out the adjustments on your own body while the client performs the exercise.

Another technique is to provide a mental image such as "squeezing the abdomen like an accordion" (Cantwell 1998).

Art of Exercise Demonstration

The skills involved in demonstration are significantly based in the psychosocial domain. Table 5.13 outlines some of these psychosocial aspects involved in the stages and activities, from the time we meet our clients for the program demonstration until later in the program follow-up.

Program demonstration is an excellent opportunity for motivation and reinforcement. Baker (2001) described three methods of reinforcing behavior.

1. Achievement reinforcement helps cultivate motivation to achieve preset goals. Recognize even a small improvement, but make sure it is praiseworthy because clients will know if you are sincere.

2. Sensation motivation comes from the feeling of execution excellence and, if reinforced immediately, will remain clear in the kinesthetic memory.

3. Verbal reinforcement should be positive and specific to the performance. To correct a client error, avoid negative phrases such as "No . . . that's not right," "That's too fast," or "Don't lock your elbows." Instead try more positive corrective cues such as, "If you adjust that position, you should feel the difference," "Keep that cadence of 1 up and 3 down," or "Keep your elbows soft . . . good."

Table 5.12   Spotting Guidelines for Monitoring Lifting Techniques

Area	Spotting guidelines
Upper body	• Position yourself close to the client where you have the most effective position for assistance. • Assist the client with heavier weights to bring the weight to the starting position. • Position your hands on the barbell. • During dumbbell exercises, position your hands at the joint that is immediately below the weight. • Assist the client at the end point of a movement during the final reps.
Lower body	• Position yourself close to the client where you have the most effective position for assistance. • Assist the client to bring the weight to the starting position for squats and lunges. • Position your hands just above the waist for squats and lunges. • Position your hands on the machine or the involved limb for pulley, machine, or hand exercises. • Assist the client at the end of a movement or if the speed decreases because of fatigue.
Trunk	• Use the assistance of gravity by using incline or decline positions of the bench. • Teach a pelvic stabilization to minimize low back curvature and strain. • Manually assist when client has difficulty with correct movements. • Manually assist at the ends of normal range of motion once fatigue has occurred.

Table 5.13 Psychosocial Aspects in the Program Demonstration and Follow-Up Model

Step	Activities
1. Predemonstration	• Reassess and discuss client goals, values, motivational interests, and fitness assessment results. • Reconnect: Re-create and further build a positive climate. • Give clients permission to be themselves; show pleasure in what they are doing; provide protection from negative forces (e.g., negative self-talk, interruptions, intimidating atmosphere). • Ensure that clients' needs are being met.
2. Demonstration	• Base delivery of the information on clients' preferred learning styles. • Use an experiential learning approach. • Provide precise and appropriate verbal instructions. • Be time efficient with descriptions and explanations.
3. Client trials	• Provide feedback to the client that is specific, positive, and helpful (provides success). • Focus on the behavior, not the person. • Use verbal skills such as cues during execution, paraphrasing, and summarizing. • Use nonverbal skills to show engagement.
4. Follow-up	• Determine level of comfort and understanding. • Obtain feedback from client (specific probing). • Use active listening skills and respond to feedback. • Modify design if necessary; make sure the client accepts the exercise. • Make an appointment for connection in 2 to 3 days. • Move toward using intrinsic motivators.

Reinforcing the client during this demonstration and follow-up stage is an effective means of motivating him to continue with positive behaviors or to modify incorrect techniques. Westcott and colleagues (2003) found that high levels of focused trainer–client interaction should address major aspects of proper exercise performance without being too technical during the first few weeks of training. They further suggested that comments should not disrupt exercise flow and should be exercise-focused, reinforcing the client's training efforts.

Connecting With Your Client

Try to get a broad picture of the human side of program demonstration. Imagine that you are demonstrating a modified squat to a novice middle-aged client. In the following, a description of your role in each stage precedes a brief sample statement appropriate for that stage of the exercise demonstration.

- **Predemonstration.** This first step requires a sales technique. You need to sell the benefits and show your client how the exercise is relevant to him.

By doing the squats regularly, you will be better able to climb longer flights of stairs, lift heavier objects from the floor, and walk farther without fatigue.

- **Demonstration.** You are the role model, yet you must be sensitive to your client's style of learning—tactile, auditory, or visual.

Stand with feet shoulder-width apart, knees slightly bent; your back is pushed flat against the wall with your arms on your thighs for support like this.

- **Client trials.** Your focus is on your client's behavior. Leave him with a feeling of success and an idea of how to do better.

As you bent your knees to lower your body, your knees moved beyond the line of your toes initially, but then you pressed your hips farther back as you lowered your body and realigned . . . that's good.

- **Follow-up.** Ask for your client's feelings. If you have rapport with him, you will gain valuable insights. Knowing that you are there for him gives him the confidence for greater autonomy.

Are there any aspects of the exercise you are unsure of or want to clarify? Which part of the program are you most looking forward to?

JAM (Joint–Action–Muscle) Charts

Table 5.14 Shoulder Joint Muscles and Their Actions

Muscle	Flexion	Extension	Abduction	Adduction	Medial rotation	Lateral rotation	Horizontal adduction	Horizontal abduction
Anterior deltoid	PM		AM				PM	
Middle deltoid			PM					PM
Posterior deltoid		PM						PM
Supraspinatus			PM					
Pectoralis major[a]	PM						PM	
Pectoralis major[b]		PM		PM			PM	
Subscapularis					PM		AM	
Infraspinatus						PM		PM
Teres minor						PM		PM
Latissimus dorsi		PM		PM				AM
Teres major		PM		PM	PM			

Note. PM = prime mover; AM = assistant mover.
[a]clavicular; [b]sternal.

Table 5.15 Shoulder Girdle Muscles and Their Actions

Muscle	Elevation	Depression	Abduction	Adduction	Upward rotation	Downward rotation
Pectoralis minor		PM	PM			PM
Serratus anterior			PM		PM	
Trapezius I	PM					
Trapezius II	PM			AM	PM	
Trapezius III				PM		
Trapezius IV		PM		AM	PM	
Levator scapulae	PM					
Rhomboid	PM			PM		PM

Note. Large muscles of the shoulder joint can influence shoulder girdle actions. PM = prime mover; AM = assistant mover.

Table 5.16 Elbow and Radioulnar Joint Muscles and Their Actions

Muscles	Flexion	Extension	Pronation	Supination
Biceps brachii	PM			AM
Brachialis	PM			
Brachioradialis	PM		AM	AM
Pronator quadratus			PM	
Pronator teres			AM	
Supinator				PM
Triceps brachii		PM		
Wrist extensors (posterior forearm)		AM		
Wrist flexors (anterior forearm)	AM			

Note. PM = prime mover; AM = assistant mover.

Table 5.17 Hip Joint Muscles and Their Actions

Muscles	Flexion	Extension	Abduction	Adduction	Medial rotation	Lateral rotation
Iliacus	PM[a]					AM
Psoas	PM[a]					AM
Rectus femoris	PM[a]					
Pectineus	PM[a]			PM	AM	
Sartorius	AM		AM			AM
Tensor fasciae latae			PM		AM	
Gluteus medius			PM			
Gluteus minimus			AM		PM	
Gluteus maximus		PM	AM			PM
Semitendinosus		PM				
Semimembranosus		PM				
Biceps femoris (LH)		PM				
Adductor longus				PM		
Adductor brevis				PM		
Adductor magnus				PM		
Gracilis				PM		
Six lateral rotators						PM

PM = prime mover; AM = assistant mover; LH = long head.

[a]These muscles may indirectly cause hyperextension of the low back by tilting the pelvis forward.

Table 5.18 Knee Joint Muscles and Their Actions

Muscles	Flexion	Extension	Medial rotation	Lateral rotation
Semitendinosus	PM		PM	
Semimembranosus	PM		PM	
Biceps femoris	PM			PM
Rectus femoris		PM		
Vastus lateralis		PM		
Vastus intermedius		PM		
Vastus medialis		PM		
Sartorius	AM		AM	
Gracilis	AM		AM	
Popliteus			PM	
Gastrocnemius	AM			

Note. PM = prime mover; AM = assistant mover.

Table 5.19 Ankle and Foot Muscles and Their Actions

Muscles	Dorsiflexion	Plantar flexion	Inversion	Eversion
Gastrocnemius		PM		
Soleus		PM		
Tibialis posterior[a]		AM	PM	
Peroneus longus [a]		AM		PM
Peroneus brevis		AM		PM
Flexor digitorum longus[a]		AM	AM	
Flexor hallucis longus[a]		AM	AM	
Tibialis anterior	PM		PM	
Peroneus tertius	PM			PM
Extensor digitorum longus	PM			PM
Extensor hallicus longus	AM		AM	

Note. PM = prime mover; AM = assistant mover.

[a]These muscles also support the arch.

Table 5.20 Spinal Muscles and Their Actions

Muscles	Flexion	Extension	Lateral flexion	Rotation (same side)	Rotation (opposite side)
Lumbar and thoracic spines					
Rectus abdominis	PM		AM		
External oblique	PM		PM		PM
Internal oblique	PM		PM	PM	
Psoas	AM	[a]			
Quadratus lumborum		AM	PM		
Erector spinae group		PM	PM	PM	
Deep posterior group		PM	PM		PM
Cervical spine					
Sternocleidomastoid	PM		PM		PM
Scaleni group	AM		PM		
Erector spinae group		PM	PM	PM	
Deep posterior group		PM	PM		PM

Note. PM = prime mover; AM = assistant mover.

[a]The psoas may pull the spine into hyperextension without balance from the abdominals, especially if the iliacus tilts the pelvis forward.

Highlights

1. **Anatomically analyze the joint movements, muscles used, and types of contraction for exercises and activities common to fitness programming.**

   Analysis of an exercise allows us to select or modify it. The **five-step approach of anatomical analysis** can be applied to a variety of exercise movements.

   1. Analyze phases: Most exercises have two discernible phases: up and down, in and out, push and pull. Some complex sports skills have preparatory, power, and follow-through phases.

   2. Analyze joints and movements: Determine which joints are involved and what movements they are performing.

   3. Analyze types of contractions: The up phase of calisthenics, free weights, sports skills, and many resistance machines involves concentric contraction of the muscles producing joint movements in that direction. Eccentric contractions occur when the body or a limb is lowered or muscles attempt to counter the force of momentum by slowing down the action. Identify the major muscles involved in any isometric contraction where stabilization is a critical part of your client's activity.

   4. Analyze which muscles are being used: Muscles affect movement of the joints that they cross. If alignment of the muscle–tendon unit is in the direction of the movement, the influence of that muscle will be optimal. To facilitate this step, the end of the chapter presents **JAM** charts: quick references indicating joint, actions, and muscles (tables 5.14-5.20).

   5. Evaluate purpose, effectiveness, and risk: Evaluate the effectiveness of the exercise, how well it fills its purpose, and the degree of personal risk it carries with it.

2. **Apply biomechanical principles to optimize exercise benefits for your clients and at the same time attend to their limitations through biomechanical alterations of the exercise.**

   Biomechanical analysis examines the method of execution of an exercise. Such analyses enable us to advise our clients concerning

   - the best starting position for an exercise,
   - the optimal speed for their objectives,
   - the position of joints to isolate specific muscles,
   - how to align the movement to the muscle,
   - how to combine muscles for optimal results, and
   - how to modify the leverage to gain a greater strength output.

   The purpose, effectiveness, and safety of an exercise or sport skill may be affected by any or all of the following:

   - Muscle length and force
   - Biarticular (two-joint) muscle action
   - Composition of forces
   - Leverage and strength
   - Direction of force application/alignment
   - Alignment of external resistance

3. **Describe and use the five-step exercise design model.**

   Step 1: Identify the component and training method: Your client's objectives may also involve multiple components. Select a training method that balances several components.

   Step 2: Target the muscles: Identify the goal area of the body and then target the primary muscle groups.

   Step 3: Determine the appropriate joint movements or position—read the JAM (joint–action–muscle) charts in reverse to determine the movement needed for an exercise design.

Step 4: Design and modify: To generate creative ideas, consider changes in body position, joint angle, or range of motion; the addition of other body segments, stages of the exercise, or combining movements; or simulation of a work task or sporting skill. Describe the exercise from the initial body position, through all sequenced movements.

Step 5: Finish with a safety check: Check for high risk in the design and later in the execution. Give helpful cueing such as what to stabilize and include all relevant safety precautions.

4. **Use the client-centered exercise demonstration model to provide personal exercise demonstrations involving preexercise explanations, trainer demonstration, client trial, performance feedback, and follow-up.**

Clients need to understand how an exercise will help them. They need to see it demonstrated and then to try it with some expert feedback. Finally, the exercise may need to be modified or integrated into a full prescription. One-on-one exercise demonstration represents a core element of client-centered services. The *Exercise Demonstration Model Checklist* lists the steps to the model and identifies more than two dozen critical behaviors that will guide you through this process.

5. **Apply the technical knowledge and the people skills called for in the client-centered exercise demonstration model: (1) Predemonstration, (2) demonstration, (3) client trial, and (4) follow-up.**

Apply exercise biomechanics to design multiple variations in technique to suit the abilities of your clients and reinforce good technique as they demonstrate new exercises. Quality and safety of an exercise demonstration will come when you focus on the initial body alignment, movement patterns, verbal cueing, and your positioning or spotting.

The skills involved in the client-centered exercise demonstration model are also based in the psychosocial domain. Program demonstration is an excellent opportunity for motivation and reinforcement. Base the amount of information you share with your client on his current stage of learning as well as his preferred learning style.

PART II

Client-Centered Exercise Prescription

The counseling stage of the prescription journey has provided us with a picture of our client's history, needs, and hopes as well as potential sources of motivation. We have helped our clients to clarify priorities by refocusing on what is important. We understand our clients' needs; we have learned about their areas of interests and expectations; we have a very clear picture of what and how our clients want to change; and we have selected assessment items that best match our clients' priorities. We will create exercise strategies based in large part on our interpretation of the counseling and assessment results. The key to a successful program lies in our ability to help clients maintain the conviction that our prescription will bring about the changes they want. Exercise will be a high priority if this personalized connection is maintained. We must provide constant support and reinforcement for this action–benefit relationship.

In this second stage of our journey, we select appropriate exercises and elements of the exercise prescription, from a wide menu of choices, according to how they fit our client's goals. A variety of training methods allows us to match specific benefits to specific clients. It is because of this variety that the client-centered approach to prescription is safe and effective. The details of the personalized exercise prescription are based

on two main criteria: the physiological rationale and the client's willingness to accept the program. Knowing this in advance of our prescription design is a powerful tool.

We can prescribe exercise programs to produce three potential outcomes: increased general fitness, performance improvements, or health enhancement. Part II of the book details four prescription models: cardiovascular conditioning, resistance training, muscle balance and flexibility, and weight management. These models show how adaptation can be manipulated through prudent selection of appropriate exercises, prescription factors, machines, and training methods.

Although cardiovascular fitness is still the foundation of most exercise prescriptions, the client-centered approach can adjust the outcome to suit more personal goals such as improved performance or reduction of stress or heart disease risk factors. The challenge with resistance training is to shape the overload to suit your client by manipulating the prescription factors according to the principle of specificity—namely, that gains in muscular fitness are specific to the muscle group, training method, and exercise volume. Our concern with muscle balance is multifaceted: It is not limited to strength, flexibility, or endurance but may involve strength of one muscle group and flexibility of an opposing muscle group. The unique role of exercise in energy balance is the backdrop for discussion of client issues in weight management.

Each prescription model is followed by case studies, which deal with specific client situa-tions and demonstrate the application of many of the prescription tools. Within each case study, physiological justifications or client-centered (behavioral) justifications are presented for each design decision.

6

Client-Centered Cardiovascular Exercise Prescription Model

Chapter Competencies

After completing this chapter, you will be able to demonstrate the following competencies:

1. Use a seven-step prescription process to guide you through decisions when designing a cardiovascular prescription.

The remaining competencies reflect the seven steps of the model for cardiovascular exercise prescription.

2. Consider client needs and goals.

3. Select activities and equipment.

4. Select training method and mode.

5. Set intensity and workload.

6. Set volume (duration and frequency).

7. Address progression and monitoring.

8. Design a warm-up and a cool-down.

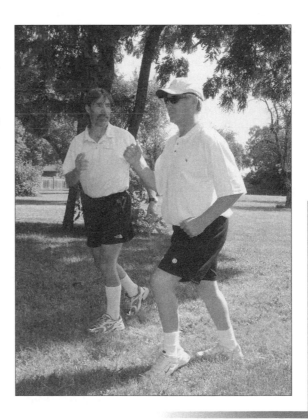

Although cardiovascular fitness is still the foundation of most exercise prescriptions, you can use the client-centered approach to adjust the outcome to suit more personal goals (e.g., reduction of stress or of risk factors for coronary heart disease, improved performance). Explaining to a client that in 4 months of aerobic exercise she can increase her maximum oxygen uptake by 15% may be realistic, but if her goal is to reduce stress, knowing about the oxygen uptake increase will provide scant encouragement. Always explain potential benefits and interpret observed results in terms of the client's goals.

The cardiovascular prescription model uses a seven-step prescription process to guide you through decisions concerning exercise intensity, volume, and progression based on access to test data, past experience, availability of monitoring equipment, and the client's exercise needs and level of fitness. Physiological justifications and client-centered (behavioral) justifications for each choice made in the prescription model are reinforced with several case studies.

The Cardiovascular Prescription Model

Following is the Client-Centered Cardiovascular Exercise Prescription Model, which will serve both as an overview of what is to come and as a useful tool for review (table 6.1). It outlines a seven-step model for physiologically sound and client-centered exercise prescription for cardio-vascular fitness. Each step describes a decision that you will face. Many of the choices available for each decision are listed for each step. Following a brief background for each step, sample case studies are presented including the choices that were made for the client and a justification for those choices.

Step 1: Consider Client Needs and Goals

As noted in part I, client needs may be related to medical or high-risk (e.g., elevated blood lipids, hypertension), educational (e.g., shoe features), or motivational (e.g., lack of self-esteem) factors. Client needs also can be determined by results of fitness assessments (e.g., oxygen uptake) or by physical limitations attributable to weight or orthopedics. Careful screening procedures can identify when medical intervention is warranted. Often the client is unaware of emerging needs such as borderline hypertension or lack of core strength. Gathering information on her activity profile can establish current levels of energy expenditure.

Recall that goal setting involves specifying what needs to be done, when and how to do it, and the anticipated outcomes. Integrating needs, wants, and lifestyle will increase the probability of compliance with any prescription. It is often easier to begin with long-term goals that are more global and then direct the client's attention to formulating several shorter-term goals that could be accomplished before major changes in assessment measures. You can play a vital role by helping your client set realistic, measurable goals and posting them for regular review. The client's goal has a direct influence on the design of the program in many ways. The case studies in this chapter demonstrate this diversity dramatically whether the client is concerned about health, fitness, or athletic performance. Explaining to your client how your prescription decisions suit her goals will significantly affect her compliance in the early stages of exercise. Because this step is so important, periodically review part I until you are sure that you have a firm grasp of the principles of counseling, motivating, and enhancing adherence and of client-centered assessment and prescription.

Step 2: Select Activities and Equipment

Your reflective listening, probes, and clarification will give your client a clearer picture of the type of activity he would like to do and any equipment he may need. Clients select their activities based on the benefits they see from their own perspective, not necessarily yours. The challenge is to demonstrate clearly how an activity will fill their wants and needs. As outlined in part I, three steps will increase your chances of demonstrating this: (1) Come up with options, (2) analyze the options, and (3) lead the client to commitment. Select the activities of highest priority, determine those that present the best combination of options, and discuss the most effective strategy for integrating the new activity or equipment.

Select Cardiovascular Activities

It is often easier for your client to talk about his needs and goals than it is to select an activity or exercises, because the latter is the start of a specific commitment. Some clients may be so overwhelmed by the whole exercise thing that

Table 6.1 Client-Centered Cardiovascular Exercise Prescription Model

Decisions	Choices
1. Consider client needs and goals.	Screening—medical history: intervention needed (e.g., meds)
	Limitations (e.g., CV risk, orthopedic issues, injury, test results)
	Activity profile and history (review current energy expenditure)
	Design considerations or preferences (e.g., time, equipment availability, location)
	Priorities: health, fitness, performance
	Motivational strategy, personality, learning style
	Stress management issues
	Assessment interpretation:
	• Functional capacity (e.g., maximum oxygen uptake, Aerobic Fitness Score) and normative or health rating
	• Heart rate, blood pressure, and perceived exertion responses (recovery rate, steady states, termination criteria)
	• Visual signs, symptoms, comments
2. Select activities and equipment.	Equipment (and brand) pros and cons
	Equipment features (e.g., info display, braking mechanism)
	Treadmill, run, walk
	Bicycle, ergometer
	Elliptical trainer
	Rower
	Stepper
	Swim
	In-line
	Group classes, sports
	ACSM group I and II—aerobic
	Specific exercises (order)
3. Select training method and mode.	Continuous
	Interval
	Circuit
	Plyometrics (see chapter 7)
	Cross-training, sports
	Fartlek
	Active living
4. Set intensity and workload.	Recommended training zone:
	• % $\dot{V}O_2$ reserve, % max METs, % HRR, perceived exertion (e.g., 40/50 85% $\dot{V}O_2$ reserve/HRR . . . sufficient to complete duration and tolerate the exercise without risk)
	• Calculate corresponding workload (e.g., ACSM metabolic formulas) or select a workload that elicits an appropriate HR (e.g., 40/50-85% HRR); verify selection during demo-client trial
	• Calculate kcal/min (e.g., chart or L/min × 5 kcal)
	• Recreational sport and active living (MET/kcal chart)
	• Manipulate balance with duration and frequency
	• Confirm consistency with goals and needs

(continued)

Table 6.1 *(continued)*

Decisions	Choices
5. Set volume (duration and frequency).	Total work per session (intensity and duration) Intervals: duration of work and rest 20-30 min, progressing to 45-60 min 250-500 kcal/session Minimum 2 ×/week; recommend 3-5 ×/week (daily active living) Total work/week (intensity, duration, and frequency) – 1,000-2,000 kcal/week Supplement with active living recommendations
6. Address progression and monitoring.	Stage of progression (ACSM: initial, improvement, maintenance) Stage of training (periodization) Methods of progression—FITT (e.g., increase time initially) Rate of progression (1-3%/week; e.g., 10-12% in first month) Monitoring to cue progression timing Monitoring to suit client's objectives but avoid overtraining Monitoring to motivate Follow-up checks established Primary safety precautions listed
7. Design warm-up and cool-down.	CV warm-up and cool-down transitions Specific joint and muscle stretching before and after Suits nature of the prescription and client specifics (e.g., mode, time, intensity, monitoring)

Note. CV = cardiovascular; MET = metabolic equivalent; HR = heart rate; HRR = heart rate reserve; FITT = frequency, intensity, time, and type.

even basic exercises or the simplest of equipment intimidates them at first. Others may hate the idea of exercising indoors and only want to do sports or aerobic exercise outside. You need to anticipate this reaction and be ready to accommodate those needs. Situations often change as well. Substituting an indoor cardio circuit for an outdoor run during a bad storm, switching to a rower or recumbent bike during a bout of shin splints, or advising a client on breathable rainwear for his new walking program will modify the activity selection and remove those barriers to regular exercise.

Your clients generally will be most satisfied with modes of exercise that allow them to sustain intensity with some variability and with ease of monitoring. These modes include walking, jogging, running, swimming, cycling, cross-country skiing, ice skating, in-line skating, stepping, skipping, and rowing. Cardiovascular improvements are comparable for most modes of aerobic exercise as long as intensity, frequency, and duration of exercise are prescribed in accordance with sound scientific principles (Heyward 2002).

Select Aerobic Equipment

Most people will eventually use some form of aerobic exercise equipment. Thus we must understand the features as well as the design, manufacture, safety, cost, and serviceability of a variety of aerobic equipment.

Accurately assessing your clients' needs is the most important part of equipment selection. This is particularly important when your client selects outdoor or sporting activities that you will not attend. You must be prepared to provide guidance on appropriate quality equipment and maintenance: for example, a mountain bike that suits the challenge of the terrain, running shoes that won't cause shin splints, in-line skates that are well made and that fit, or a good quality life jacket for rowing. Have a list of trusted retail stores and experienced proprietors who can assist you with this service. Equipment should suit the anatomy, interests, and fitness levels of your clients. They want equipment that will not cause overuse injuries, is low impact, provides well-rounded fitness, and, most of all, makes efficient use of their time.

Even though the client's preferences and availability of equipment will usually narrow the choices, you probably will need to show your clients how certain equipment can contribute to their goals. Because boredom and lack of comfort are the reasons people give most often for not using aerobic equipment (Dishman 1990), you must be proactive in preventing frustration and providing stimulation (through equipment change or use of video) as you work through questions of equipment use with your client.

Nonportable Equipment

The following examines the design and safety features of a variety of common machines and identifies the type of client for which these features are most beneficial (table 6.2). Although comfort, appearance, durability, and cost are important factors in exercise machines, the mechanism that provides resistance and the mechanics of the movement are the most critical features to scrutinize.

Table 6.2   Equipment–Client Match-Up

Design and safety features	Client match-up
Treadmills	
• Provide alternative to the hazards of outdoor running and walking	Are useful in inclement weather (e.g., too hot, cold, stormy) or unsafe times, locations, health conditions
• Allow precise measurement	Are useful for stress testing, rehab, and medical assessments (prescription is more accurate if the treadmill was also used for the assessment)
• Provide fingertip control of speed and elevation	Allow personalized, fine-tuning
• Allow user to set course and pace according to stature and condition	Allow prescription to be fed into the electronic circuitry to control workout
• Are easy to learn and use	Can feel awkward to mount and control the panel while using the machine
• Provide reduced impact vs. outdoors for runners	Are useful for clients with lower extremity or back problems or those who are overweight
• Have monitoring features	Are helpful for higher risk clients or for feedback and motivation
• Have preprogramming capabilities	Encourage proper warm-ups and cool-downs because they are part of the program; provide interval and continuous options
Stationary bicycles	
• Are long-lasting, heavy-duty, affordable (nonelectronic bicycles)	Are suitable for home programs; are space efficient and portable
• Often have exciting computer graphics (electronic bicycles)	Can increase motivation through immediate feedback (e.g., simulated hills)
• Offer option to control pedaling effort by heart rate response to the ride	Optimize training level and a safety feature
• Allow precise measurement	Are useful for stress testing, rehab, and medical assessments (prescription is more accurate if the bike was also used for the assessment)
• Provide preprogramming capabilities on most electronic models	Encourage proper warm-ups and cool-downs; provide interval and continuous options
• Offer greater comfort (recumbent bikes)	Are suited to clients with back problems; provide greater loading for gluteals and hamstrings; and reduce lower-leg weight bearing

(continued)

Table 6.2 *(continued)*

Design and safety features	Client match-up
Rowers	
• Provide low impact, especially for the lower body	Provide good aerobic alternative if weight bearing is a problem
• Provide quality simulation via the air and flywheel	Are affordable for home use and comfortable to use
• Work muscles of the legs, shoulders, back, and arms	Provide overall muscular endurance benefits for large muscle groups of the body
• Cause some compression and shearing forces in the lower back	Are not suitable for clients with low back pain
• Can be smaller than other types of equipment (some home models)	Are space efficient and portable
• Can have color TV, audio, and modulation of workout variables (e.g., competition, time, speed) (some electronic models)	Increase motivation through immediate feedback; provide interval and continuous options
Stair climbers	
• Foot platforms must hinge to remain parallel to the floor.	Clients with ankle or knee problems will have added stress if platforms don't hinge (e.g., knee hyperextension).
• Independent step allows both steps to go up or down whereas dependent step has one go up when the other comes down.	Independent takes a little more practice to learn but offers more control and often less weight shifting.
• Electronic models offer programming and monitoring displays.	Provide tracking of floors climbed, floors per minute, calories, and elapsed time, which increase interest and motivation
• Motor skill and balance are an issue with some models.	May be inappropriate for some seniors or clients with a balance or coordination problem; weight bearing with arms may cause elbow overuse injuries.
• Some models have an aerobic self-test option.	Care should be taken not to place too much confidence in the self-test results.
Elliptical trainers	
• Provide lower impact forces because feet never leave footpads	Are suitable for clients with higher risk of lower extremity orthopedic injury
• Offer wide range of intensities with low impact	Provide a good substitute for jogging
• Are able to go backward as well as forward	Backward direction may not burn more calories but it adds variety and appears to involve the hip extensors more actively.
• At similar RPEs (13), elliptical has similar heart rates and oxygen consumption values as running but less than half the ground reaction force (Porcari, Foster, and Schneider 2000).	Provide high aerobic benefit with decreased impact-related risks
• Shape of ellipse can vary on different machines and change the "feel" of the movement.	Clients should always try the machine first especially if purchasing for home use.
• Energy expenditure is higher than walking yet still low impact.	Are well suited to overweight clients and fit seniors

- **Treadmills.** In 1994, 16.2 million Americans walked for fitness at least twice a week; nearly half that number jogged or ran (Sillery 1996). This adds up to the largest identifiable group of exercisers. It is not surprising that treadmills have become so popular. Treadmills burn more calories than any other simulator at heart rates of 65%, 75%, and 85% of age-adjusted maximum (Allen and Goldberg 1986).

- **Stationary bicycles.** The choices here include electronic, in which the pedaling effort is controlled electronically, and nonelectronic, in which the resistance mechanism is a belt circling a heavy flywheel. Your clients may choose either an upright or a recumbent style bike. The upright bike is the most common piece of equipment in most centers.

- **Rowing machines.** Rowers have come a long way since the squeaky spring-loaded models tucked away in attics and garages. Except for a few designs like the hydraulic-resistance rowers, most provide a realistic feel to the rowing action. Most nonelectronic machines use a flywheel for resistance; many people like the feel of the air machines more than the more expensive electronic models. The upper-body workout provided by rowing machines is an attractive added benefit for many clients. Because these machines permit such great freedom of technique, however, clients risk injuring themselves. Show your clients how to use their legs to push off, not their backs, and to maintain a smooth pull with the arms in and just below chest level.

- **Stair climbers.** An attractive feature of these machines is that, in addition to providing excellent aerobic benefits, they provide muscular conditioning to the lower body. Many people should begin with a short range of motion and a slow stepping rate. To reduce stress on the knees, clients should not lean into the machine or move their knees forward over their toes during stepping. Leaning forward also increases strain on the low back.

- **Elliptical trainers.** Elliptical trainers involve a lower-body motion that is a cross between an upright stationary cycle and a stepper, except that the feet move in an elliptical pattern as opposed to a circular path. The low impact forces and wide ranges of aerobic intensity are good news for clients looking for a high-intensity, low-impact substitute to jogging.

Transportable Aerobic Home Equipment

The most effective, versatile, and portable piece of equipment you own is yourself. You are the computer, the feedback display, the variable resistance, the monitor, and the motivation machine. Still, you need some equipment that will enable you to deliver the best possible workout to each client. Whether advising a client about a purchase or building your own collection, strongly consider adding some affordable and transportable pieces of aerobic equipment.

- **Bench step.** Steps have probably done more to change the industry than most other equipment. Not only have the inexpensive platforms brought more men into the aerobics circle, but steps have expanded the concept of methods of training. They are effective tools for interval and circuit training, particularly when step training and conditioning exercises are combined (Brooks and Copeland-Brooks 1991). Bench steps are a good alternative for people who would rather not walk or jog or invest large sums of money in aerobic machinery.

- **Slide.** This 8-ft piece of plastic, with angled bumpers and low-friction slippers, allows for a reasonably intense lower-body and aerobic workout. Various slide techniques and arm movements can increase variety and can be combined with step or other exercises for an interval or circuit design. Slides can be adapted for sports such as hockey. Clients with ankle or knee instability should be cautious when using slides.

- **Videos.** Commercial fitness videos have expanded to the point where they are targeting specific groups and needs. Whether your client is a senior, is an athlete, is overweight, or wants to work her heart, buttocks, or thighs, there is something she can buy! Help her screen videos for the appropriate intensity level, style, and degree of safety. Consider videotaping a workout for your client to use during travel, during vacation, or when you can't get together.

- **Recreational and sporting equipment.** Any equipment that helps your client associate fitness with fun will serve you both well. There are many opportunities for one-on-one basketball, in-line skating, throwing Frisbees, and even shadow boxing.

- **Home swimming pool.** The buoyancy of water reduces the impact of land-based aerobic exercise. Older adults, obese individuals, clients with arthritis or back pain, and rehabilitating athletes will gain major benefits from aquatic exercise. Basic aquatic exercise movements include walking, jogging, kicking, jumping, and scissors against the resistance of the water. The client may also wear paddles on her hands, devices to increase drag through the water, or flotation devices used in the deep end to keep the head above water while moving.

• **Skipping ropes.** A recent survey of personal trainers found that the skipping rope was the least used piece of portable aerobic equipment (Fair 1992). Rope skipping is quite intense, can be high impact, and takes some skill; however, various techniques of lower-intensity and lower-impact skipping can make it a viable station within a circuit. The rope also can be used as a source of resistance or as a stretching device.

• **Music and CD players.** Building a client's endurance or time at an activity is a challenge. Music does more than distract from sweat and pain. Studies on perceived exertion have shown that music makes an exercise session feel easier and extends the time required to reach exhaustion (Iknoian 1992). Preparing music for your client is greatly simplified by the availability of commercial speed-adjusted recordings from funky exercise to soft stretch.

Cardiovascular Endurance Activities Grouped by Intensity

Any activity that uses large muscle groups, can be maintained, and is rhythmic and aerobic in nature can increase cardiovascular endurance. The American College of Sports Medicine (1995) classifies cardiovascular endurance activities into three groups:

• **Group 1:** Physical activities in which exercise intensity is easily sustained with little variability in heart rate response: walking, aerobic dancing, swimming, jogging, running, and cycling

• **Group 2:** Physical activities in which energy expenditure is related to skill but for a given individual can provide a constant intensity: figure skating, swimming, highly choreographed dance exercise, cross-country skiing, and skating

• **Group 3:** Physical activities that are quite variable in intensity and skill: soccer, basketball, and racquetball

Group 1 activities are most appropriate for beginning clients who need to carefully control intensity.

Group 2 activities are often outside of the gym, providing an enjoyable venue. Combining a group 1 and 2 activity can reduce boredom and attrition and improve skill levels.

Group 3 activities may be the most fun and provide variety and cross-training opportunities. They are often group-oriented, adding a social element. The sporadic changes in intensity demand caution: People should spend time in a group 1 activity (e.g., preseason conditioning) before entering a group 3 activity.

Step 3: Select Training Method and Mode

Select a training method or exercise mode based on your conversations with your client about

• stated preferences and interests,

• goals and objectives,

• availability and convenience (facility, equipment, time),

• skills and background,

• suitability (e.g., level of fitness, risk), and

• other desired benefits (e.g., enhanced skills, social opportunities, targeted energy system).

Although some training methods rely mainly on one energy system, usually they use a combination of two or even three (see Backgrounder on *Energy Systems Used by the Body*). Consequently, different types of exercises and training methods will be needed to maximize your client's use of the required system.

Energy Systems Used by the Body

1. Adenosine triphosphate (ATP) is the immediately usable form of chemical energy stored in muscle cells and used for muscular activity. The ATP–PC system is an anaerobic energy system that resynthesizes ATP from energy released when phosphocreatine (PC) is broken down. This energy system is a very rapid but limited source of ATP that is used predominantly during high-power, short-duration activities. PC is restored for reuse during each relief interval (50% in 30 s, 75% in 60 s, 95% in 2 min), thereby reducing reliance on the lactic acid system.

2. The lactic acid (LA) system, also anaerobic, resynthesizes ATP from energy released during the breakdown of glyco-

gen (sugar) to lactic acid. Accumulation of the latter causes muscular fatigue. This system is used mainly during activities that require between 1 and 3 min of maximum effort.

3. The oxygen system uses both glycogen and fats as fuels for ATP resynthesis. By a series of reactions that take place in the mitochondria of the cells, the system yields large amounts of ATP but no fatiguing by-products. The aerobic system is used predominantly during endurance tasks or low power output activities (Fox 1979).

Continuous Versus Interval Training

The two broad categories of aerobic methods are continuous and interval training. Research indicates that both are effective in improving cardiovascular fitness (Heyward 2002). The methods differ in their physiological bases, types of demand, and benefits. You must select the method and the training factors that match your client's needs.

Continuous Training

Continuous training (CT) involves exercise (walking, jogging, in-line skating, cycling, stair climbing, swimming) at a moderate intensity with no rest intervals. Runners often call this LSD, or long, slow distance training.

There are many advantages to continuous training for certain clients:

- Low to moderate intensities (e.g., 40-70% $\dot{V}O_2$max or 60-80% maximum heart rate [HRmax]) are safe, comfortable, and able to produce health and cardiovascular benefits for less fit individuals.

- CT is generally well-suited for clients initiating an aerobic exercise program.

- Dropout rates for adults may be half those for high-intensity interval programs (Dishman 1990).

- A prescribed exercise intensity is easily maintained in an evenly paced workout.

- More easily than with interval training, your client can maintain a training effect simply by reducing the training load (Brynteson and Sinning 1973).

- CT is generally less taxing physiologically and psychologically and therefore requires minimal motivation.

- Daily workouts are possible, because glycogen is not sufficiently depleted so that it cannot be replenished within 24 hr (Wilmore and Costill 2004).

- Continuous submaximal training is appropriate for athletes during off-season and during the competitive season as a light day alternating with heavier interval days.

- Benefits to the oxygen transport system from continuous training are more easily transferred from one mode of training to another or to a specific sport. This provides a variety of training activities and is well-suited to incorporation of cross-training techniques.

- Fewer injuries are reported in CT than in interval training (Pollock et al. 1977).

Depending on the client and the desired outcome, the optimal prescription can vary considerably based on the following guidelines:

- **Athletes and well-conditioned clients.** Continuous exercise involving large muscle groups at 75% of the client's aerobic capacity or $\dot{V}O_2$max (around 85% HRmax) optimally trains the central oxygen transport system (Wilmore and Costill 2004).

- **Average client.** Training gains for the average client initiating a program may start at 50% to 70% $\dot{V}O_2$max or 65% to 80% HRmax (Heyward 2002).

- **Sedentary client.** Health benefits may be seen at as low as 40% of $\dot{V}O_2$max (60% HRmax) (ACSM 2000).

When the intensity level causes a sharp increase in lactic acid production and in fatigue, your client has reached the ***anaerobic threshold***. The duration of the training session will be shortened dramatically if she exercises above this intensity level. The greatest benefits without early fatigue are provided with intensities just below the anaerobic threshold. Anaerobic threshold can be measured accurately in a laboratory. With some guidance, however, your client can learn to recognize the abrupt increase in ventilation and rating of perceived exertion (RPE; p. 173) that occur when she exceeds her threshold.

If you have not determined an anaerobic threshold through aerobic assessment or a submaximal test, you can calculate a crude but generally effective target heart rate (THR) from the equation

$$THR = RHR + 75\% \ (HRmax - RHR),$$

where RHR = the resting heart rate and HRmax = the maximum heart rate (estimated as 220 – age). The percentage is based on the client and outcome guidelines listed earlier in this chapter. Use the target heart rate initially as an approximate guide. Then by trial and error adjust the intensity to keep your client just below the anaerobic threshold. Your client can maintain or adjust the intensity level for continuous training by monitoring her peak training heart rate and her perceived exertion level.

Interval Training

In interval training (IT), periods of low-intensity exercise (which use the body's aerobic energy system) are alternated with periods of higher-intensity exercise (which use anaerobic energy systems). Interval training is a high-intensity effort designed to enhance performance, usually in a competitive sport. Because one energy system can recover while the other is being used, your client is able to exercise for long periods of time with a greater total amount of work performed.

Interval training improves the body's ability to adapt and recover. Like continuous training, it improves cardiorespiratory fitness (Heyward 2002). It also provides paced training that athletes can monitor and modify to suit their training phase and purpose. These and many other advantages make interval training attractive for many people:

- When you know which energy systems you want to emphasize, interval training allows for great variations. You can regulate it to develop mainly aerobic, anaerobic, or muscular systems. You can target specific energy systems for improvement.
- IT often stimulates the aerobic system without producing the high levels of lactic acid that occur with continuous higher-intensity exercise. During the recovery phase of IT, heart rate declines at a proportionately greater rate than the return of blood to the heart, resulting in brief increases in stroke volume many times during a workout. This process increases myocardial strength and enables the muscles to be quickly cleared of waste products (lactic acid) (Wilmore and Costill 1999).
- IT achieves the greatest amount of work possible with the least fatigue (although longer workout times are usually necessary).
- By examining the requirements of a particular event and the energy systems used,

you can design an IT program that provides specificity of training.

- If used late preseason and selectively during the season, IT can peak an athlete's performance.
- For clients in poor condition who have trouble maintaining their training intensity, the work–relief intervals of IT allow them to complete more total work.
- The ACSM (2000) recommends IT for symptomatic individuals who can tolerate only low-intensity exercise for short periods of time (1-2 min).
- The frequent breaks in activity allow you to monitor your client and make appropriate adjustments.
- The possibility of greater variety is a motivating factor.

To prescribe interval training, you will need to know the following terms (Karp 2000):

- *Work interval:* That portion of the interval training program consisting of the work effort (e.g., a 220-yd run performed within a prescribed time).
- *Relief interval:* The time between work intervals in a set. The relief interval may consist of light activity such as walking (rest relief) or mild to moderate exercise such as jogging (work relief).
- *Work–relief ratio:* The ratio of the work and relief intervals. A work–relief ratio of 1:2 means that the work interval is half as long as the relief interval.
- *Set:* A group of work and relief intervals (e.g., six 220-yd runs, each performed within a prescribed time, separated by designated relief intervals).
- *Repetition:* The number of work intervals per set. Six 220-yd runs would constitute six repetitions.
- *Training time:* The rate of work during the work interval (e.g., each 220-yd run might be performed in 28 s).
- *Training distance:* Distance of the work interval (e.g., 220 yd).
- *IT prescription:* Specifications for the routines to be performed in an IT workout. For several sample prescriptions, see page 164, *Sample Interval Training Prescriptions.*

Table 6.3 shows which energy system athletes should develop, according to their sport (Fox

1979). For example, because a basketball player relies heavily on anaerobic systems for ATP energy, his IT program should focus on anaerobic systems.

Match your interval training prescription to your client's outside activities. For a specific sport, for example, find out the typical length of time during which your client puts in continuous, strenuous effort. Consider ice hockey, which typically has players on the ice for about a 45- to 90 s shift. Use tables 6.3 and 6.4 together. According to table 6.3, ice hockey predominantly uses the ATP–PC–LA energy system. Therefore your hockey-playing client's prescription should emphasize this same system. Now go to table 6.4, find ATP–PC–LA in the left column, and note the training time that is closest to the range of a hockey shift (i.e., 1:00-1:10 min). According to table 6.4, the prescription for your client should include 5 repetitions and 3 sets, with a work–relief ratio of 1:3 or perhaps 1:2. The relief interval should be of the work-relief type.

These IT prescription factors may need fine-tuning if

- the work is not difficult or is too difficult,
- your client is in poor or very good condition,
- your client is fresh or near the end of the workout, or
- the training signs (e.g., recovery heart rates) do not seem appropriate.

Two of the most important considerations with an IT prescription are sufficient work rate and sufficient relief and recovery. For short, highly intensive performance, the relief interval may be three times as long as the work interval. For longer, less intensive work periods, the relief interval may be equal to or less than the work interval. When the work interval has produced lactic acid, the most rapid removal rate occurs during continuous aerobic activity.

Table 6.3   Various Sports and Their Predominant Energy Systems

Sport or activity	% Emphasis of energy system:		
	ATP–PC and LA	LA and O$_2$	O$_2$
Basketball	85	15	—
Ice hockey	80	20	—
Recreational sports	—	5	95
Skiing, downhill	80	20	—
Skiing, cross-country	—	5	95
Swimming, 100 m	80	15	5
Swimming, 1,500 m	10	20	70
Tennis	70	20	10

Note. ATP = adenosine triphosphate; PC = phosphocreatine; LA = lactic acid.

Adapted from E. Fox and D. Mathews, 1974, *Interval Training* (All rights reserved to author: Ohio State University), 60.

Table 6.4   Guidelines for Writing Interval Training Prescriptions

Major energy system	Training time (min:s)	Reps per workout	Sets per workout	Reps per set	Work–relief ratio	Type of relief interval
ATP–PC	0:10	50	5	10	1:3	Rest relief (e.g., walking, stretching)
	0:15	45	5	9		
	0:20	40	4	10		
	0:20	32	4	8		
ATP–PC–LA	0:30	25	5	5	1:3	Work relief (e.g., light exercise, jogging)
	0:40-0:50	20	4	5		
	1:00-1:10	15	3	5		
LA–O$_2$	1:30-2:00	8	2	4	1:2	Work relief Rest relief
	2:10-2:40	6	1	6	1:1	
	2:50-3:00	4	1	4		
O$_2$	3:00-4:00	4	1	4	1:1	Rest relief
	4:00-5:00	3	1	3	1:1/2	

Note. ATP = adenosine triphosphate; PC = phosphocreatine; LA = lactic acid.

Adapted, by permission, from E. Fox 1979, *Sports physiology* (New York: McGraw-Hill Companies), 205. With permission of The McGraw-Hill Companies.

Steps for Constructing the IT Prescription

Review the steps for constructing an appropriate IT prescription:

1. Using table 6.3, determine which energy system is to be improved.

2. Select the type of exercise to be used during the work interval (e.g., running, cycling, stair climbing, a sport).

3. From table 6.4, select the training times (per work interval), the number of repetitions and sets, the work–relief ratio, and the type of relief interval.

4. Fine-tune the prescription based on your observations of your client's first few workouts.

The intermittent nature of interval training allows you to monitor the client's heart rate at the end of work intervals and relief intervals. Table 6.5 provides some guidelines for suitable target heart rates for different ages at the conclusion of different intervals.

Sample Interval Training Prescriptions

Moderately Fit 34-Year-Old Female

This client wants to follow her favorite aerobic video while interval training for cardiovascular condition. The prescription is as follows:

4 × 4:30 (4:00) where

4 = number of repetitions,

4:30 = training time in minutes and seconds, and

(4:00) = time of relief interval in minutes and seconds.

Each work interval consists of following the video for 4-1/2 min followed by a relief interval of walking on the spot and stretching while the video is on pause for 4 min. Four repetitions of this sequence constitute a set. The prescription works the oxygen system, with a work-to-rest-relief interval of 1:1. For most moderately fit clients, exercise intensities should fall within the range of 70% to 85% of $\dot{V}O_2$max (80-90% of HRmax), starting at the lower end of this range. Create the initial overload by progressively increasing the length of the work period; later, you can decrease the length of the rest-relief interval.

Competitive Squash Player

This client complains of fatiguing too early. The ATP–PC and LA systems are predominant (table 6.3). It is preseason, so you decide to start by working his LA–O_2 system. You design a series of carefully timed, on-the-court drills:

- **Set 1: 6 × 2:30 (3:45)** in which each of six drills lasts 2-1/2 min (high intensity) with a 3 min, 45 s light exercise (jogging, or using a nearby bike or treadmill)

- **Set 2: 8 × 1:30 (3:00)** in which the drills are slightly shorter but use the same format, intensity, and energy system

Because the recovery intervals will be incomplete, the client will increase his tolerance to

Table 6.5 Monitoring Target Heart Rates in Interval Training Prescription (Men and Women)

Age (years)	Work HR (beats/min)	Relief HR (between reps)	Relief HR (between sets)
Under 20	190	150	125
20-29	180	140	120
30-39	170	130	110
40-49	160	120	105
50-59	150	115	100
60-69	140	105	90

Note. HR = heart rate.

From E. Fox and D. Mathews, 1974, *Interval training* (Philadelphia, PA: W.B. Saunders), 60. By permission of Donald Mathews.

lactic acid as well as his anaerobic capacity—important for a squash player. As the season approaches, you progress to a more intense workout of his ATP–PC–LA system. According to the guidelines in table 6.4, this progression will mean shorter (more intense) training intervals and more repetitions per workout, so you will need to prescribe a slightly longer work–relief ratio.

Other Aerobic Training Methods

Although continuous and interval training are two of the most popular training methods, it may be more suitable for your clients to use circuit training, cross-training, Fartlek training, or simply active living.

Circuit Training

Circuit training usually consists of 10 to 15 different exercise stations with the circuit repeated two or three times.

The following advantages of circuit training will make it particularly suitable to certain clients:

- Makes efficient use of time for the benefits obtained
- Provides moderate gains in aerobic fitness, muscular strength, and endurance
- Can be adapted for beginners or athletes
- Provides a focus and a challenge to the training
- Can maintain fitness levels when client is recovering from an injury

The stations are either calisthenics (such as stride jumps, stepping, sit-ups, high knee hops, push-ups, pull-ups, skipping), resistance equipment (such as machines, free weights, bands), or a combination. Stations are near one another to facilitate efficient movement. The exercises are selected to avoid repeated use of the same muscle group and early fatigue.

When you prescribe weights, select a moderate intensity (40-60% of maximum capacity) with either a repetition limit such as 15 reps or a timed limit around 30 s. The relief periods between the stations are an important part of the design. For example, with lighter-intensity exercises (or lighter weights), rest periods between stations need be only 15 s—or about the time to move to and get set up at the next station. Circuit weight training typically has an exercise-to-rest ratio of 1:1 (Baechle and Earle 2000). Greater aerobic gains

are achieved when relief times involve aerobic activities such as jogging or use of aerobic machines (space and facilities permitting). A client training at home can use the stairs, a skipping rope, an aerobic video, or any number of aerobic calisthenics such as stride jumps, high knee hops, or leg exchange lunges between the weight stations.

Circuit weight training is a compromise between muscular conditioning and aerobic conditioning. Monitoring target heart rate is important. The metabolic requirements of circuit weight training usually meet minimum requirements for the development of aerobic capacity with an aerobic cost of 40% to 60% $\dot{V}O_2$max or 60% to 75% HRmax (ACSM 2000). In a review of research, Gettman and Pollock (1981) reported that circuit weight training produced a 5% to 11% increase in aerobic capacity, compared with a 15% to 20% increase with other methods of aerobic training over the same period.

Sample Calisthenic Training Circuit

Circuit training does not need weights or machinery. A circuit of 8 to 10 aerobic calisthenics will elevate and maintain a heart rate more effectively than weights. For this sample circuit, a 4- to 6-ft piece of surgical tubing or exercise band can provide added resistance but is not necessary. The compact versatility of this circuit is a major advantage for clients working in their home with little space or equipment.

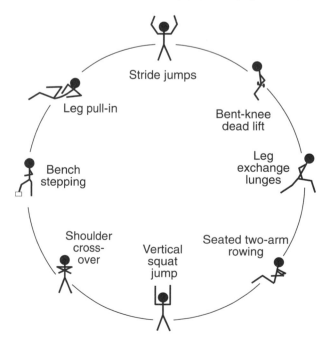

In the first or second workout, and then about every tenth workout, you should assess each exercise. Establish the client's starting level by noting, with ample time for recovery between each exercise test, the maximum number of perfectly executed exercises done at each station during 30 s. Watch for excessive momentum, incomplete ranges of motion, and poor alignment. Allot your client 1 min at each station to do the number of repetitions performed on the assessment. With 15 s between each station, one full circuit should take 10 min. After the first circuit trial, you can fine-tune the number of reps. Start with two sets or circuits per session and progress by adding reps to selected stations; you can also progress by including the surgical tubing or exercise band or by adding a third circuit. The following calisthenics involve large muscle groups, including most of the major groups, and should minimize local muscle fatigue.

Cross-Training

Cross-training involves a variety of fitness activities. It provides the flexibility of mixing activities, allowing joints and soft tissues to rest without stopping workouts. Appropriate for the beginner as well as the athlete, cross-training can expand the training benefits of a single-sport exerciser.

Yacenda (1995) explained how runners can use aerobics and swimming to shorten the duration of fatigue in their legs. Runners typically have a high incidence of lower-leg overuse problems, but missing workouts means losing an acquired level of aerobic conditioning. Their chronic knee and shin problems may also be mediated with complementary cycling or circuit weight-training workouts. Swimmers can gain endurance and joint stability from low-impact aerobic classes. The contrasting stresses are a positive challenge. Cross-training is often selected at a time of injury recovery, because most aerobic training gains are maintained if another mode of activity is substituted for several weeks while an injury is allowed to heal. If your client maintains the cross-training after the injury recovery, it will protect against other single-activity overuse injuries.

The four primary prescription factors for cardiovascular fitness (FITT: Frequency, Intensity, Time, Type) can be approximately duplicated regardless of the activity selected. Table 6.6 will help you select aerobic activities based on intensity levels. You can calculate the intensity of exercise as a percentage of your client's maximum metabolic equivalent (MET) value (chapter 3). If you don't know the appropriate MET training level, start by identifying the activity level that your client can consistently maintain and move across the row to the workload. Any other activity in this column should be close to what your client can perform. Kosich (1991) and the ACSM (2000) have published extensive lists of activity energy expenditures.

Fartlek Training

Fartlek (translation of Swedish term that means "speed play") is a form of training developed in Sweden. It combines elements of continuous training with interval training. Although Fartlek is timed and formalized by athletes as a serious mode of training, you can adapt it as an interesting change to a fitness program that can be a lot of fun alone or in a small group.

Fun is the main goal, and distance and time are secondary. People are relatively free to run whatever course and speed they prefer, although the speed should periodically reach high intensity levels. Fartlek involves fast-paced accelerations interspersed with endurance running. The accelerations vary in distance, and the "form" may be a sport-specific action, straight running, or simply playful activity. Fartlek training is often performed in the countryside where there are a variety of hills and terrain. Warm-up is important for this type of training. More than 10 min of jogging and long static stretches of the running muscles are necessary. Runs may last for 40 min or longer.

Here are the advantages of Fartlek training that can help you match it to appropriate clients at appropriate stages in their programs:

- The break in monotony from changing speeds and scenery makes it psychologically stimulating.
- It improves both anaerobic and aerobic capacity.
- It is an enjoyable means of achieving cardiovascular fitness and to a lesser extent other health-related aspects of fitness.
- It is a good training break for a small group of athletes and a welcome addition to a serious training program.
- If your client lives in a rural area, the match is a natural one.

Many city parks have fitness trails with exercise stations spread along the pathway. Whereas the true cross-country speed play of Fartlek may prove to be too intense for many exercisers, a customized park fitness trail is well suited for many clients.

Table 6.6 Intensity Levels of Aerobic Activity

Activity								
	METs	3-4	4-5	5-6	6-7	7-8	8-9	10+
	kcal/min	4-5	5-6	6-7	7-8	8-10	10-11	11+
Walking	mph	3.0	3.5	4.0	5			
	min/mile	20	17	15	12			
Jogging	mph					5	5.5	6, 7, 8
	min/mile					12	11	10, 8-1/2, 7 1/2
Stationary bicycle (tension Kp)	130 lb (59 kg)	1/2	1	1-1/4	1-3/4	2	2-1/4	3+
	175 lb (79 kg)	3/4	1-1/4	1-3/4	2-1/4	2-3/4	3-1/4	4+
Outdoor cycling	mph	6	8	10	11	12	13	15
	min/mile	10	7:30	6	5:30	5	4:40	4
Swimming	mph		0.85	1.0	1.25	1.5	1.7	2.0
	s/25 yd (23 m)		60	50	43	35	30	25
Bench stepping (70 kg/154 lb)		8 in. × 12/min	8 in. × 18/min	8 in. × 24/min 11 in. × 18/min	11 in. × 24/min 12-6 in. × 18/min	8 in. × 30/min 12-6 in. × 24/min	11 in. × 30/min 15-8 in. × 24/min	(11 METs) 15 in. × 30/min
Recreational sports		Bowling Golf (pulling a cart) Light calisthenics Light games	Table tennis Volleyball Golf (carry clubs) Tennis doubles Badminton doubles Most calisthenics	Ice- and roller-skating Badminton singles Moderate dancing Jogging in place (60-70 steps/min)	Tennis singles Water-skiing Group aerobic exercise class Jogging in place (90-100 steps/min)	Downhill skiing Paddleball Basketball Fast and hard dancing Jogging in place (120 steps/min)	Squash Handball Cross-country skiing Rope skipping (<75 rpm)	Most competitive sports, if continuous activity Rope skipping (>75 rpm)
Other activities		Cleaning windows Mopping floors Light gardening Painting Active child care and play	Scrubbing floors Mowing lawns Chopping wood	Shoveling Manual labor Hand sawing				

Note. MET = metabolic equivalent.

Sample Fartlek Prescription

To simulate a Swedish Fartlek, the athlete can start in the country by a lake. After a walk–jog warm-up and some lower-body static stretching, the athlete begins with a moderately paced 1 km (0.62-mile) run on flat paths. Coming to a hill, she should attack it at near top speed, walk back down the hill, and repeat this four or five times. She should follow this with a level run at about 75% speed for 3 to 4 min and repeat this sequence two or three times. A few short sprints over local obstacles and an easy jog will bring her back to the lake. Follow with a social sauna, fluid replacement, some stretching, and a plunge in the lake!

Active Living

Gord Stewart (1995) described active living as an enhancement of the simple activities in a daily routine, like walking to the corner store instead of taking the car, or climbing stairs instead of riding the elevator. At first sight, this may not seem like a method of training; but for a majority of adults, the leap into an aerobic class, weight room, or running track is too large a step (see discussion of stages of change in chapter 1).

Recent research has shown that regular, moderately intense activity can provide impressive health benefits (Blair et al. 1989; Haskell 1985; Kesaniemi 2001). Active living is particularly well suited for a previously sedentary or older client concerned about blood pressure, blood lipids, heart health, and preventive medicine. Active living can relieve stress, improve energy, inject enjoyment, and provide feelings of well-being.

In a recent study with adolescents, Horswill and colleagues (1995) demonstrated how the choice of a leisure activity such as playing a musical instrument rather than watching television can increase energy expenditure by 41%. Even these small changes in lifestyle habits can have a substantial, cumulative effect on long-term energy balance and weight management. For your older clients, the benefits of active living translate to greater independence and the prevention of disabilities.

If your client is inactive, initially prescribe an expenditure of 1,000 kcal/week, striving eventually for 2,000. Any one of the following will burn about 1,000 kcal:

- 5 hr of housework
- 5 hr of active child care and play
- 3.5 hr of gardening or yard work
- 3 hr of dancing
- 3 hr of walking
- 2.5 hr of ice-skating
- 2.5 hr of manual labor
- 2 hr of tennis

The variety is limited only by your ingenuity. Help your clients see their opportunities: stationary cycling while watching television, finding alternatives to the car for transportation, using more manual tools for daily chores, playing with the kids, taking an active vacation, playing cartless golf, or walking at lunchtime.

Active living extends beyond the physical and has the potential of becoming a way of life. Your clients may need some initial guidance, but active living is about making choices—it is truly client-centered.

Client-Centered Tips for Setting Cardiovascular Mode or Training Method

Whenever possible, the test mode should be specific to the training mode—if your client will be training on a bicycle, test her on a bicycle. Monitor your clients to verify that the workload you prescribed is eliciting the desired heart rate. This is especially important if no assessment was done or if the training mode is different from the assessment mode.

If the total work (intensity × duration × frequency) and initial fitness status are similar, the mode of activity does not significantly influence the cardiovascular training effect. However, each activity has some local or specific muscle benefits. Therefore, consider selecting a mode that will enhance other objectives such as isolating a body area or pursuing cross-training benefits for a sport.

Consider the possibility of overuse or acute injury when selecting the mode. For athletes, this may mean selecting a fitness mode that provides some rest for overused joints. You can use metabolic calculations and charts (table 6.7) to match activities with energy costs, but you will need to monitor and fine-tune the results (see *Metabolic Calculations*, p. 170).

 ## Step 4: Set Intensity and Workload

We have discussed the first three steps of the Client-Centered Cardiovascular Exercise Prescription Model:

- Step 1: Consider client needs and goals.
- Step 2: Select cardiovascular activities and equipment.
- Step 3: Select training method and mode.

Now we are ready to discuss setting the intensity and the corresponding workload on a specific exercise mode for your client. Intensity is probably the most important and complex determinant of the cardiovascular exercise prescription. If it is set too high, our clients will be discouraged and will risk injury. If it is set too low, results may be deferred and objectives not met. Before we can prescribe a client's exercise intensity, we must know how to calculate intensity. After you have learned how to calculate exercise intensity, we will discuss how to set the target intensity for given segments of your prescription, for example, the warm-up, the cool-down, the plateau to be reached in constant training, and the peaks and valleys in interval training.

Calculating Exercise Intensity

The most direct way of calculating intensity is to use a percentage of the measured functional capacity (e.g., percent of maximum oxygen consumption). If, however, a graded exercise test was not performed, there are several indirect methods to estimate a training zone. The method selected will depend not only on your access to test data but also on your experience as an exercise professional, the availability of monitoring equipment, and the client's exercise program and level of fitness.

The following are the primary methods of calculating and prescribing exercise intensity:

- Methods with assessment:
  - MET level
  - Graph method
  - Percentage of maximum heart rate
- Methods without assessment:
  - Percentage of maximum heart rate (estimated)
  - Heart rate reserve (HRR)

MET Level Method (VO$_2$ Reserve)

The MET level method uses a percentage of the client's measured VO$_2$ reserve (VO$_2$R; i.e., functional reserve) converted to MET equivalents (1 MET = 3.5 ml · kg^{-1} · min^{-1}). Although exercise intensity has traditionally been expressed as a percentage of a client's maximum oxygen consumption (VO$_2$max), ACSM now recommends using

the percent VO$_2$R instead. VO$_2$R is the difference between VO$_2$max and resting VO$_2$. Therefore

$$VO_2R = VO_2max - VO_2 \text{ rest (ACSM 2000)}.$$

With this change, %VO$_2$R and %HRR methods for prescribing intensity are much closer.

Calculate a target intensity of 50% to 85% of functional reserve, given a VO$_2$max = 35 ml · kg^{-1} · min^{-1}.

Example:

$$VO_2max = 35 \text{ ml} · kg^{-1} · min^{-1}$$

$$\text{Therefore, } VO_2R = VO_2max - VO_2 \text{ rest}$$

$$VO_2R = 35 \text{ ml} · kg^{-1} · min^{-1} - 3.5 \text{ ml} · kg^{-1} · min^{-1}$$

$$= 31.5 \text{ ml} · kg^{-1} · min^{-1}$$

$$\text{or METs} = 10 - 1$$

$$= 9 \text{ METs is functional reserve}$$

If the intensity prescription is set at 50% to 85% of functional reserve:

$$[50\% \text{ of } (10 - 1 \text{ METS})] + 1 \text{ MET} = 5.5 \text{ METs;}$$

$$[85\% \text{ of } (10 - 1 \text{ METS})] + 1 \text{ MET} = 8.6 \text{ METs}$$

Therefore, the client should select activities with similar energy expenditures that require 5.5 to 8.6 METs. Table 6.7 (ACSM 2000) indicates that possible activities include aerobic dance, badminton, conditioning exercise, downhill skiing, hiking, or tennis. Wilmore and Costill (2004) provided a more exhaustive list of physical activities and their respective MET values.

The section *Metabolic Calculations* (p. 170) will allow you to progress from a target MET level to a corresponding workload on a specific exercise mode.

When you are deciding whether to use the MET level method, consider the following points:

- The MET level method is useful for clients selecting activities like racket sports or horseback riding, who want approximate energy costs.
- This method can be used for weight loss programs (e.g., 1 MET is 1 kcal/kg × hr). Therefore, an 80 kg (176 lb) client in average condition, working at 6 METs, would expend 480 kcal/hr or 8 kcal/min.
- MET is a commonly used measure with referrals.
- The MET level method can be used when the test mode is different from the training mode.

Table 6.7 Leisure Activities in METs: Sports, Exercise Classes, Games, Dancing

Activity	MET range	Average METs	Activity	MET range	Average METs
Badminton	4-9+	5.8	Running		
Basketball	7-12+	8.3	12 min/mile	–	8.7
Canoeing, rowing	3-8	–	10 min/mile	–	10.2
Calisthenics	3-8+	–	8 min/mile	–	12.5
Cross-country skiing	6-12+	–	Skating	5-8	–
Cycling (recreation)	3-8+	–	Skipping: 60-80/min	8-10+	9
Dance (aerobic)	6-9	–	Squash/racquetball	8-12+	9
Downhill skiing	5-8	–	Swimming	4-8+	–
Golf (walking)	4-7	5.1	Tennis	4-9+	6.5
Hiking	3-7	–	Volleyball	3-6+	–

Note. MET = metabolic equivalent.

- Assessment in other modes may be difficult and costly.
- The actual energy cost of activity may be affected by environment, weather, clothing, diet, mechanical efficiency, or fatigue.
- When used in conjunction with perceived exertion, "talk test," or heart rate, the MET level method allows fine adjustments to be made.

Metabolic Calculations

You can use ACSM equations (2000) to calculate the speed or workloads corresponding to a specific MET intensity for walking, jogging, running, cycling, and bench stepping activities.

Example 1: How fast should a client jog on a level route to be exercising at an intensity of 8 METs?

$$VO_2 = 8 \text{ METs} \times (3.5 \text{ ml} \cdot kg^{-1} \cdot min^{-1})$$
$$VO_2 = 28 \text{ ml} \cdot kg^{-1} \cdot min^{-1}$$

ACSM running equation:

$$ml \cdot kg^{-1} \cdot min^{-1} = [\text{speed (m/min)} \times 0.2 \, ml \cdot kg^{-1} \cdot min^{-1}] + 3.5 \text{ ml} \cdot kg^{-1} \cdot min^{-1}$$

$$28 \text{ ml} \cdot kg^{-1} \cdot min^{-1} - 3.5 \text{ ml} \cdot kg^{-1} \cdot min^{-1} = \text{speed (m/min)} \times 0.2 \text{ ml} \cdot kg^{-1} \cdot min^{-1}$$

$$24.5 \text{ ml} \cdot kg^{-1} \cdot min^{-1} = \text{speed (m/min)} \times 0.2$$

$$122.5 \text{ m/min} = \text{speed}$$

If 1 mph = 26.8 m/min, 122.5 m/min ÷ 26.8 m/min = 4.57 mph.

If pace = 60 min/hr ÷ mph; pace = 60 min/hr ÷ 4.57 mph; pace = 13.1 minutes per mile.

Example 2: What workload should be set for an 80 kg (176 lb) client on a bicycle ergometer, exercising at an intensity of 4.3 METs?

$$VO_2 = 4.3 \text{ METs} \times (3.5 \text{ ml} \cdot kg^{-1} \cdot min^{-1})$$
$$VO_2 \text{ (ml/min)} = 15 \text{ ml/kg} \cdot min \times 80 \text{ kg}$$
$$VO_2 \text{ (ml/min)} = 1200 \text{ ml/kg}$$

ACSM leg ergometer equation:

$$VO_2 = 1.8 \text{ (work rate)/(body mass)} + 7$$
$$15 = 1.8 \text{ (work rate)}/80 + 7$$
$$8 = 1.8 \text{ (work rate)}/80$$
$$640 = 1.8 \text{ (work rate)}$$
$$355 \text{ kg} \cdot m/min = \text{work rate}$$

Graph Method

Plot your client's steady-state heart rate response to each stage of a graded maximal or submaximal exercise test. Heart rate is linearly related to metabolic load (energy cost) and therefore can be plotted on a graph against oxygen consumption equivalents (or METs). Do this for each stage of the test, and then draw a "best fit" line between the points. Now at any oxygen consumption or MET level, a corresponding heart rate can be read from the graph. Determine the training zone range by taking appropriate percentages of the functional reserve (e.g., %VO$_2$R) and finding the heart rate responses at those points.

Figure 6.1 provides an example of using the graph method. The five plots on the graph represent the five steady states obtained during the assessment. The final stage elicited a heart rate of 170 beats/min, which corresponded to an energy cost of 10 METs. Remember, the functional reserve is the level from rest to functional capacity (1 MET up to 10 METs), so the reserve is that area above 1 MET. Once the percentage of the functional reserve has been calculated, the actual energy cost includes the resting MET, so it is added back on.

If the intensity prescription is set at 60% to 80% of functional reserve:

[60% of (10 − 1 METs)] + 1 MET = 6.4 METs

[80% of (10 − 1 METs)] + 1 MET = 8.2 METs

The broken lines on the graph show these levels correspond to heart rates of 132 and 152 beats/min, respectively.

Consider the following client issues as you decide whether to use the graph method of calculating intensity:

- If test mode is the same as training mode, the relationship of the prescribed workload and heart rate should be very close.

- Assessment may be difficult and costly, but this method is the most reliable for prescription.

- There may be a loss of accuracy if the test mode differs from training mode (modulate the intensity with RPEs and monitor more often).

- Exercise can be prescribed at a training heart rate range that is below the point of adverse signs or symptoms experienced by the client during the test.

Percentage of Maximum Heart Rate

Maximum heart rate can be determined directly through a maximal functional capacity test using a treadmill or bicycle ergometer and going to a point of fatigue or a limiting symptom. Determine the training zone by taking a percentage of the measured HRmax. This method is based on the fact that the %HRmax is related to %VO$_2$R and %HRR (figure 6.2 and table 6.8).

Example: ACSM (2000) recommends an exercise intensity of 55% or 60% to 90% HRmax. If the measured maximum heart rate is 180 beats/min, then

60% of 180 = 108 beats/min;
90% of 180 = 162 beats/min.

Consider the following issues as you decide whether to use the HRmax method of calculating intensity:

- This method has been validated across many populations.

- If the test mode is the same as the training mode, the relationship of the prescribed workload and heart rate should be very close.

- Assessment may be difficult and costly, but it is accurate with use of an electrocardiogram.

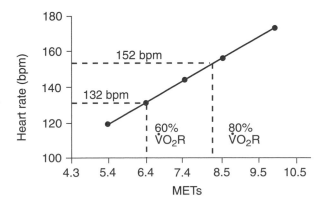

Figure 6.1 Direct method of determining the target heart rate zone. MET = metabolic equivalent; V̇O$_2$R = functional reserve.

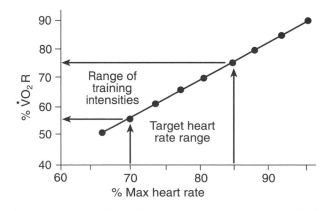

Figure 6.2 Relationship of percentage of maximum heart rate (%HRmax) and percentage of maximum aerobic power.

Table 6.8   Methods of Classification of Exercise Intensity

%HRmax	% $\dot{V}O_2R$/%HRR	RPE (Borg scale)	Class of intensity
<35	<20	<10	Very light
35-54	20-39	10-11	Light
55-69	40-59	12-13	Moderate
70-89	60-84	14-16	Hard
≥90	≥85	17-19	Very hard

Note. %HRmax = percentage of maximum heart rate; %$\dot{V}O_2R$ = percentage of $\dot{V}O_2$ reserve; %HRR = percentage of heart rate reserve.

- Discomfort and some risk during this test are possible with the average client (ensure that the certification you have allows maximal assessments).

Percentage of Maximum Heart Rate (Indirect Estimate)

Traditionally, maximum heart rate has been estimated as 220 – age. Although the traditional formula is still widely used, a new formula has been proposed to estimate maximum heart rate based on broad age and fitness-level ranges of healthy subjects:

HRmax = 208 – 0.7 × age (Tanaka et al. 2001)

The old formula underestimated HRmax in those older than 40 years, a group in higher need of exercise prescription (Schnirring 2001). The training zone is determined by taking a percentage of the estimated HRmax.

Example:

Heart rate training zone = [(208 – 0.7 × age) × training zone %]

For a 50-year-old client training between 60% and 70% HRmax,

[(208 – 0.7 × 50) × 60%] = (208-21) × .6 = 173 × .6 = 104 beats/min

[(208 – 0.7 × 30) × 70%] = 173 × .7 = 121 beats/min

Consider the following client issues in deciding whether to use the %HRmax method:

- The formula (HRmax = 208 – 0.7 × age) is conservative and variable (±10 beats/min) (Tanaka et al. 2001).
- You should use RPE and subjective exercise comments to guide this method.

Heart Rate Reserve (HRR)

As noted, heart rate reserve is the difference between the maximum heart rate and the resting heart rate. To use the HRR method, determine at what intensity you want the client to exercise. Take that percentage of the "reserve" and add it to the resting HR to determine the heart rate training zone. The percentage of HRR is approximately equal to the percentage of $\dot{V}O_2$ reserve (Swain et al. 1998) (figure 6.3). Example:

Heart rate training zone = [(HRmax – HRrest) × (50-85%)] + resting HR (ACSM 2000).

For a 40-year-old client with a resting heart rate of 70 beats/min at an intensity of 60%,

[(180 – 70) × 60%] + 70 = 66 + 70 = 136 beats/min.

Consider the following client issues in deciding whether to use the HRR method:

- This method is very popular. A well-informed client may be familiar with or already using this method.
- True resting HR is not always available, but this does not seem to introduce a serious error.
- HRmax estimates may be inaccurate.
- This method physiologically represents reserve of the heart for increasing cardiac output.

General Guidelines for Selecting Intensity

You can vary the prescribed intensity level for your clients, depending on their fitness level, exercise history, objectives, and risk factors. Chapter 3 discussed health gains possible at lower levels of intensity (Haskell 1995; Kesaniemi et al. 2001). Intensities that provide adequate cardiovascular improvement for most of the population are in the following ranges:

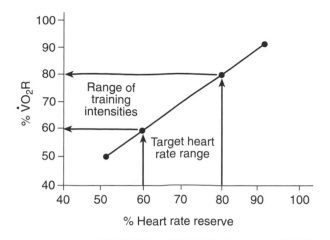

Figure 6.3 Relationship of percentage of heart rate reserve and percentage of maximal aerobic power.

- 60% to 80% of VO$_2$R (ml · kg^{-1} · min^{-1} or METs)
- 60% to 80% of HRR
- 70% to 85% of HRmax

These ranges are narrower than but still within the ACSM guidelines (2000). Intensity guidelines can be further personalized when they are based on client descriptions (table 6.9)

Rating of perceived exertion (RPE) is a subjective measure of exercise intensity that takes into account the client's feelings of exercise fatigue, including musculoskeletal, psychological, and environmental factors. The Borg scale of RPE assigns a numerical value between 6 and 20 (figure 6.4). You can use RPEs from a graded exercise test independently or in combination with heart rate to prescribe exercise training intensities. For example, a client had reported an RPE of 13 (somewhat hard) at a stage of the assessment that you selected as the target intensity for his prescription. Then regardless of the mode of activity, whenever he perceives an intensity level of "somewhat hard" (13), he is at the correct level of exertion. To extend the prescriptive and monitoring value of RPEs, Heyward (2002) showed the relationship of perceived exertion and relative intensity (table 6.9).

Client-Centered Tips for Setting Cardiovascular Intensity

Here are some practical considerations to help you set the correct intensity for a client. Following these principles will put you well on the way to successful prescription.

1. Consider the information gained from the cardiovascular assessment. Graded exercise tests provide general categorizations of fitness status to help you select the training zone. For example, table 6.9 shows an intensity of 50% to 65% HRR

6	No exertion at all
7	
8	Extremely light
9	Very light
10	
11	Light
12	
13	Somewhat hard
14	
15	Hard (heavy)
16	
17	Very hard
18	
19	Extremely hard
20	Maximal exertion

Borg RPE scale
© Gunnar Borg, 1970, 1985, 1994, 1998

Figure 6.4 Borg's rating of perceived exertion scale.

Reprinted, by permission, from G. Borg, 1998, *Borg's Perceived Exertion and Pain Scales* (Champaign, IL: Human Kinetics), 47.

Table 6.9   Client-Centered Intensity Prescription

Zone	Client description	Intensity (%HRR/%VO$_2$R)	Beats ± AT	RPE
1 Aerobic base	Low fitness status, inactive, several risk factors, wants lower intensity, longer duration	50-65%	30-20 beats below AT	13-14
2 Steady-state tempo	Average fitness status, normal activity, few risk factors	65-80%	20-10 beats below AT	14-16
3 Threshold	Excellent fitness status, very active, low risk, an athlete, interval training	80-90%	10 beats ± AT	16-18

Note. %HRR = percentage of heart rate reserve; %V̇O$_2$R = percentage of V̇O$_2$ reserve; AT = anaerobic threshold; RPE = rating of perceived exertion.

for a client in a low fitness category and 65% to 80% for an average fitness category. The following "flags" identify the point just *above* which you should set the intensity:

- A sudden jump in heart rate, blood pressure, or physical effort during a test (or supervised change in workload if a test was not done)
- Systolic blood pressure rising significantly or rapidly
- A long time to steady state
- A slow recovery

Often it is helpful to start at a lower intensity and increase the volume of work gradually. Also consider using intervals to encourage adaptation in smaller increments. Set relief times based on recovery heart rates. The final cool-down should be gradual.

2. Consider the relationship of intensity to the other prescription factors. Duration, frequency, and mode interact with intensity in terms of total work and the stage of progression. Duration and frequency are often chosen to accommodate the selected intensity: Intensity may be dangerously high if selected to accommodate low duration or low frequency. Extending the duration of the work (or the work interval) provides the safest initial progression. Wider intensity ranges may be appropriate for some interval training programs. For example, you may prescribe an upper heart rate limit slightly beyond the standard aerobic training zone because the work interval is short, or you may prescribe a lower heart rate limit below the standard zone because it represents an interval recovery rate (see discussion of interval training, p. 164). The aerobic warm-up intensity at the beginning of a workout should approach the lower end of the heart rate training zone.

3. Consider the personal goals of your clients. What your clients want must be balanced against your physiological objectives. Although the most rapid improvements usually occur when intensity is increased, the type of improvement your clients want (e.g., sport specific) should influence intensity selection. High-intensity intervals will produce aerobic and anaerobic benefits; moderate, steady intensities improve stamina and aerobic endurance. Listen to your clients and their perceptions of the intensity. The Borg scale (RPE) is an excellent tool for tracking your clients' adjustments to their workloads, whether you are present or the ratings are logged.

Step 5: Set Volume (Duration and Frequency)

We have considered the first four steps in the client-centered model for cardiovascular exercise prescription:

1. Consider client needs and goals
2. Select activities and equipment
3. Select training method and mode
4. Set intensity and workload

Now we are ready to discuss setting the desired duration and frequency of exercise, referred to as the weekly "volume" of activity and often measured in calories per week.

Duration

The optimal duration of an exercise session for a particular client depends on her prescribed intensity. Generally, the higher the intensity, the shorter the duration. You must know your clients well enough to prescribe an appropriate mix of intensity and duration to challenge their cardiovascular systems without overexertion.

Total Work Done

The most important variable for cardiovascular gains is the total work done. Although other health gains are possible at quite low intensities, cardiovascular improvements appear to require a minimum threshold for the total work done in an exercise session. So if your client is working at a low intensity, the duration must be longer to achieve the same amount of total work done as another client who is working at a higher intensity.

The body responds well to workouts lasting 20 to 30 min, with benefits leveling off after this time. Figure 6.5 shows that improvements in oxygen uptake increase with the duration of the exercise session. But figure 6.5 also shows that, with moderate intensity, workouts much longer than 40 min increase the risk of orthopedic injury. This being the case, you must adjust your client's workout duration to accommodate his fitness level. Here are ranges of duration that generally work well:

- Low fitness: 10-20 min (100-200 kcal/workout)
- Average fitness: 15-40 min (200-400 kcal/workout)
- High fitness: 30-60 min (>400 kcal/workout)

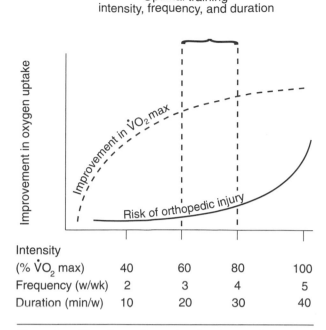

Optimal training intensity, frequency, and duration

Intensity (% V̇O₂ max)	40	60	80	100
Frequency (w/wk)	2	3	4	5
Duration (min/w)	10	20	30	40

Figure 6.5 The effects of intensity, duration, and frequency on cardiovascular improvements. w = workout.

Total work may be expressed in terms of the caloric cost of an activity. The caloric equivalent of 1 MET is 1 kcal/kg × hr. For example, if an 80 kg client in average condition works at 6 METs, he expends 480 kcal/hr (6 METs × 80 kg) or 8 kcal/min (480 kcal/hr/60 min).

If this same 80 kg client's initial recommended workout load includes expending 200 kcal, working at an intensity of 6 METs he would need to work out for 25 min (200 kcal/workout/8 kcal/min). If the duration gradually increased to 40 min at the same intensity, the total work per session would be 320 kcal.

Client-Centered Tips for Setting Cardiovascular Duration

If your client's objective is cardiovascular improvement, "duration" should refer to the time within the training zone. Activity below the training zone still may positively affect body composition or decrease risk factors. Longer durations can help your client tolerate submaximal challenges, but they are less effective in changing maximum oxygen uptake.

Determine the duration of higher-intensity "spurts" of activity in those sports that demand cardiovascular endurance; then design interval training programs with similar durations.

Duration is an important prescription factor for clients who have symptoms that limit their level of intensity. Because such people have less chance of intensity-related injury, you can progressively

increase the duration of their activities. If recovery is incomplete within 1 hr, or heart rate is still more than 20 beats/min above the preexercise level after 10 min of recovery, then either total work or duration may be too high.

Frequency

The frequency of exercise depends on the duration and intensity of the session. If the intensity is kept low and duration is short, plan more sessions per week.

Being Realistic

Frequency may be the most difficult factor in the fitness formula. The number of sessions per week is limited by your clients' lifestyle—but it also depends on how motivated the client is. Your key role in motivation, then, may be one reason for the growth of the personal fitness training field.

The American College of Sports Medicine (2000) recommends 3 to 5 days a week for most aerobic programs.

Recommendations

Very low fitness	1-2 days/week (if intensity and duration low)
Low fitness	3 days/week
Average fitness	3-5 days/week
Maintenance	2-4 days/week

Figure 6.5 shows that improvements in oxygen uptake (cardiovascular endurance) increase with the frequency of the exercise sessions. These benefits begin to level off after 4 days/week. In fact, if a client has been previously sedentary, exercising more than 4 days per week seems to be too much, and the incidence of injuries and dropouts increases (Powers and Howley 1990). If sessions are shorter and less intense, frequency can safely increase.

Client-Centered Tips for Setting Cardiovascular Frequency

Frequency is a key prescription factor in building a habit. Daily walking routines appear to have lower attrition than less frequent programs, because walking becomes part of your clients' lifestyles. Daily doses of lower-intensity activity for those with a lower functional capacity will minimize fatigue and help build muscular endurance.

The work-a-day then rest-a-day routine will improve cardiovascular health, lower the incidence of injury, and achieve weight-loss goals (ACSM 2000). If aerobic improvement is a primary objective, there should be no more than 2 days between workouts.

Although exercising only twice a week may cause some cardiovascular improvements, the higher intensity necessary to bring about the improvements can be hazardous. If your client is just beginning a weight-bearing activity such as jogging or aerobic classes, suggest 36 to 48 hr of relative rest between aerobic workouts to prevent overuse injuries. The rest is even more important for overweight people or those who have lower-leg alignment problems. Lower-body stretching before and after the aerobic workout will improve safety and performance, but you must instruct your client about the dangers of overstretching and how to avoid this.

Step 6: Address Progression and Monitoring

The previous steps involved selecting

1. needs and goals,
2. activities and equipment,
3. training method and mode,
4. intensity and workload, and
5. volume (duration and frequency).

These steps lead us to the ongoing process of progression and monitoring, the sixth step in the Client-Centered Model for Cardiovascular Exercise Prescription.

The perpetual challenge for fitness professionals is to find a rate of progression that builds aerobic capacity without overtraining or reducing compliance. Monitoring progress at follow-up sessions should begin by reviewing the steps taken toward goals. If the goals were specific and measurable, it is easy to focus on the projected outcomes. Feedback should go beyond recognition and encouragement. Involve clients in taking ownership of their program and in strategizing for change.

Progression

The rate of improvement depends on an individual's age, functional capacity, health status, and objectives. Clients who are more fit or closer to their genetic potential and some older individuals will not improve as much as those who are less fit (Heyward 2002). The fastest rate of progression is during the first 6 to 8 weeks, when physiological changes enable clients to significantly increase the total work performed. According to Sharkey (1984), aerobic endurance may improve as much as 3% a week during the first month, 2% a week during the second month, and 1% a week or less thereafter. Your clients can achieve safety and comfort by building a level of endurance before initiating higher-intensity workouts or engaging in competitions.

Stages of Progression

The three stages of progression for cardiovascular exercise programs are

- initial conditioning,
- improvement conditioning, and
- maintenance conditioning (ACSM 2000).

The *initial conditioning stage* usually lasts 4 to 6 weeks and is characterized by longer warm-ups and cool-downs, intensities of 40% to 60% of HRR, durations of 12 to 15 min progressing up to 20 min, and frequencies of three times per week on nonconsecutive days. Active clients with better than average fitness may skip this stage.

The *improvement conditioning stage* usually lasts 16 to 20 weeks and is characterized by more rapid progressions, intensities moving from 50% to 85% of HRR, durations increasing every 2 to 3 weeks up to 30 continuous minutes, and frequencies of three to five times per week.

The *maintenance conditioning stage* usually begins after 6 months of training. It is characterized by maintenance of an energy cost comparable to that of the conditioning stage. However, the workout is altered to include some cross-training activities, more Group 2 or 3 activities (see *Cardiovascular Endurance Activities Grouped by Intensity*, p. 160) involving skill and variety, a change of training method for some of the workouts, or a change of goals.

Client-Centered Tips for Setting Cardiovascular Progression

Table 6.10 will help you establish prescription factors appropriate to your clients' stages of cardiovascular progression. During the first few weeks, move your clients through gradual increases in duration, holding intensity nearly constant until they have achieved 20 to 30 min of endurance in the training zone. Building frequency and duration will increase workout volume, with resulting beneficial changes in body composition, reduction of risk factors such as blood lipids, and physiological changes at the submaximal levels (McArdle et al. 1991).

With an interval training program, you can maintain the total duration of the workout but prescribe progression by changing the ratio of work time and relief time. Base your progressions on data from regular monitoring. For example, monitoring resting (morning) heart rate over a 4- to 5-week period of aerobic endurance training should reveal a decrease of about 5 to 10 beats/min. An increase in resting heart rate over several days, however, may indicate physical or mental fatigue. Suspect overtraining or possible illness in such a case, and adjust the workouts accordingly.

Small alterations to the prescription factors (intensity, mode, duration, frequency, and progression) can favor different aerobic objectives in different clients. Table 6.11 illustrates how you can manipulate the prescription factors to highlight the potential gains for specific aerobic objectives.

Monitoring

Follow-up and monitoring provide

- regular feedback for clients
- a basis to judge the effectiveness of your prescriptions, and
- trends that are invaluable for planning changes or progressions.

Recording Data

Some data, such as heart rates, times, perceived exertions, training loads, and other fitness mea-

sures, are best collected during the workout on a monitoring form or program card. This may involve keeping a multipurpose exercise diary or plotting recovery heart rates after a standardized work segment. The charts on pages 178 and 180 may be copied for your clients' use.

Monitoring Heart Rate

Heart rate has long been a key physiological parameter. It is reliably used to estimate the relative intensity of an exercise and to quantify training loads. Following are guidelines for heart rate monitoring and advantages of using a heart rate monitor rather than relying on manually taking a pulse.

- Training intensities should be determined on an individual basis. Time spent at a specific heart rate can vary considerably among clients exercising at the same workload.

Table 6.10   Cardiovascular Progressions

Stage	Week	Frequency (workouts/week)	Intensity (%HRR)	Duration (min)
Initial stage	1	3	40-50	12
	2-5	3	50-70	15-20
Improvement stage	6-10	3-4	70-80	20
	11-24	3-5	70-80	20-30
Maintenance stage	25+	3	70-85	30-45

Table 6.11   Prescription Factors for Specific Aerobic Objectives

Aerobic objective	Selection of prescription factor
1. Ability to do prolonged work (>30 min); development of aerobic capacity and lactic acid tolerance	• Alternate increasing intensity and then duration • Apply these progressions regularly (approximately every 2 weeks during improvement stage) • Encourage supplemental activity and cross-training
2. Ability to resist fatigue and maintain high energy	• Use interval training (e.g., upper to lower levels of training zone) • Gradually decrease time of relief • Use active recovery
3. Ability to rapidly recover from higher rates of work; preparation for sports	• Include very hard work for short intervals (<2 min) of work • Allow quite a lengthy and yet active recovery
4. Ability to adapt to psychological stress and gain a feeling of well-being	• Incorporate low to moderate intensity of a longer, continuous nature (no fatigue) • Use a lengthy, gradual recovery • Provide positive mood and climate (e.g., music, voice, lighting, smile)
5. Weight loss	• Avoid lactic acid buildup by keeping client below the anaerobic threshold • Use nonfatiguing, longer activity to better mobilize fats and continue to burn calories

Exercise Diary—Multipurpose

Date	Type of exercise	Distance (km/miles)	Duration (min)	Pulse/RPE before/after	Observations/comments

Note. RPE = rating of perceived exertion.

From *Client-Centered Exercise Prescription, Second Edition,* by John C. Griffin, 2006, Champaign, IL: Human Kinetics.

- Training zones should be established from the results of graded exercise tests. The tests should use the same modes of exercise as you will be prescribing for the clients.
- At a given submaximal workload, heart rate will tend to be higher in children and females than in adult males (on whose data most heart rate norms are based!).
- Because of dehydration and increased core temperature, heart rate tends to be higher toward the end of a prolonged exercise even though the intensity remains constant (Marion et al. 1994).
- Overdressing or protective equipment (e.g., while hiking or engaging in sports such as lacrosse) will cause higher heart rates at submaximal exercise and recovery.
- Day-to-day variations can account for up to ±5 beats/min for the same individual at identical submaximal workloads (Åstrand and Rodahl 2003).
- During interval training, a pulse rate check at the end of the relief period can verify if the client is ready to repeat the work interval.
- Your client's heart rate can tell you when it is time to apply the progressive overload principle. Record the heart rate at the end of a standardized workload on a daily basis. As the heart rate decreases (figure 6.6), increase the intensity of the workout.

Although it is helpful for clients to take their own heart rate, using a heart rate monitor has a number of quantifiable advantages. Heart rate during exercise is intermittent, and heart rate readings may be inaccurate by as much as ±15 beats/min (Black 2001). Other muscle movements and heavy breathing can make a pulse difficult to count. Howard (2003) listed some of the benefits associated with the industry's most widely used portable exercise devices:

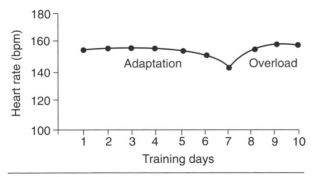

Figure 6.6   Progression based on heart rate adaptation.

- Provide immediate, individual feedback
- Are relatively inexpensive (lower-end models)
- Provide precise measure of intensity
- Can be used to monitor and measure progress
- Regulate quantity and intensity of workouts
- Add motivation by indicating improvements
- May boost exercise adherence

Other Effective Means of Monitoring

Unfortunately, many adults—particularly those just starting an exercise program—find it difficult or inconvenient to monitor their heart rate. Ratings of perceived exertion and the talk test are remarkably effective in keeping clients within safe yet productive intensity levels. Pedometers help monitor volume with the incentive of continuous feedback.

- **Ratings of perceived exertion (RPE).** We saw earlier how RPEs could be used for exercise prescription. You can also use ratings of perceived exertion (RPE) to monitor exercise intensity (figure 6.4). This approach is very client-centered; it sensitizes people to judge local cues (such as muscular discomfort) as well as central cues (such as breathing and heart rates). Table 6.12 uses heart rate and RPE to provide guidelines for either the adjustment of an exercise session or the progression of the prescription after a training effect has taken place. There is a bit of a learning curve with RPE because it is subjective. You will need to help your clients understand how to match their body feelings with the RPE scale.

- **The talk test.** When using the talk test, clients should exercise at an intensity where they can still carry on a normal conversation and maintain a steady state. When this point is exceeded, the body cannot supply enough energy and must supplement the energy needs through anaerobic mechanisms. This is called the anaerobic threshold (AT). A convenient way to estimate AT is to assess ventilatory (breathing) patterns during exercise, because they are affected by lactic acid buildup. The increase in respiration often coincides with the AT (Porcari, Foster, and Schneider 2000) making the talk test a simple, noninvasive way to individualize exercise intensity.

- **Pedometers.** America on the Move, a national program launched in 2003, is a pedometer-based walking program designed to get Americans

Recovery Heart Rate Progress Chart

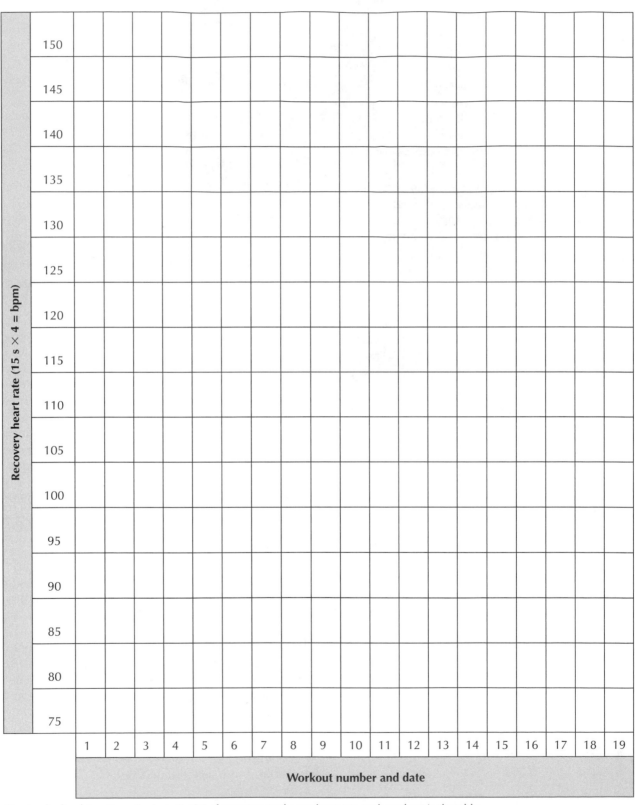

At a standardized time (e.g., 1 min or 3 min) of recovery, mark your heart rate each workout in the table.

From *Client-Centered Exercise Prescription, Second Edition,* by John C. Griffin, 2006, Champaign, IL: Human Kinetics.

Table 6.12 Interpretation of Intensity Monitoring

Intensity monitoring method		
%HRR	RPE	Exercise prescription
>85	>16	Decrease intensity, duration, or both. Continue to monitor at the reduced intensity.
80-85	15-16	Use caution, and monitor heart rate. Make sure client is working at the prescribed workload. Use for a client with good fitness status.
60-80	12-15	Use for clients with average fitness status and few risk factors. Increase duration when RPE remains lower for consecutive workouts. Increase intensity instead of duration every third and fourth progression.
<60	<12	Use for clients with low fitness status or several risk factors. Progress with longer durations. Usually means intensity or duration need to increase.

Note. % HRR = percentage of heart rate reserve; RPE = rating of perceived exertion (figure 6.4).

to walk an additional 2,000 steps per day. Pedometers measure distance traveled and can also provide motivation—particularly for beginning clients who prefer to be exact. Positive cardiovascular and health benefits have been seen in pedometer-based programs for sedentary adults, those with type 2 diabetes or osteoarthritis, moderately hypertensive people, and obese children (Gaesser 2003).

Step 7: Design Warm-Up and Cool-Down

The prescription model reaches full circle with this final, seventh step. Within the client's needs and goals (step 1), we have selected the activity and equipment (step 2), determined a training method and mode (step 3), and specifically set intensity and workload (step 4) and volume through duration and frequency (step 5), while putting in place methods for progression and monitoring (step 6).

The cardiovascular prescription model suggests that the warm-up and cool-down should be designed last. These components must be prescription-specific and client-centered. You need to understand the purpose as well as the methods of both warming up and cooling down.

Warm-Up

The warm-up should increase heart rate, blood pressure, and oxygen consumption; dilate the blood vessels; and increase elasticity of muscle and connective tissue in a gradual fashion. As seen in table 6.13, range of motion exercises, stretches, and gradual low-level aerobic exercise are essential for safety, delay of fatigue, and economy of movement.

Your client's warm-up activities should provide a graduated level of activity mechanically similar to that within the aerobic segment. This will improve mechanical efficiency and facilitate the transmission of neural impulses that augment coordination and power (Nieman 1999).

- Participants in racket sports should begin with a light jog or brisk walk, followed by a gradually increased tempo of volleying.
- Swimmers should begin with a slow crawl (perhaps in intervals) and gradually increase stroke pace.
- Outdoor cyclists should begin on flat terrain in lower gears.
- Stationary cyclists should begin at half the intended work setting and a slower speed.
- Joggers should warm up with a walk–jog interval or a slower-paced jog.

Duration of the warm-up should be longer if the intensity of the aerobic segment is high or your client's fitness level is low.

Cool-Down

The cool-down should gradually decrease the cardiac work and metabolism with low-level aerobic activity similar to the preceding aerobic segment. For clients with higher cardiovascular risk, the cool-down is crucial. Lower-extremity blood pooling and high concentrations of exercise hormones can significantly strain the heart. Table 6.14 shows that circulatory cool-down should be followed by stretching—particularly of the active muscles.

The length of the cool-down segment is proportional to the intensity, mode, and duration of the aerobic activity and to your client's level of fitness.

Table 6.13 Warm-Up (Preparation) Segment Design

Prescription	Design issues
Range of motion (moving major joints through their range of motion)	• Use warm-up to increase joint lubrication and synovial fluid (protect joints). • Have client check on how body feels before work. • Use warm-up to provide some flexibility gains.
Circulatory warm-up (light aerobic; same mode as cardiovascular work)	• Continue warm-up to increase tissue temperature and synovial fluid in preparation for stretching. • Use segment to gradually prepare heart and circulatory system. • Simulate joint mechanics with low trauma.
Stretching (emphasizing static stretching)	• Promote flexibility gains. • Target muscles used, especially if used eccentrically. • Include dynamic stretches for sport preparation.
Transition (easing into next segment)	• Add a light overload in the activity to follow (start of progressive overload). • Look for opportunities to do a mini-warm-up and skill practice (especially in intermittent sports such as baseball).

After a moderate-intensity workout, most people should allot for their cool-down a period equal to about 15% of the time they spent exercising. Ensure that heart rate is below 100 beats/min or within 20 beats/min of the original HR and that your client looks and feels recovered.

Case Studies

The following case studies deal with specific client situations and demonstrate the application of many of the cardiovascular prescription tools. A reproducible blank cardiovascular card is provided for your use (see p. 192). It follows the 7-step prescription process and will guide you through recording the decisions that you have made when designing the cardiovascular prescription. Complete prescription samples using the template are provided for case #1 (Ingrid) and case #3 (Rory).

Case study 1 involves a 37-year-old woman in good condition who was interested in cycling and wanted to improve her cardiovascular conditioning. The second case involves a 27-year-old male for whom no fitness assessment was administered. The third client is a sprint athlete interested in a long-term plan.

Case Study 1: Well-Conditioned Woman

Ingrid was a 37-year-old woman in good condition, interested in cycling. She was at a maintenance stage but was interested in a progressive prescription that would get her over her fitness plateau.

Assessment

Ingrid had set a goal of cycling 50 km (31 miles) in a single day, and although training results were leveling off, I could sense her determination. During our counseling, I learned that when Ingrid was single, she had played some racquetball and participated a couple of years in aerobic dance classes. We decided to stick with just cycling as long as no overuse patterns emerged. As the weather got warmer, we could move outside with some street cycling. But the big challenge was to work around her busy schedule. We agreed that a very specific prescription based on the cardiovascular assessment would yield the best results.

I assessed Ingrid on a bicycle ergometer using a multistage graded exercise protocol. Her blood pressure, perceived exertion, and other signs were within normal ranges. The following is a summary of the assessment data.

Figure 6.1 plots heart rate against MET levels. Ingrid's final heart rate was 170 beats/min. Using the plotted curve, the point on the horizontal axis that coresponds to 170 beats/min is 10 METs.

Prescription

With her needs and goals well established from the counseling and assessment, we selected a bicycle ergometer to easily measure the workload and found a comfortable gel seat and her favorite music to lessen the load. A continuous training method suited her goal of amassing 50 km. The following calculations demonstrate how we established a starting intensity and workload. The duration (20 min) and frequency (3 days/week) reflected the time she had on lunch break.

Table 6.14 Cool-Down Segment Design

Prescription	Design issues
Circulatory cool-down and transition	• Make sure cardiovascular indicators (e.g., heart rate, depth of breathing, blood pressure) are reduced. • Ensure that muscles feel worked but not sore or tight. • Ice any "hot spots" or minor injuries. • Tier down gradually; avoid final sprints or sudden stops (better cardiovascular adaptations permitted).
Stretching (emphasizing static stretching)	• Use this segment for greatest flexibility gains—tissue is warm. • Have client hold stretch for up to 30 s. • Use target muscles, especially if used eccentrically • Consider proprioceptive neuromuscular facilitation if flexibility is a priority.

Calculation of Exercise Intensity

Given Ingrid's "good" rating (Howley and Franks 1997), I selected a training zone of 60% to 80% of max METs. With the intensity, prescription is set at 60% to 80% of functional reserve:

[60% of (10 − 1 METS)] + 1 MET = 6.4 METs;

[80% of (10 − 1 METS)] + 1 MET = 8.2 METs

The graph in figure 6.1 shows that these levels correspond to heart rates of 132 beats/min and 152 beats/min, respectively.

At an initial intensity of 60% of the functional capacity:

$$VO_2 = 6.4 \text{ METs} \times (3.5 \text{ ml} \cdot \text{kg}^{-1} \cdot \text{min}^{-1})$$

$$VO_2 = 22.4 \text{ ml} \cdot \text{kg}^{-1} \cdot \text{min}^{-1}$$

$$VO_2 \text{ (ml/min)} = 22.4 \text{ ml} \cdot \text{kg}^{-1} \cdot \text{min}^{-1} \times 70 \text{ kg}$$

$$VO_2 \text{ (ml/min)} = 1{,}568 \text{ ml/min}$$

The American College of Sports Medicine (2000) provides an equation for calculating work rate on the bicycle ergometer.

$$VO_2 \text{ (in ml/min)} = 1.8 \times \text{work rate} + 3.5 \text{ [body weight (in kg)]}$$

where work rate (WR) is in kg · m/min. Substituting the measurements for Ingrid:

$$1{,}568 = 1.8 \text{ WR} + 3.5(70)$$

$$1.8 \text{ WR} = 1568 − 245$$

$$WR = 735 \text{ kg} \cdot \text{m}^{-1} \cdot \text{min}^{-1}$$

It is most practical to assign a 600 kg · m⁻¹ · min⁻¹ workload (i.e., 2 kg at 50 rev/min). Although Ingrid was not primarily concerned with burning calories, it may be useful to remember that the caloric equivalent of 1 MET is 1 kcal/kg × hr. For example, if our 70 kg (154 lb) client worked at 6.4 METs, she would expend 6.4 × 70 = 448 kcal/hr, or 7.5 kcal/min.

General Prescription

The general prescription is summarized next (see figure 6.7), with Ingrid starting at the lower levels for each of the prescription factors. The essential segments of a cardiovascular exercise program include warm-up and cool-down, aerobic segment prescription factors (intensity, mode and training method, duration, frequency), and a progression plan.

The warm-up I prescribed was standard: range of motion (lower-body joints moved through their range of motion), circulatory (light aerobic activity, such as stationary cycling, walking, or calisthenics), stretch (emphasis on static stretching legs and trunk), and transition (easing into the aerobic segment with easy cycling).

The prescribed cool-down also was rather standard: circulatory cool-down (light cycling), transition (reverse of warm-up parts), and stretch (emphasis on static stretching of the legs to work on whole-body flexibility).

During the initial stage of the exercise program, I assigned Ingrid a workload corresponding to 60% of VO₂max (6.4 METs or 600 kg · m⁻¹ · min⁻¹) for 3 weeks. The workload is calculated using the ACSM formula for leg ergometry (see p. 170). Her heart rate was near or slightly above 132 beats/min, duration was 20 min, and frequency was three times per week.

Results

Ingrid was very keen, worked out regularly, and recorded her heart rates and RPEs when I was not

Cardiovascular Prescription Card

Client name	Trainer name
Ingrid	JG

Client goals	Special considerations
• Progress beyond her earlier fitness plateau • 50 km (31 miles) cycling in 1 day • Maintenance	• Variety to maintain interest

Circulatory Warm-Up

Equipment and mode	Workload	Time	HR/PE objective
Stationary cycling (walking and calisthenics)	1 kg at 50 rev/min (brisk walk, light exercise)	3-5 min	HR >90, <120 beats/min

Stretching Warm-Up

Name and brief description	Guidelines
• Range of motion (lower-body joints moved through their ROM) • Stretch (emphasis on static stretching legs and trunk)	

Cardiovascular Workout

Intensity training range

Lower limit: 60% HRR ($\dot{V}O_2R$) 132 beats/min 12 RPE 6.4 (METs)

Upper limit: 80% HRR ($\dot{V}O_2R$) 156 beats/min 15 RPE 8.2 (METs)

	Equipment	Training method	Frequency	kcal/session
1	Bicycle ergometer	Continuous	3	150
2				

Phase	Workload	Time	Phase	Workload	Time
Warm-up	Ease into peak work with 1 kg at 50 rev/min	3-5	Warm-up		
Peak	600 kg · m^{-1} · min^{-1} workload (i.e., 2 kg at 50 rev/min)	20	Peak		
Cool-down	Taper to 1 kg then 1/2 kg, ensure HR <90 beats/min	3-5	Cool-down		

Interval Training Prescription

Set	Reps	Work time	(Relief time)	Ratio	Intensity

Progression and Monitoring

Phase (weeks):

• See Summary of Progressions

(continued)

Figure 6.7 Ingrid's cardiovascular prescription card.

Cool-Down

Name and brief description	Guidelines
• Circulatory cool-down (light cycling) • Transition (reverse of warm-up parts) • Stretch (legs)	• Emphasis on static stretching of the legs—good opportunity to work on whole-body flexibility

Summary of Progressions

Phase (weeks)	Intensity (% $\dot{V}O_2R$)	Intensity (METs)	Workload (kg · m⁻¹ · min⁻¹)	Duration (min)	Frequency
			Initial		
1	60	6.4	600	20	3
2	60	6.4	600	25	3
3	60	6.4	600	30	3
4	60-65	6.4-7.0	600-660	30	3
			Improvement		
5-6	65-70	7.0-7.5	660-720	30	3
7-8	70-75	7.5-8.0	720-800	30	3
9-10	70-75	7.5-8.0	720-800	35	4
11-12	75-80	8.0-8.5	800-880	35	4
13-14	75-80	8.0-8.5	800-880	40	5
15-16	80	8.5	880	40	5
			Maintenance		
17	+80	8.5	880	40-45	3
	80-85	8.5-9.0	Squash	40-50	1
	80-85	8.5-9.0	Aerobics	40-50	1

Note. HR = heart rate; PE = perceived exertion; ROM = range of motion; HRR = heart rate reserve; $\dot{V}O_2R$ = $\dot{V}O_2$ reserve; RPE − rating of perceived exertion; MET = metabolic equivalent.

Figure 6.7   continued

there. After a few weeks, Ingrid's heart rates were regularly below 132 beats/min, even with slight increases in duration. I increased the workload about 10% in the fourth week. With gradual increases in duration during this initial stage, her energy expenditure progressed from 150 to 250 kcal per workout (7.5 kcal/min), excluding warm-up and cool-down.

As the summary of progressions segment of the cardiovascular prescription card indicates, I progressively increased intensity, duration, and frequency during the improvement stage. Although I varied the prescription factors to suit Ingrid's schedule, the total work per week remained the same. In this stage, the caloric expenditures ranged from 250 to 400 kcal per workout. Within 8 to 10 weeks, she reached her objective of progressing beyond her earlier fitness plateau and was doing

some extra mileage outdoors. Ingrid eventually did a total of 50 km (31 miles), 25 km in the morning and 25 km later that same summer day. To add variety and keep Ingrid's interest high in the maintenance stage, after about 4 months I had her supplement the cycling with racquetball and aerobic dancing.

Justification of Cardiovascular Prescription

Each personal fitness trainer will have a slightly different approach to the case study prescription. However, as you make choices, be sure you have a strong rationale for each one. The following provides physiological justifications and client-centered (behavioral) justifications for each choice made.

Physiological and Client-Centered (Behavioral) Justification of Ingrid's Cardiovascular Exercise Prescription

Below each step are the justifications for the prescription decisions made in that step.

1. **Consider Client Needs and Goals**
   - The client was willing to increase work even at her maintenance stage.
   - Intensities based on assessment results should use limited time optimally.
   - The client's highest priority was to get over a fitness plateau in cycling.
   - Racquetball or aerobic dance could be considered later as alternatives.
   - The client was motivated to cycle 50 km (31 miles) in a day.

2. **Select Activities and Equipment**
   - Ingrid found cycling fun.
   - She had access to a bicycle ergometer and a road bike.
   - Cycling could serve as transportation, making it time efficient.
   - The gel seat will add comfort and may increase exercise time.

3. **Select Training Method and Mode**
   - Cycling is continuous, and the client had sufficient fitness and exercise tolerance.
   - Cycling suits the objective of 50 km in a day.
   - Cycling is safe, well tolerated, and convenient.

4. **Set Intensity and Workload**
   - Workload was calculated using ACSM formula and assessment results.
   - Heart rate was easily maintained in appropriate range for objectives.
   - RPEs were helpful.

5. **Set Volume (Duration and Frequency)**
   - A schedule of 20 min and 3 ×/week suited her lunch hour availability.
   - Cycling is an active lifestyle integration.
   - Volume progression was needed to reach her 50 km goal.

6. **Address Progression and Monitoring**
   - Progressive overload would improve cardiovascular conditioning at same RPE.
   - The chart provided was quite detailed and easy to self-administer.
   - Increasing time and pace would rapidly increase cardiovascular improvements.
   - Monitoring would guide time and extent of cardiovascular overload.
   - Cycling was easy to monitor.
   - A 10% increase in workload was based on monitoring and was reasonable.

7. **Design Warm-Up and Cool-Down**
   - Range of motion and stretching focused on joints and muscles used in cycling.
   - Circulatory warm-up was used to increase muscle temperature.
   - Transitions would allow her to ease into aerobic workout intensities and clear metabolic wastes in cool-down.
   - Stretches targeted previously active muscles.
   - The cool-down provided a gradual return to the preexercise state.

Case Study 2: Prescribing Without Cardiovascular Assessment

I met Josh while I was working with a fitness center that does not offer cardiovascular fitness assessments, claiming they were too expensive—an unfortunate but not uncommon situation. When hard data are in short supply, we have to be creative in obtaining information that will guide us in our prescription designs.

Assessment

Josh wanted to improve his cardiovascular fitness significantly. More extensive questioning during the counseling stage revealed the following:

- This 27-year-old had been active in several aerobic sports but in the last 4 months had only been using a home exercise bicycle once or twice a week.
- He did not mind the cycling but found it hard to motivate himself.
- After only 10 to 12 min on his bike, his legs were tired—and he believed it took him a long time to recover.
- On the rare occasions when he did a warm-up, it consisted of two or three stretches that were completed in less than a minute; he never did a cool-down.
- He was interested in improving his squash game and in beginning to compete.
- He had no injuries or other health problems, and his weight was controlled.
- Most days he had an hour to work out and was confident he could work out four times per week.

I had to use an indirect method to estimate a training zone. Heart rate reserve (HRR) physiologically represents the reserve of the heart for increasing cardiac output. I had Josh monitor his resting heart rate on three consecutive days before he got up in the morning, and I found a consistent 62 beats/min.

Josh was young and healthy and was still somewhat active. Some of his early fatigue appeared to be caused by an inappropriate intensity (workload setting) and the lack of proper warm-ups or cooldowns. His history of involvement in multiple sports suggested that he would enjoy the squash competition, and I considered the intensity level and interval nature of squash in the program design.

Prescription

Josh's goals were split between aerobic fitness and squash. Some of his needs involved getting assistance on the use of equipment and better guidance with a minimum of information about his physical condition. Although Josh had access to an exercise bicycle at home and at the fitness center, the method of establishing intensity and workload differed at each location. We started with 25 min of continuous cycling but eventually moved to an interval training program more representative of a game of squash. He was quite open to change and trying new exercises. Warm-up and cool-down were important to add to Josh's activity, especially at the higher intensities.

Calculation of Exercise Intensity

$$HRmax = [208 - (0.7 \times age)] = (208 - 19)$$
$$= 189 \text{ beats/min}$$

I used the HRR method and a moderate to high training zone of 70% to 80% HRR:

$$\text{Heart rate reserve} = [(HRmax - HRrest) \times \%\text{training zone}] + HRrest$$

$$= [(189 - 62) \times 70\text{-}80\%] + 62$$

$$= [127 \times 70\text{-}80\%] + 62$$

$$= (89\text{-}102) + 62$$

$$= 151 \text{ to } 164 \text{ beats/min}$$

General Prescription

One of the difficulties of prescription without assessment is allocation of a workload. Sometimes Josh used his home exercise bicycle and sometimes the bicycle ergometer at the fitness center. At home I had him cycle at a load and speed about half of what he had been using and then check his heart rate after 3 min of steady cycling. If his heart rate was less than 151 beats/min, he increased the workload for another 3 min and monitored heart rate again. He continued this process until his heart rate was between 151 and 164 beats/min, at which point he recorded the tension setting and speed for the next session. The ergometer at the center gave a more precise measure of work. I informed him that his perceived exertion should be "somewhat hard" (about 13-14 on the Borg scale).

Josh's warm-up included light cycling for 5 min followed by static stretches for his quadriceps, hamstrings, calves, shins, and low back. The first 3 min of the cycling were at one half to two thirds of the training zone. For the cool-down, he tapered the cycling for the final 3 to 5 min and redid the warm-up stretches—holding them longer, because tissue temperature was high, for added flexibility gains.

Results

Once Josh began to tolerate intensity levels closer to his upper limit for 25 to 30 min, I introduced him on alternate days to some interval training. He started with 3 min periods of cycling at his upper limit load but at a faster speed and then did 3 min of cycling at his warm-up level. He repeated this cycle six to eight times. Squash eventually became his primary focus, and I adjusted the intervals accordingly. To more intensely work the ATP–PC–LA System, I designed an ITP with 3 sets of 5 repetitions, each being 2 minutes in length. Exercise heart rates started around 160 beats/min but crept up to 170 beats/min by the fifth repetition. During the 3 minute relief period between repetitions, heart rates came down to 120-130 bpm. This interval training program for Josh successfully prepared him to be in better condition for squash.

Case Study 3: 23-Year-Old Male Sprinter

A serious 23-year-old male sprinter, Rory specialized in the 200 m event. He wanted to train all year long and was looking for a safe, progressive program.

Assessment

I used the treadmill for Rory's aerobic assessment because I want him to achieve his highest measurable oxygen uptake, because he was familiar with the device, and because he wanted a prescription for running. Not surprisingly, his results ($\dot{V}O_2$max = 60 ml · kg^{-1} · min^{-1}) were in the excellent category. His maximum measured heart rate was 196 beats/min. And when the assessment was redone in 3 months, we had a benchmark for comparison. Perhaps most valuable for a client-centered prescription was Rory's personal best in the 200 m (219 yd) at 24 s. This time was used as a basis for building times for the interval training programs. Percentage of HRmax and adequate heart rate recovery helped monitor and fine-tune the prescription.

Prescription

Rory's program would span three phases: preparation, competition, and transition. Rory's goal was performance based, and although he was motivated, he needed to work smarter and more systematically. Running was the activity, but the venue varied from cross country to treadmill to track. Continuous and Fartlek training would strengthen his aerobic base followed by various interval prescriptions with some plyometrics. Intensities will be discussed. However, in combination with duration and frequency of the workouts, the volume increased during the preparation phase and then tapered into the competition phase. Warm-ups were progressive and cool-downs were long, and both had lots of lower-body stretching.

Phases of Training

Periodization is the process of dividing the annual training plan into shorter, more manageable phases. Each phase can be further subdivided to allow the planning of specialized training with each phase and cycle ordered to ensure proper peaking for competition.

- **Preparation phase.** The early portion of Rory's preseason effort emphasized aerobic training, flexibility and strength balance, and muscular endurance. The volume of training was high and the intensity low. As the preseason progressed, however, I had him ease up on volume and increase intensity. The technical skill preparation involved drilling fundamental techniques such as running the turn. The progression was from simple to complex skills as the preseason advanced. For example, he practiced with basic acceleration form before proceeding to block form.

- **Competition phase.** Rory's next phase included high intensity and a decline in volume. The training was specific, concentrating on fitness and motor components that simulated sprinting. Adequate recovery from workouts was important. As is true in many sports at this stage, Rory needed increased emphasis on speed of movement, reactive training (e.g., plyometrics), and technique work.

- **Transition phase.** The off-season provided an opportunity for Rory to recover physiologically and psychologically, through a period of active rest that involved lower-intensity activities that required motor skills similar to those needed for sprinting.

Calculating Intensity

During the continuous work of the preparation phase, we aimed for heart rates of 156 to 175 beats/min (80-90% HRmax). During the interval work of the late preparation and competitive phases, heart rates would routinely reach the 180 to 190 beats/min range with relief heart rates dropping to at least 140 to 150 beats/min.

General Prescription

In the early preseason, the preparation was general: continuous runs, Fartlek, or cross-country runs. I prescribed specific times, not distances, such as starting with 20 min and building up to 45 min. In the late preseason, the volume or total work was double that of the competitive phase. For Rory, this was a mixture of continuous and interval work. A 400 m runner typically may be given a volume of 2,400 m (4 × 600 m) (2,624 yd, 4 × 656 yd). Because Rory ran 200 m (219 yd), I gave him a volume of 1,200 m (6 × 200 m or 4 × 300 m). The intensity at the start was 60% of his personal best of 200 m/24 s, or 24 s × (100/60) = 40 s for 200 m. He worked up to 70% (34-35 s) in 5 to 6 weeks. After this time, I increased the intensity by 5% and decreased the volume by 10% (20 m for every 200 m) every 2 to 4 weeks.

In the competitive phase, interval training was at a 1:3 or 1:4 work–relief ratio. The volume was about half that of the late preseason or about three to four times the racing distance. For example, I prescribed a volume of 600 m (3 × 200 m) (656 yd, 3 × 218 yd) at 90% intensity. Because his personal best in the 200 m was 24 s, 24 × (100/90) = 26.6 s was the workout time. Therefore, the prescription was 3 × 200 m at 26.6 s with a walking recovery lasting 1-1/2 to 2 min or until his heart rate returned to 120 to 130 beats/min.

Results

Initially, Rory needed a longer recovery time near the end of a workout than I expected. As the volume decreased and his condition improved, he no longer needed to extend his recoveries. In the competitive season, Rory ran better than his personal best in all but one competition. He never sustained a serious injury the whole year, and his personal best dropped to 22.6 s.

In the off-season, Rory jogs at his family's cottage and plays some recreational soccer.

Highlights

1. **Use a seven-step prescription process to guide you through decisions when designing a cardiovascular prescription.**

   The Client-Centered Cardiovascular Exercise Prescription Model outlines a seven-step model for physiologically sound and client-centered exercise prescription. Each step describes a decision that you face concerning exercise intensity, volume, and progression based on access to test data, past experience, availability of monitoring equipment, and the client's exercise needs and level of fitness.

   Each personal fitness trainer will have a slightly different approach to prescription; however, it is important that you have a strong rationale for each choice that you make.

   The remaining competencies reflect the seven steps of the model for cardiovascular exercise prescription.

2. **Consider client needs and goals.**

   Client needs may be related to medical or high risk (e.g., elevated blood lipids, hypertension), educational (e.g., shoe features), or motivational factors. They also can be defined by results of fitness assessments (e.g., oxygen uptake), by lack of self-esteem, or by special designs necessitated by physical limitations attributable to weight or orthopedics.

3. **Select activities and equipment.**

   Cardiovascular improvements are comparable for most modes of aerobic exercise as long as intensity, frequency, and duration of exercise are prescribed in accordance with sound scientific principles. Even though the client's own preferences and availability of equipment will usually narrow the choices, you probably will need to educate your clients and show how certain equipment can contribute to their goals. Tables 6.2 through 6.6 identify the design and safety features of a variety of common machines and activities and the type of client for whom these features are most beneficial. Although comfort, appearance, durability, and cost are important factors in exercise machines, the mechanism providing the resistance and the mechanics of the movement are the most critical features.

4. **Select training method and mode.**

Select a training method or exercise mode by drawing on your conversations with your client about preferences and interests, goals and objectives, availability and convenience (facility, equipment, time), skills and background, suitability (e.g., level of fitness and risk), and other desired benefits (e.g., skills, social opportunities, targeted energy system). The two broad categories of aerobic methods, continuous training and interval training, are both effective in improving cardiovascular fitness. Benefits to the oxygen transport system from continuous training are more easily transferred from one mode of training to another, and continuous training is well suited to incorporation of cross-training techniques. Interval training improves the body's ability to adapt and recover. It provides paced training that clients can monitor and modify to suit their training purpose. Match your interval training prescription to the reality of your client's outside activities. For a specific sport, for example, find out the typical length of time during which your client puts in continuous, strenuous effort. Circuit training usually consists of 10 to 15 different exercise stations with the circuit repeated two or three times. Circuit weight training is a compromise between muscular conditioning and aerobic conditioning. The compact versatility of this circuit is a major advantage for clients working in their home with little space or equipment. Cross-training involves a variety of fitness activities and provides the flexibility of mixing activities, allowing joints and soft tissues to rest without stopping workouts. Fartlek training combines elements of continuous training with interval training. Participants are relatively free to run whatever course and speed they prefer, although the speed should periodically reach high intensity levels. Active living is an enhancement of the simple activities in a daily routine, like walking to the corner store instead of taking the car, or climbing stairs instead of riding the elevator.

5. **Set intensity and workload.**

After you calculate what a given exercise intensity is, set the target intensity for given segments of your prescription, for example, the warm-up, the cool-down, the plateau to be reached in constant training, and the peaks and valleys in interval training. The primary methods of calculating and prescribing exercise intensity are the graph method and percentage of maximum heart rate (with assessment) and the percentage of maximum heart rate (estimated) and heart rate reserve (without assessment). You can vary the prescribed intensity level for your clients, depending on their fitness level, exercise history, objectives, and risk factors. Practical considerations to help you set the correct intensity for a client include the information gained from the cardiovascular assessment, the relationship of intensity to the other prescription factors, and the personal goals of your clients. Although the most rapid improvements usually occur when intensity is increased, the type of improvement your clients want should influence intensity selection.

6. **Set volume (duration and frequency).**

The weekly volume of activity involves setting the desired duration and frequency of exercise. The most important variable for cardiovascular gains is the total work done. Although health gains are possible at quite low intensities, cardiovascular improvements appear to require a minimum threshold for the total work done in an exercise session. The frequency of exercise depends on the duration and intensity of the session. If the intensity is kept low and duration is short, plan more sessions per week.

7. **Address progression and monitoring.**

Your perpetual challenge is to find a rate of progression that builds the aerobic capacity without overtraining or reducing compliance. Monitor progress at follow-up sessions by reviewing the steps taken toward goals. The three stages of progression for cardiovascular exercise programs are initial conditioning, improvement conditioning, and maintenance conditioning. Follow-up and monitoring allow you to give your clients regular feedback, judge the effectiveness of your prescriptions, and track trends that are invaluable for planning changes or progressions.

8. **Design warm-up and cool-down.**

The prescription model reaches full circle with this final step, the design of the warm-up and cool-down. The warm-up should increase heart rate, blood pressure, and oxygen consumption; dilate the blood vessels; and increase elasticity of muscle and connective tissue in a gradual fashion. The cool-down should gradually decrease the cardiac work and metabolism with low-level aerobic activity similar to the preceding aerobic segment.

Cardiovascular Prescription Card

Client name	Trainer name
Rory	JG

Client goals	Special considerations
• Safe, progressive annual program for 200 m sprint • Early portion of preseason, emphasize aerobic training, flexibility and strength balance, muscular endurance, and technical skill preparation	• Personal best in the 200 m = 24 s

Circulatory Warm-Up

Equipment and mode	Workload	Time	HR/PE objective
Track and park (treadmill in bad weather)	Light cross country pace (60-70% HRmax)	7-10 min + stretching (longer in competitive phase)	117-136 beats/min

Stretching Warm-Up

Name and brief description	Guidelines
• Combination of static and PNF stretching • Emphasis on hips and lower leg	• Vary with the current workout emphasis or injury

Cardiovascular Workout

Intensity/training range

Lower limit: 80% HRmax 156 beats/min _____ RPE _____ (METs)

Upper limit: 90% HRmax 175 beats/min _____ RPE _____ (METs)

	Equipment	Training method	Frequency	kcal/session
1	Track and park	Preparation phase (P): (a) continuous runs, Fartlek, or cross country runs; (b) ITP—higher volume	5×/week	NA
2	Track	Competitive phase (C): ITP—higher-intensity sprints including plyometrics	4×/week	NA

Phase	Workload	Time	Phase	Workload	Time
Warm-up			Warm-up		
Peak	(P) Continuous 75-80% HRmax, 150 beats/min	30-40 min	Peak		
Cool-down			Cool-down		

Interval Training Prescription

Set	Reps	Work time	(Relief time)	Ratio	Intensity
(P)1 (P)2	6 3	200 m at 40 s 400 m			60% of PB
(C)1	3	200 m at 26.6 s	1½ to 2 min walk (120-130 beats/min)	1:3 or 1:4 work-to-relief ratio	90% (PB) intensity

Progression and Monitoring

Three phases (weeks):

• (P) Preparation: work up to 70% of PB (34-35 s) in 5 to 6 weeks
• (C) Competition: increase intensity by 5% and decrease the volume by 10% (20 m for every 200 m) every 2 to 4 weeks
• (T) Transition: jog at family's cottage and play some recreational soccer

Cool-Down

Name and brief description	Guidelines
• Light jog • Combination of static and PNF stretching • Emphasis on hips and lower leg	• Vary with the current workout emphasis or injury

Note. HR = heart rate; PE = perceived exertion; HRR = heart rate reserve; $\dot{V}O_2R$ = $\dot{V}O_2$ reserve; PNF = proprioceptive neuromuscular facilitation; RPE = rating of perceived exertion; MET = metabolic equivalent; ITP = interval training program; NA = not applicable; PB = personal best.

Figure 6.8 Rory's cardiovascular prescription card.

Cardiovascular Prescription Card

Client name _____   Trainer name _____

Client goals	Special considerations

Circulatory Warm-Up

Equipment and mode	Workload	Time	HR/PE objective

Stretching Warm-Up

Name and brief description	Guidelines

Cardiovascular Workout

Intensity training range:

Lower limit: ____%HRR ($\dot{V}O_2R$) ___ beats/min ____ RPE _____ (METs)

Upper limit: ____%HRR ($\dot{V}O_2R$) ___ beats/min ____ RPE _____ (METs)

	Equipment	Training method	Frequency	kcal/session
1				
2				

Phase	Workload	Time	Phase	Workload	Time
Warm-up			Warm-up		
Peak			Peak		
Cool-down			Cool-down		

Interval Training Prescription

Set	Reps	Work time	(Relief time)	Ratio	Intensity

Progression and Monitoring

Phase (weeks):

Cool-Down

Name and brief description	Guidelines

Note. HR = heart rate; PE = perceived exertion; HRR = heart rate reserve; $\dot{V}O_2R$ = $\dot{V}O_2$ reserve; MET = metabolic equivalent; RPE = rating of perceived exertion.

From *Client-Centered Exercise Prescription, Second Edition,* by John C. Griffin, 2006, Champaign, IL: Human Kinetics.

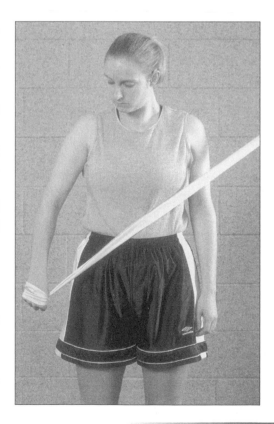

Client-Centered Resistance Training Prescription Model

7

Chapter Competencies

After completing this chapter, you will be able to demonstrate the following competencies:

1. Shape the resistance training overload to suit your client's objectives and training level.

2. Decide on the best type of resistance and equipment and the interface of equipment with the client.

3. Select the resistance training methods that will meet your client's needs, time constraints, experience, motivation, and level of condition.

4. Design a physiologically sound and client-centered exercise prescription for resistance training using the eight-step model of sequenced decisions.

   Step 1. Assess needs and formulate goals

   Step 2. Select resistance equipment

   Step 3. Select resistance training method

   Step 4. Select exercises and order of performance

   Step 5. Assign resistance intensity and weight

   Step 6. Establish resistance volume

   Step 7. Assign and monitor resistance progression

   Step 8. Design warm-up and cool-down

This chapter outlines an eight-step model for the design of a physiologically sound and client-centered exercise prescription for resistance training. Each step presents you with several choices. The correct amount of overload depends on your client's objectives and training level. The challenge is to shape the overload to suit your client by manipulating the prescription factors according to the principle of specificity—namely, that gains in muscular fitness are specific to the muscle group, training method, and exercise volume. After the client-centered prescription model is introduced, a case study illustrating its application is presented.

Principles of Client-Centered Resistance Training Prescription

Muscular strength is required for fitness, performance, health, and a good quality of life. Resistance training not only increases muscular strength but can also enhance muscle endurance, power, hypertrophy, and muscle balance. A number of principles will allow you to effectively design and implement a prescription for resistance training.

Specificity of Resistance Training

At the core of resistance training is the body's ability to adapt to the demands placed on it. The kinetic chain on which we place these demands will respond in a fashion that reflects the demands themselves. Knowing this in advance of our prescription design is a powerful tool. The desire to seek an adaptation, whether it is fitness related (muscle strength or endurance), health related (bone density or back care), or performance related (speed or power), is the primary motivation of most clients. The type of adaptation resulting from resistance training is related to the type of resistance, the metabolic demands, and the neuromuscular nature of the recruitment. These factors can be manipulated through prudent selection of appropriate exercises, prescription factors, machines, and training methods. The training benefit is directly related to the nature of the training. Your clients may desire enhanced muscle size, strength, power, balance, recoverability, movement pattern, rate of force production, energy system, tension through range of motion, or posture, and all of these can be enhanced with an appropriate prescription.

Facts About Strength Training

- Strength is the maximum force generated during muscle contractions.
- Strength can be exerted without joint movement (isometric) or with joint movement (isotonic).
- Power is the ability to exert strength quickly.
- Muscular endurance is the ability to apply force repeatedly or sustain a contraction for a period of time.
- Muscle hypertrophy refers to an increase in muscle size.
- A repetition is the completion of a designated movement through a full range of motion. A set is a specified number of repetitions attempted consecutively. Intensity is the power output of an exercise and is dependent on the resistance and the speed of the movement.
- Low-repetition, high-resistance weight training favors strength and hypertrophy gains.
- Low-resistance, high-repetition training favors muscular endurance gains and possibly some aerobic gains if rest periods are brief.
- High-speed specific tasks can enhance power outputs.
- With a concentric contraction, the muscle shortens as it exerts a force to overcome a resistance. With an eccentric contraction, the muscle lengthens as it exerts a force.
- A closed kinetic chain exercise involves the foot or hand being in contact with the ground or some other surface. The ankle, knee, and hip joints form the kinetic chain for the lower extremity. Here the forces begin at the ground and work their way up through each joint.

Factors in Muscle Conditioning Prescriptions

To be genuinely client-centered, you must control each prescription factor to meet specific client needs. Table 7.1, although only a guideline, shows how manipulation of prescription factors can affect the specificity of training effects.

Table 7.1 Prescription Factors for Resistance Training

Component factor	Preparation	Hypertrophy	Strength-hypertrophy	Strength	Strength-endurance
Intensity and load	Low 60-69% of 1RM	Moderate 70-76% of 1RM	Moderate–high 77-84% of 1RM	High 85-100% of 1RM	Low–moderate 60-69% of 1RM
Reps	13-20	9-12	6-8	1-6	13-20
Sets	1-4	3-5	3-5	2-4	1-3
Rest between sets	60-120 s	30-60 s	30-120 s	1.5-3 min	10-60 s
Frequency	2-3	5-6 (split)	5-6 (split)	5-6 (split)	3
Volume	Medium	High	Medium	Low	Medium–high

Adapted from S.J. Fleck & W.J. Kramer, 2004 and V. Heyward, 2002.

For example, a client interested in general conditioning may have a prescription outline as follows:

- **Goal and component need:** Fitness, general conditioning, strength–endurance
- **Equipment:** Stack weights and free weights
- **Training method:** Standard sets (i.e., set–rest–set)
- **Selection of exercises:** 10 to 12 basic exercises for all major muscle groups, plus selected exercises for areas of weakness or imbalance
- **Order:** Large-muscle, multijoint exercises (all sets) before small-muscle, single-joint exercises; lighter warm-up set for each large muscle exercise
- **Resistance intensity or loads:** Seventy percent of maximum
- **Resistance volume (sets, reps, frequency):** Two sets; 12 to 15 repetitions; 60 s rest between sets; slow–moderate speed; 3 days/week
- **Resistance progression and monitoring:** Increase repetitions up to 20; then increase load by 10% while reducing reps to 12; log workouts and reassess after 6 to 8 weeks.

The American College of Sports Medicine (2000) has guidelines for the development of muscular fitness in healthy adults. They include strength training of a moderate intensity, sufficient to develop and maintain a healthy level of fat-free weight (FFW). As a minimum, ACSM recommends 1 set of 8 to 12 repetitions of 8 to 10 exercises that condition the major muscle groups,

at least 2 to 3 days per week. Muscular strength and endurance are the most common component goals for fitness and health programs. More detail and further examples are discussed later this chapter (pp. 206-208).

Matching Resistance Equipment to the Client

When you prescribe resistance training, you must make some important decisions—in consultation with the client—about the best type of resistance and equipment and the interface of equipment with client (ergonomics).

Most fitness centers have several types of machines along with free weights and benches. Moreover, resistance equipment is increasingly popular in the home market. Any type of resistance will affect muscle conditioning. Table 7.2 summarizes the advantages and disadvantages of free weights and machines, but there are many other decisions you must make about the type of resistance. This section examines the advantages and client suitability of specific types of resistance: body weight, free weight, constant resistance, variable resistance, hydraulics and pneumatics, electronics, isokinetics, and others. The best workout for your client will include the equipment that meets his needs.

Body Weight

Body weight is the most versatile source of overload and is truly "client-centered"! It provides a load that often reflects the real demands placed on the body. Lifting your body weight or a segment of your body against gravity demands a concentric contraction of the muscles (i.e., shortening of

Table 7.2   Advantages and Disadvantages of Free Weights and Machines

Advantages	Disadvantages
Free weights	
• Weights can be tailored to specific demands of individual clients and permit unlimited variety of exercises. • Supporting muscles are also used, which should assist with muscle balance. • Free weights may be more effective in increasing muscle mass (O'Hagan et al. 1995).	• Safety is a consideration for the novice (i.e., proper execution and slippage). • A spotter is needed with heavier weights. • There is a learning curve where technique may initially impair performance.
Machines	
• Machines can isolate a single large muscle group. • Machines provide greater safety because they guide the movement, remove the concern for balance, and make it more difficult to use bad form. • Machines are easier to use than free weights, are appropriate for beginners, and guide clients through a full range of motion. • It's easy to change loads (e.g., pin placement). • The lifter can move quickly from one exercise to another; machines are well-suited for circuit training. • Certain machines may be able to adjust resistance to suit the force output, control resistance to suit the force output, control speed of movement, dictate type of muscle contraction, simulate a sport skill, or provide electronic feedback.	• Exercise is restricted to predetermined movement patterns (i.e., less versatility). • Exercise is restricted to predetermined joint angles. • Cost and space restrict home use. • Machines do not train balance of movement or supportive muscle action. • Machines do not teach coordinated power movements that are often needed for sports. • Many machines (especially home models) have insufficient adjustments to comfortably and safely fit a small or large client.

the muscle under tension). The lowering action involves an eccentric contraction of the same muscles (i.e., lengthening of the muscle under tension). Examples include chin-ups, dips, curl-ups, aerobic floor exercises, calisthenics, and plyometrics. The Gravitron is a specialized piece of equipment that uses a percentage of your body weight to do exercises such as chin-ups and dips. Body weight resistance is well-suited to clients recovering from an injury (chapter 11).

Free Weight

Dumbbells and barbells are probably the oldest and most easily understood forms of resistance. Bars come in 5-, 6-, and 7-ft (Olympic) lengths and are straight, cambered, or angled for arm curl work (EZ Curl). A stable adjustable-incline bench allows a large range of exercises and joint angles. Free weights may be the obvious choice for the client who has no access to a larger facility, has a limited budget, and has limited space at home. Free weights are also the method of choice for many bodybuilders interested in muscle isolation and hypertrophy. Free weights lend themselves to single-joint exercises such as the biceps curl and to multijoint exercises such as a squat. Free weights are categorized as constant resistance (i.e., weight

does not change through the range of motion). Although the load remains the same, the perception of effort changes as the biomechanical leverage changes through the range of motion. As with calisthenics, the muscles work concentrically when lifting and eccentrically when lowering. Safety is a consideration for the novice, such as when the client hits a sticking point with no spotter. Proper instruction and supervision are critical.

Machine Resistance

Beyond the debate between free weights and machines, you must understand the use, applications, and benefits of various machine resistance modalities. Generally, machines are safer to use and easier to learn and, if available, should be used to complement training programs at all levels.

Constant Resistance

Constant resistance machines generally duplicate free weight exercises and offer both concentric and eccentric contractions. Although the machine may alter the direction of motion required, the resistance is still the movement of weight against gravity. Popular machines include selectorized, multigym, plate-loaded, and pulleys. The cable system used simply redirects gravity, and with some cable crossover alignments a person can cut in half the stack resistance, permitting the exercise of smaller muscle groups in more gradual increments.

Variable Resistance

Variable resistance equipment is designed around the principle that the force a muscle produces during contraction is not constant. In fact, muscles produce the greatest force in the middle of the range of motion and the least force at either extreme (Wolkodoff 1989). Most often a cam-shaped pulley alters the effective resistance of the weight stack to match the strength curve of the muscle. Some believe that such equipment provides particularly high training efficiency: With optimal resistance through a full range of motion, the client can get an intense workout quickly. One of the difficulties with cam equipment is that no two people are alike in their muscle strength curves, so the machines are built for an average force curve. Nonetheless, many clients prefer the comfortable lift provided by variable resistance equipment. Devices such as springs, rubber bands, or sliding fulcrums increase the resistance through the range of motion, which is not how most muscles actually work. Through hands-on experience, you should get acquainted with the feel of different brands of variable resistance equipment. Also look for devices that limit range of motion and that allow users of different size to fit comfortably and safely. Equipment examples include Nautilus, David, Polaris, Cybex, and Eagle.

Hydraulics and Pneumatics

Alternatives to weight stacks include hydraulics and pneumatics. **Hydraulics** use a cylinder of compressed water or oil to vary the resistance. They offer concentric–concentric work where the muscles on one side of the joint raise the weight and the antagonist muscles on the other side of the joint pull it down. With both the agonist and antagonist working, these machines are efficient, because only half the number of machines is needed. One advantage is reduced muscle soreness for the novice exerciser; a disadvantage, however, is that many daily activities and sport skills involve eccentric contractions. **Pneumatics** use compressed air and make the muscle work eccentrically (i.e., the muscle is developing tension while it is being elongated). Hydraulic and pneumatic machines differ from weight stacks in that the client does not have to deal with overcoming the inertia of the weight or the momentum created once the machines are moving. These machines are quite safe, are good for higher-speed training, and can be adapted for clients interested in sport training. Hydra-Gym is a manufacturer of hydraulic equipment, and Keiser is an example of pneumatic equipment.

Electronics

Computerized equipment can offer a number of different exercise modes: isometrics, isotonics, or isokinetics. Such equipment usually has an integrated display panel, and the detail and immediacy of the feedback are very motivating.

Isokinetics

Isokinetic machines mechanically control the speed of movement. The resistance is accommodating and matches the force produced by the muscle group throughout the entire range of motion. Although some hydraulic and pneumatic machines simulate isokinetics, they allow some acceleration through the initial range of motion (O'Hagan et al. 1995). In contrast, electronic resistance machines, particularly dynamometers, provide true isokinetic conditions. Some electronic machines provide resistance only during concentric contractions, whereas others offer resistance during both concentric and eccentric phases. Advantages of isokinetic devices include accommodating forces, reduced muscle soreness (concentric only), display feedback, collection of data, high- or low-speed training, and development of muscular power, strength, and endurance (Heyward 2002). These devices also offer a great deal of safety, because resistance dissipates with the onset of pain, injury, or fatigue. Machines with high-speed settings are appropriate for clients training for sports with high-speed skills (e.g., football or track). Disadvantages include cost, accessibility, need for motivation, and a constant-speed action that is not natural to most activities. Equipment examples include Cybex, Orthotron, Omni-tron, and Kin-Com. On the low-tech/high-touch side, as a personal fitness trainer you can offer manual, accommodating resistance. However, this resistance cannot be precisely controlled.

Other

Other types of resistance are possible: elastic bands and tubing, water, and manual resistance.

- **Elastic.** Some home multigyms use various thicknesses of tubing as a basis of resistance. Surgical tubing or commercial bands (e.g., Dynaband) are popular and come in a variety of thicknesses that offer a range of resistance. The effective resistance increases as the device is elongated. By carefully positioning both your client and the secured end of the tubing, you can obtain a variety of movements and joint angles. For about two dollars, you can supply your client with a personal home gym or a hotel workout! Elastic has a short life, however—beware of breakage or release while bands are under tension. To extend their longevity, the bands need to be dusted with talcum powder after each use; place the bands in a bag, sprinkle with powder, and stir with your hand. Avoid exposing the bands to extended periods of sunlight, and store them in a cool, dry location.

- **Water.** In water, gravity and impact are not issues. Water controls speed and offers a natural, accommodating resistance. Your client can vary the resistance by trying different body segments, body positions, or specialty devices. The enveloping resistance allows for an endless combination of joint angles and simple and complex movements. The multiplane movements possible with water exercise are particularly appropriate for older clients and those with arthritis or joint problems. Community pools usually have an assortment of aquafit classes and other water activities with specialized instructors. However, you can also provide aquatic exercises using the resistance of the water. These may include calisthenic-type exercises or simulated weight training movements like squats, lunges, or arm raises. Aquatic resistance equipment worn on the arms or legs can increase intensity and resistance.

- **Manual resistance.** You can simulate many of the principles of exercise machines by working as a training partner. Knowing what muscles cause specific joint movements, you can position yourself to provide manual resistance. If the resistance is greater than your client's force, the contraction will be eccentric; if the resistance equals that of the client, the contraction will be isometric; if the resistance is less than the client's force, the contraction will be concentric. You can also control the speed of movement to simulate isokinetic training. With creativity, you can mold the nature of the resistance to the direct needs of the client.

Resistance Training Methods

You must select muscular conditioning methods that meet your client's needs, time constraints, experience, motivation, and level of condition. Your design can become quite distinctive when you manipulate prescription factors within a system.

Standard Set System

The standard set system consists of one (single set) or more sets (multiple set) of each exercise. This system usually demands 8 to 12 repetitions with a weight that elicits a point of momentary failure. A standard set system can be performed at any resistance, for any number of repetitions or sets, to match the client's goals. This system is very versatile, allowing the beginner and advanced client enough variation to suit their needs. Novice exercisers can use either single- or multiple-set programs for the first 3 to 4 months, but data indicate that for continued progress, multiple-set programs should be used (ACSM 2002).

Pyramid System

The pyramid system begins by working a specific muscle group using a relatively light weight so that about 10 to 12 repetitions can be performed. After each set the weight is increased so that fewer and fewer repetitions can be done, until only 1 or 2 repetitions can be performed. The resistance is then progressively decreased each set, and the session ends with a set of 10 to 12 repetitions (e.g., table 7.3). The system can be modified to include any number of reps for the desired number of sets and is favored by many bodybuilders for its potential hypertrophy gains. The first half of the pyramid is called the **light-to-heavy system**. The reverse **heavy-to-light system** is preferred over the former in producing strength gains (Fleck and Kraemer 2004). For an example, see table 7.3.

Superset System

The superset system uses several sets of two exercises performed one after the other with little or no rest. The two exercises are for the same body part but for antagonistic muscles. For example, you might follow a bench press with rowing exercise, arm curls with triceps extensions, or leg curls

Table 7.3 Pyramid System

Sets	Reps	Weight
1	10	
1	8	
1	6	
1	4	
1	1-2	
1	4	
1	6	
1	8	
1	10	

with leg extensions. Have your client rest for 1 or 2 min after both exercises are complete and then complete the remaining 2 to 5 sets. The repetitions are usually limited to 8 to 10. Supersets can lead to significant increases in strength (Riley 1982), and, if your client is fit and motivated, he can reduce his workout time by including more exercises in a given training session.

A variation of the superset system uses 1 set of several exercises for the same muscle group performed one after another with little rest. For example, this may include bench press, military press, and incline flys, or one set of lat (latissimus dorsi) pull-down, seated rowing, and bent-over rowing. This variation is also effective in improving muscular strength and hypertrophy.

Table 7.4 prescribes a sample superset program. Your client should do the first set of exercise 1(a), followed immediately by the first set of exercise 1(b). Have him rest 1 to 2 min and then go on to second sets of 1(a) and 1(b). Follow this format for the prescribed number of sets and reps.

Table 7.4   Superset Program

Exercises	Reps (sets)	Exercises	Reps (sets)
1(a) Leg extensions (quadriceps)	10-8-6 (3)	4(a) Bench press (pectoralis major)	10-8-6 (3)
1(b) Leg flexions (hamstrings)	10-8-6 (3)	4(b) Lat pull-down (latissimus dorsi)	10-8-6 (3)
2(a) Resisted hip abduction (hip abductors)	10-8/leg (2)	5(a) Dumbbell flys (anterior deltoid and pectoralis major)	10-8 (2)
2(b) Resisted hip adduction (hip adductors)	10-8/leg (2)	5(b) Reverse flys (posterior deltoid and latissimus dorsi)	15-15 (2)
3(a) Standing toe raise— calf machine (gastrocnemius)	8 to 12 (1)	6(a) Standing barbell curl (biceps)	10-8 (2)
3(b) Seated barbell toe raise (soleus)	15 to 20 (1)	6(b) Dips (triceps)	up to 15 (2)

Compound or Tri-Set System

A compound set involves two exercises, and a tri-set is a group of three exercises for the same body part, one done after another with little or no rest between exercises or sets. Use tri-sets to work three different muscle groups, to work the same muscle from three different angles, or to work the same area of the muscle (from the same angle). Three sets of each exercise are usually performed. Fleck and Kraemer (2004) reported that tri-sets are good systems to increase local muscular endurance. A tri-set might include lateral raises, arm curls, and triceps extensions all working the upper arms and shoulder area but distinctly different muscles. A tri-set for the same muscle group (different angles) may comprise decline flys, bench presses, and incline flys. This can be a useful change of pace for a client who has hit a training plateau.

Plyometrics

Although weight training can produce gains in strength, the speed of movement is limited. Because power combines strength and speed, many athletes need to decrease the amount of time it takes to produce muscular force. A form of training that combines speed of movement with strength is plyometrics.

Principles of Plyometrics

Plyometric training involves rapid eccentric lengthening of a muscle followed immediately by rapid concentric contraction of that muscle to produce a forceful explosive movement. The increase in explosive power comes in part from the storage of elastic energy within the prestretched connective tissue tendon. The concentric contraction can be magnified only if the preceding eccentric contraction is of a short range and is performed quickly and without delay (Voight and Tippett 1994). Plyometrics emphasizes this speed of the eccentric phase and control in dynamic movements.

Examples of plyometric exercises for the lower extremity include hops, bounds, and depth jumping. In depth jumping, your client jumps to the ground from a specified height and then quickly jumps again as soon as she makes ground contact. For the upper extremity, you can prescribe medicine balls or other weighted equipment.

Sample Plyometric Circuit

One benefit of plyometric training is that it can be organized into circuits. The program shown in figure 7.1 describes a high-volume circuit designed to improve both vertical and linear power patterns (Chu 1992).

Guidelines for Using Plyometrics

Plyometrics is a very valuable tool, but you must use it judiciously according to your client's tolerance. Demonstrate all movements, provide adequate recovery, avoid overtraining, and match the activity to your client's abilities. The following guidelines will help you avoid injuries and maximize your client's improvement:

- Precede each workout with an extended warm-up and gradual buildup. Plyometrics involves a lot of eccentric (i.e., ballistic) actions, and the muscles must be stretched and exposed to light eccentric movements in the warm-up.
- Remember that the greater the intensity, the longer the recovery. This guideline applies both between sets during the workout and between workouts.
- Emphasize proper technique and explosive intensity. Stop the exercise if your client's form begins to fail.
- Train specific movement patterns for specific activities.
- Modify prescription factors for progressive overloads by increasing the number of exercises, increasing the number of repetitions or sets, or decreasing the rest periods between sets. Discourage use of ankle or wrist weights because they may cause excessive momentum.
- Carefully observe, monitor, and test your client to gain important feedback for motivation and progression.
- Assign a frequency of no more than three times per week in the preseason (higher volume) and less during the season (higher intensity).
- At the end of a workout, use a plyometrics segment that is shorter and less stressful than that at the beginning, because your client is partially fatigued.

Circuit Weight Training System

Chapter 6 described circuit training under *Other Aerobic Training Methods* (p. 165). Circuit weight training consists of a series of resistance exercises in a multiple station system: approximately 10 to 15 repetitions of each exercise, at a resistance of 40% to 60% of maximum (RM), with 15 to

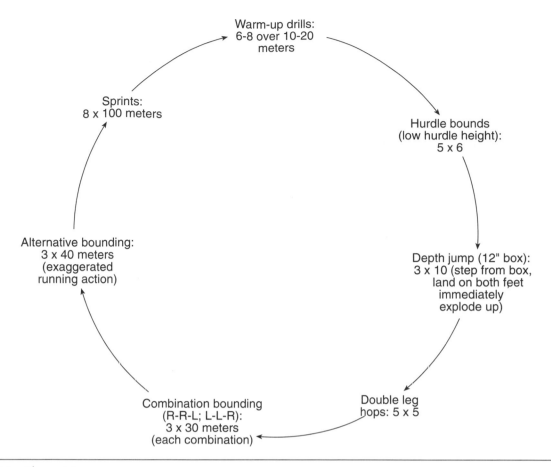

Figure 7.1   Plyometrics program.

30 s rest between exercises (Fleck and Kraemer 2004). Design the circuit to meet specific goals or use available equipment. This is a very efficient method of developing strength and endurance (with some aerobic and calorie-burning benefits). It can be a good way to add variety to traditional cardiovascular training and resistance training. Heyward (2002) presents a sample circuit weight training program in figure 7.2.

Systems That Are Extended Forms of Other Systems

Some systems of resistance training are extensions of other systems or can be used within an existing system. They allow further manipulation of the prescription factors that allow individual needs to be addressed. The following are examples of such extensions.

Split Routine System

Developing hypertrophy is a time-consuming process for bodybuilders. Not all body parts can be covered in one training session. The split routine system trains various body parts on alternate days—arms, legs, and abdomen on 3 days per week, for example, and chest, shoulders, and back on alternate days. Variations in this example may allow a reduction of training days. Calder and colleagues (1994) found that split routines (four sessions/week) produced results that were similar to whole routines (two sessions/week) over 5 months of training. The increased time for recovery helps reduce overuse injuries and overtraining and allows for a more intense training level.

Exhaustion Set System

Momentary failure is the point at which another full repetition is not possible—that is, the set has been done to exhaustion. You can incorporate sets to exhaustion into almost any training system. This system appears to recruit a large number of motor units and to produce significant strength gains (Baechle and Earle 2000). An added "burn" can be achieved by performing 5 or 6 partial repetitions after exhaustion.

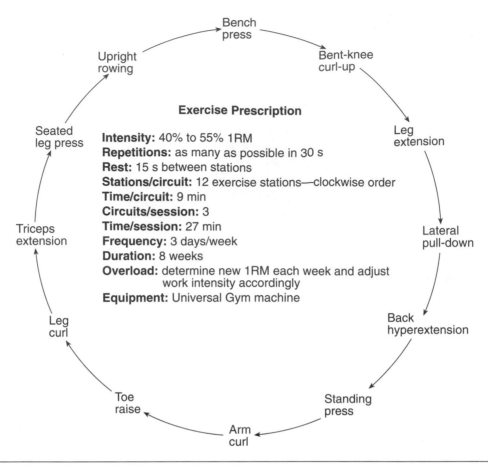

Exercise Prescription

Intensity: 40% to 55% 1RM
Repetitions: as many as possible in 30 s
Rest: 15 s between stations
Stations/circuit: 12 exercise stations—clockwise order
Time/circuit: 9 min
Circuits/session: 3
Time/session: 27 min
Frequency: 3 days/week
Duration: 8 weeks
Overload: determine new 1RM each week and adjust work intensity accordingly
Equipment: Universal Gym machine

Figure 7.2   Circuit weight training.

Reprinted, by permission, from V. Heyward, 2002, *Advanced fitness assessment and exercise prescription,* 4th ed. (Champaign, IL: Human Kinetics), 141.

The weight used to reach momentary failure is called a repetition maximum (RM). If eight repetitions of 150 lb (68 kg) are done to exhaustion, the 8RM is 150 lb. If you have assessed your client's 1RM (chapter 4), the following chart can estimate a prescription for intensity (% of 1RM) and number of repetitions that will elicit momentary failure (Fleck and Kraemer 2004, Heyward 2002):

60% 1 RM = 15 to 20 RM (i.e., 15-20 repetitions to exhaustion at 60% 1RM)

65% 1RM = 14RM

70% 1RM = 12RM

75% 1RM = 10RM

80% 1RM = 8RM

85% 1RM = 6RM

90% 1RM = 4RM

95% 1RM = 2RM

100% 1RM =1RM

Forced Repetition System

The forced repetition system allows you to work very closely with your client. After a set to exhaustion, help your client determine just the amount of weight that will permit her to do 3 or 4 additional repetitions. By demanding stimulation from a partially fatigued muscle, this approach is well suited to clients who want increased strength and muscular endurance.

Periodization

Periodization is characterized by systematic cycles of alternating prescription variables such as intensity and volume (Fleck 1999). This provides the necessary recovery time for certain muscle fibers while other fibers are overloaded. Nonlinear (undulating) periodization creates different exercise stimuli to provide variation and challenge. This concept of periodization allows you to vary intensity and volume within each 14-day training cycle by rotating different exercise protocols (Kraemer 2003). Compared with using the same repetition maximum for every workout or a lower-volume circuit design,

Table 7.5 Undulating Periodization Program

	Monday	Wednesday	Friday
Sets	3-5	3-4	5-6
Reps	6-12	12-20	2-5
Intensity/load (% of 1RM)	70-80	60-70	80-100
Rest and recovery (min)	1-2	<1	2-5

the nonlinear periodization program has shown significant superiority during a 6-month training period (Marx et al. 2001). Sorace and LaFontaine (2005) suggested using an undulating periodization program to train strength, hypertrophy, and endurance within the same cycle (table 7.5).

The Resistance Exercise Prescription Model

A resistance prescription can stand alone or can be incorporated into a cardiovascular or weight loss prescription for a number of supportive health, fitness, and performance benefits. Table 7.6 outlines an eight-step model for the design of a physiologically sound and client-centered exercise prescription for resistance training. Each step involves choices that you must make, and the table lists many of these choices. Following a brief background to each of the steps, a sample case study is presented including the choices that were made for the client.

Step 1: Assess Needs and Formulate Goals

Client needs may be related to health (low bone density or low back pain), fitness (strength and endurance), performance (sport-specific power or occupational fitness), or education (e.g., regarding diet and supplements). Your client's motivation could also be appearance (hypertrophy, weight loss or gain) or rehabilitation (injury and posture). Client needs can also be defined by results of fitness assessments (sit-ups/% 1RM), by lack of self-esteem, or by special designs necessitated by physical limitations or high-performance demands.

As discussed in chapter 1, goal setting is the process of specifying what needs to be done, when and how to do it, and what the anticipated outcomes will be. It is often easier to begin with long-term goals that are more global and then formulate several shorter-term goals that could be accomplished before major changes in assessment measures such as maximal lifts, change in body contours, or target weight gain. You can play a vital role by helping your client set realistic, measurable goals and then recording outcomes. Physical goals may need to be preceded by activity integration goals relating to flexibility in the program design, purchase of home equipment, or time management. As well, be sensitive to your client's preferences and expectations regarding outcomes, style of assistance, venue selection, and choice of equipment or training method.

Table 7.6 Resistance Exercise Prescription Model

Decisions	Choices
1. Assess needs and formulate goals	• Limitation (e.g., risk, injury) • Design (e.g., time, facility, equipment) • Health, fitness, appearance • Motivational strategy and personality—learning style • Strength, hypertrophy, muscular endurance, power • Functional needs (muscular balance, posture, occupation) • Rehabilitation • Weight loss or gain • Preferences and expectations (e.g., equipment, venue, outcomes)

(continued)

Table 7.6 *(continued)*

Decisions	Choices
2. Select resistance equipment	• Equipment (and brand) pros and cons • Constant, variable, accommodating resistance • Free weights, machines • Bands, tubes, balls, boards • Equipment features (e.g., range of motion limits, pivot locations)
3. Select resistance training method	• Standard (simple) sets • Circuit • Super sets • Compound sets or tri-sets • Pyramids (ascending or descending) • Split routine • Negatives (forced repetition) • Plyometrics
4. Select exercises and order of performance	• Large to small muscle groups • Multijoint to single joint • Agonist–antagonist (alternating push and pull) • Upper body–lower body (alternating) • Stabilizers (e.g., trunk) later in order • Complex or sport-specific exercises • Open or closed chain, functional • Exercises in more than one plane • Overdevelopment of unnecessary areas • Balanced, unbalanced (e.g., more front than back exercises) • Weak, high-need areas first • Coordinated with training method
5. Assign resistance intensity and weight	• Based on goal (e.g., strength, hypertrophy) • Established from assessment or during demo (e.g., percent of 1RM [relative intensity] or trial and error [5-10RM]) • Interdependent with volume (sets × reps × load) • Match reps to load (based on goals) • Momentary failure for trained clients (greater neural activity) • Large muscle groups may require higher percent 1RM
6. Establish resistance volume	• Sets × reps × load = volume • See table 7.8: "Volume Comparison" • Rest between sets reflects objective, size of muscle group, and reps × load • Time under tension (e.g., slower movements) • Time under tension for workout affected by rest time • Minimum 2-3/week
7. Assign and monitor resistance progression	• Volume first, intensity second • One volume factor modified at a time: (Example 1: increase reps: 2 × 12-15; then 3 × 10); (Example 2 (strength): 2 × 12 at 100; then 3 × 8 at 110; then 4 × 6 at 120) • 5% increase in load tolerable (when upper limit of reps met) • Minimum length of program 6 weeks • Periodization stages used when program duration is longer • Monitoring used to cue progression timing • Related to client's objectives (motivation) • Follow-up checks established (objective, subjective) • Primary safety precautions and execution mechanics listed and demonstrated
8. Design warm-up and cool-down	• Cardiovascular warm-up and cool-down transitions • Specific joint and muscle stretching • Suits nature of the prescription and special client considerations

Step 2: Select Resistance Equipment

Earlier in this chapter, we examined various types of resistance and how to match resistance equipment to the client. Your choices for type of resistance and equipment may be limited by various venues in which you train. It is often helpful to think in terms of selecting the equipment to cover the following body areas. For example:

- Chest (e.g., bench press, supine flys, pec deck)
- Upper back (e.g., lat pull-down, rowing, cable crossover)
- Shoulders (e.g., lateral arm raises, shoulder press)
- Arms (e.g., curls, extensions)
- Front thigh (e.g., leg press, knee extension)
- Back thigh (e.g., knee curl, deadlift)
- Calf (e.g., toe raise)

If you are setting up a training area in your own home or advising your client, your equipment list should include the following:

- Dumbbells (with at least a flat and incline bench)—good for isolation and smaller muscle groups
- Barbells (benches should have spotting racks)
- Olympic bar lifting—for more serious bodybuilders

Sometimes rather simple equipment can provide great benefit in return for very low cost:

- Pulley systems (high and low, fixed and swivel base), which allow versatile movements; good for rehab
- Bands and tubing—similar benefits as pulleys
- Body weight apparatus (e.g., chin-up bar, dips, stall bars, mats)
- Other small equipment (e.g., medicine or plyo balls, body bars, wobble boards, Theraballs, balance discs, Bosu trainer, wrist and ankle weights, boxing gloves and shields)

Step 3: Select Resistance Training Method

Your selection of resistance training method is important in shaping the prescription to meet your client's needs, time constraints, experience, motivation, and level of condition. Your design can become quite distinctive when you manipulate prescription factors within a given system.

Training methods such as standard sets, pyramid, circuit, supersets, compound or tri-sets, plyometrics, and others were covered earlier in this chapter.

Step 4: Select Exercises and Order of Performance

Knowing the purpose and benefit of each exercise can help maintain muscle balance and avoid overworking a particular body area. Keep in mind physical limitations, past injuries, and conditions such as hypertension. In most cases, and certainly with novice clients, order your selection of specific exercises (muscle groups) to meet the following criteria:

- Choose successive exercises that do not involve the same muscle group.
- Prescribe large-muscle, multiple-joint exercises (e.g., bench press, squat) to precede small-muscle, single-joint, isolation exercises (e.g., biceps curl, crunch). This will avoid early fatigue and poor performance later in the workout.
- Work areas of weakness or imbalance while your client is still fresh.
- Prioritize sport-specific movements for athletes.
- Choose exercises that are functional for the demands on the client; these often include exercises in more than one plane.
- For the large-muscle exercises, have the client perform a warm-up set with less weight.
- Prescribe one exercise for each muscle group that maintains agonist–antagonist and bilateral symmetry, which promotes a balanced development and helps prevent overuse injuries. For example, a frequent cause of shoulder rotator cuff injury is overtraining of the upper chest muscles and undertraining of the upper back and posterior shoulder muscles.
- Include stabilizers (e.g., lower spine muscles) later in the session.
- Choose exercises that complement the training method (which may be counter to some of these guidelines).

Step 5: Assign Resistance Intensity and Weight

Generally, as the intensity or load (weight) is increased, there is an increase in the motor unit activation. This results, over a period of training, in an increased force production as measured by strength or power. Encouraging trained clients to reach the muscle's threshold (momentary failure) increases the neural activity and speeds the training results. Training intensity is a critical prescription factor providing the stimulus needed for improvement in specific muscular components (table 7.7).

Without knowledge of 1RMs for each exercise, you can use an educated trial and error to determine the training zone intensity. Choose a weight that your client can do 6 repetitions to failure. This will give you a 6RM and a weight to begin strength training.

Step 6: Establish Resistance Volume

Exercise volume is one of the most important prescription factors. The intensity or load must be heavy enough to cause temporary discomfort and momentary muscle fatigue. For combined strength and endurance improvements, the resistance should be about 75% of the maximum load your client is able to lift. Baechle and Earle (2000) indicated that most people can complete 8 to 12 repetitions with about 75% load. If your client is a beginner or is training at high intensity, 1 or 2 sets are sufficient to produce excellent benefits. Prescribe a frequency of 3 days per week for strength development. At least 2 days per week are necessary for maintenance. Detraining will occur when frequency is less than 1 day per week.

Volume is often described as sets × reps × load. However, the rest between the sets and the speed of the movements all contribute to total "time under tension," which is a more complete measure of volume. The length of time you are actually working with the resistance is the time under tension. Longer rests (>3 min) may be needed to replace creatine kinase during high-

intensity strength training with larger muscle groups (Larson et al. 1997).

It is interesting to compare a prescription for hypertrophy with one for a more traditional strength–endurance component (table 7.8). Although the load is only 10% higher for hypertrophy and the rest between sets is comparable, the total lifts per workout are quite a bit greater and the lifts per week are substantially more.

Table 7.8 Volume Comparison: Hypertrophy Versus Strength–Endurance

Component factor	Hypertrophy	Strength–endurance
Intensity and load	Moderate 70-76% of 1RM	Low–moderate 60-69% of 1RM
Reps	9-12	13-20
Sets	3-5	1-3
Rest between sets	30-60 s	10-60 s
Frequency	5-6 (split)	3
Volume	High	Medium–high

In a full component workout, time is needed for a warm-up, aerobic activity, resistance work, and a cool-down. Depending on the type and availability of equipment, the time devoted to resistance training will limit the number of reps and sets and the number of exercises selected. For example, in a 30 min lunchtime workout, your client may only have 10 min for resistance work versus a 60 min session allowing perhaps 25 min for resistance work (table 7.9).

For more serious athletes, "periodization" is used in their long-term training plans. Periodization systematically varies the volume and intensity of training over units of training called mesocycles that last for a few weeks to several months (Bompa 1999). Most often, training volume progressively decreases as the intensity increases. This changes

Table 7.7 Intensity/Load

Component factor	Preparation	Hypertrophy	Strength–hypertrophy	Strength	Strength–endurance
Intensity and load	Low 60-69% of 1RM	Moderate 70-76% of 1RM	Moderate–high 77-84% of 1RM	High 85-100% of 1RM	Low–moderate 60-69% of 1RM

Table 7.9   Length of Resistance Workout

30 min workout	45 min workout	60 min workout
10 min resistance	15-20 min resistance	25 min resistance
4-5 exercises (1 set)	4-5 exercises (2 sets) or 6-8 exercises (1 set)	6-8 exercises (2 sets)

the training stimulus through each of the mesocycles and has been shown to provide peak strength and power performances at times appropriate for the competitions (Stone et al. 1999).

Step 7: Assign and Monitor Resistance Progression

The universal principle of conditioning is **progressive overload,** that is, a periodic increase in workload that increasingly overloads the muscle group. The correct amount of overload depends on your client's objectives and training level. The challenge is to shape the overload to suit your client by manipulating the prescription factors according to the principle of specificity—namely, that gains in muscular fitness are specific to the muscle group, training method, and exercise volume.

If your client is doing resistance work at least twice a week, you need to change (increase) the overload each week when possible. For example, table 7.10 shows a progressive overload at a given weight appropriate for strength and endurance gains (e.g., 70% 1RM).

To ensure safe and effective progression, modify only one volume factor at a time. For example:

1. Increase reps: 2 × 12-15; then 3 × 10-15.
2. Increase intensity: 2 × 12 at 100; then 3 × 8 at 110; then 4 × 6 at 120.

The following guidelines will assist you in monitoring progress:

- Clients interested in strength gains will continually want to increase their load.

- Monitoring girth measures will track gains in hypertrophy.
- Clients working on strength–endurance should increase their reps up to about 15 and then increase the load and drop the reps back down. As their condition improves, they may decrease the rest between sets.
- *A 5% to 10% increase in load is very tolerable (when upper limit of reps is met).*
- Clients working on muscular endurance should use repetitions or sets (volume) as a method of progression. Decreasing rest time between sets can further challenge this component.
- Monitoring total poundage per workout will easily demonstrate improved work capacity.
- Program cards that allow quick recording of these factors can save time and encourage regular recording.
- A minimum length of program is usually 6 weeks.
- *You should visually monitor primary safety precautions and execution mechanics.*

Step 8: Design Warm-Up and Cool-Down

The warm-up and cool-down should reflect the type and magnitude of the work done in the resistance training portion.

In the warm-up, introduce and progress low-impact movements to raise temperature and heart rate. After some warming, statically stretch the muscle groups to be used in the workout. Add supplemental stretches if muscles are tight or sore or if you expect higher intensity than usual. If workout is to be high eccentric, build eccentric overloading gradually.

In the cool-down, relieve muscle tightness that may result from eccentric work (e.g., in quadriceps, calves, chest, and erector spinae). Stretch tight postural muscles (e.g., anterior chest, hip flexors, hamstrings).

Table 7.10   Progressive Overload

Week	1	2	3	4
Set 1–Set 2	12 reps–12 reps	13 reps–12 reps	14 reps–13 reps	15 reps–14 reps

Case Studies

Michael was a 38-year-old male with little experience in resistance training. He was interested in feeling better and gaining general conditioning for the whole body but was particularly concerned with his upper body posture and poor abdominal tone.

Assessment

The assessment provided me with the following data:

- Weight: 85 kg (187 lb)
- Height: 180 cm (5 ft 11 in.)
- BMI: 26.2
- Resistance exercises: 10RM established for each exercise and 1RM estimated
- Circuit time: Initial time recorded for 2 circuits (10 reps) including 2 min rest between cycles

Counseling revealed that Michael was at a preparation stage. He had purchased a membership at the local YMCA and although his time was tight, he thought that he could spend 40-45 min two to three times per week. There were no overt health or musculoskeletal limitations; however, his technique during the 10RM assessments was consistent with a novice motor knowledge level.

We agreed to use some equipment that seemed appealing to Michael and complement those pieces with others that could form a circuit centered around his goals.

Resistance Training Prescription

Most of the equipment selected was variable resistance, and Michael found it quite smooth. There was a minimum of weight stack adjustment from station to station in the circuit. The equipment that Michael had chosen fit easily into the circuit. Most of the exercises were multijoint with some isolations for posture and trunk. They alternated lower body to upper body with a balance of agonist to antagonist. Precautions were listed on the program card. The abdominal and core work on the stability ball was done after the circuit and was one of Michael's favorites. The intensity (weight) and volume (sets and reps) were based on the preparation stage and his 10RM assessment. A training log was kept reflecting these primary prescription factors and Michael's subjective feelings. The progression was "volume" based, building reps from 13 up to 20 (momentary failure) then going to 3 sets of 15 (up to 20). Because of a lack of time, the stretches within the warm-up and cool-down included specific postural stretches. Details of the prescription are on the Resistance Training Prescription Card (figure 7.3).

Resistance Training Prescription Card

Client Name Michael	Trainer Name John
Client Goals	**Special Considerations**
Preparation stage—concerned with upper-body posture, abdominal tone, and feeling better.	General fitness needs—whole body • local YMCA 2-3 × per week • 40-45 min—time efficient

Circulatory Warm-Up

Equipment and Mode	Workload	Time	HR/PE Objective
Treadmill	Moderate to brisk walk; gradually increase speed	5-7 min	HR: 100-110 beats/min RPE: 11-12

Stretching Warm-Up

Stretches to include	Guidelines
• Four to six stretches for lower body after treadmill, including low back, hip flexors, hip extensors, and calf and shin muscles • One stretch each for the chest, upper back and shoulders, triceps, biceps, and hip adductors and abductors in preparation for the circuit • Stretches for pectoralis minor and shoulder medial rotators to maintain or improve posture	• Static stretches after treadmill • Hold for 15-20 s • Between the two circuit sets, redo any of the warm-up stretches of muscles that feel tight *(continued)*

Figure 7.3   Resistance training prescription card.

Resistance Workout

Equipment type (e.g., free weights)	Training method
• Selectorized equipment (variable resistance) • Theraball	• Modified circuit with standard (simple) sets • Mainly multijoint exercises, some isolations for posture and trunk

Guidelines

- Circuit fashion (i.e., perform all exercises once and then do second set)
- Rest 2 min between circuits
- 10RM established in each exercise

Exercise (brief description)	Muscles	Intensity/weight	Reps	Sets	Rest between sets	Precautions
1. Leg press (seated) 	Quadriceps, hamstrings, gluteus maximus	65-70% of 1RM	10-13	2	30 s	• Maintain alignment • Avoid full knee extension
2. Bench press 	Pectoralis major, anterior deltoid, triceps	65-70% of 1RM	10-13	2	30 s	• Use soft elbows • Avoid bounce at bottom of ROM
3. Hamstrings curl 	Hamstrings	65-70% of 1RM	10-13	2	30 s	• Stabilize low back • Maintain form even with low ROM
4. Lat pull-down 	Latissimus dorsi, pectoralis major	65-70% of 1RM	10-13	2	30 s	• Lower to top of sternum and squeeze scapulae
5. Leg abductor–adductor 	Hip abductors and adductors	65-70% of 1RM	10-13	2	30 s	• Use slow and controlled movements
6. Seated row 	Posterior deltoid, trapezius, biceps	65-70% of 1RM	10-13	2	30 s	• Squeeze scapulae together
7. Abdominal curls and twists on ball 	Rectus abdominis, obliques, spinal stabilizers	Body weight	3 × 7 (left, front, right)	2	30 s	• Maintain stable core and breathing • Keep ball on low back

Figure 7.3 *(continued)*

Progression
• Build reps from 13 up to 20 (momentary failure) then go to 3 sets of 15 (up to 20)—"volume overload." • Use log provided to record load, reps, sets, volume, and subjective feelings. • Retest 10RM in 4 weeks.

Cool-Down

Name and brief description	Guidelines
Repeat warm-up stretches.	Hold static stretches for 15-20 s.

Note. HR = heart rate; PE = perceived exertion; RPE = rating of perceived exertion; ROM = range of motion.

Figure 7.3   *(continued)*.

Justification of Michael's Resistance Training Prescription

When we design an exercise prescription, we must integrate principles of exercise science and training with the psychosocial factors of our clients and the circumstances affecting their exercise prescription. Every decision made should be based on a sound physiological justification and a rationale that is client-centered. Table 7.11 provides the critical thinking that was involved in Michael's resistance training prescription.

Table 7.11   Justification of Resistance Training Sample Prescription

Decision	Physiological justification	Client-centered rationale
1. Assess needs and formulate goals	• Client has no overt limitations. • Modified circuit will allow efficient use of time and cover whole body. • Major muscles are included. • Weaker phasic muscles (e.g., rhomboids, lower traps, abdominals) need to be strengthened.	• Length and difficulty of program suit exercise and time. • Rounded shoulders and lumbar lordosis stated as concern (exercises 6 and 7).
2. Select resistance equipment	• Multijoint exercise is more functional and efficient for only six exercises. • Choice is suitable for client's comfort and motor knowledge. • Choice provides variable resistance and smooth strength curve. • Equipment provides stabilization for novice.	• Exercises are suited to goals and time. • Equipment is readily available at YMCA. • Station switch is quick and easy.
3. Select resistance training method	• Standard sets are provided in a circuit format. • Choice is good for prep stage. • Time under tension is maximized with circuit.	• Program is fast moving, should keep interest.
4. Select exercise and order of performance	• Lower body to upper body is worked alternately. • Agonist–antagonist muscles are worked (Exercises #1 & 3, 2-4) • See specific exercise justification.	• Exercises suit circuit and there is ample recovery time. • Feedback on execution mechanics ensures personal safety and benefits.
Exercise 1	• Hip and knee extensors	• Balance with 3.
Exercise 2	• Anterior shoulder and chest (horizontal adduction of shoulder and extension of elbow)	• Balance with 4.
Exercise 3	• Knee flexors	• Balance with 1.
Exercise 4	• Posterior and anterior shoulders (adduction of shoulder and flexion of elbow)	• Balance with 2.

Decision	Physiological justification	Client-centered rationale
Exercise 5	• Outer and inner thigh (concentric in and out)	• 1-5 involve whole body
Exercise 6	• Posterior shoulders (horizontal abduction of shoulders and retraction of scapula)	• Strengthens weaker muscles to address rounded shoulders
Exercise 7	• Trunk flexors and rotators	• Client goal: abdominal tone, core stability and mobility
5. Assign resistance intensity and weight	• Resistance intensity and weight are established from assessment (i.e., 10RM is close to starting load). • Load is fine-tuned in the demonstration. • Resistance intensity and weight are interdependent with volume (sets × reps × load).	• Segment is based on preparation stage and goals (i.e., posture and abdominal tone)
6. Establish resistance volume	• Initial overload is focused on volume. • Momentary failure peaks neural stimulation. • Choice supports load setting.	• Volume is best for a beginner. • Circuit allows recovery (rest between sets). • Minimum frequency of 2 ×/week is possible.
7. Assign and monitor resistance progression	• Reps and sets (volume) adjust one factor at a time. • Training log reflects primary prescription factors. • Program provides for retesting "load" and readiness for next stage.	• Program is steady but reasonable and allows self-administration. • Review of subjective feeling is a good predictor of compliance. • Program is related to client's motivation type.
8. Design warm-up and cool-down	• Cardiovascular warm-up raises muscle temperature. • Specific joint and muscle stretching is provided for resistance exercises.	• Segment suits special client considerations (e.g., postural stretches).

Highlights

1. **Shape the resistance training overload to suit your client's objectives and training level.**

   The most suitable overload involves manipulating the prescription factors of resistance training according to the principle of specificity—namely, that gains in muscular fitness are specific to the muscle group, training method, and exercise volume. At the core of resistance training is the body's ability to adapt to the demands made on it. The desire to seek an adaptation, whether it is fitness related (muscle strength or endurance), health related (bone density or back care), or performance related (speed or power), is the primary motivation of most clients. To be genuinely client-centered, you must control each prescription factor to meet specific client needs (table 7.1).

2. **Decide on the best type of resistance and equipment and the interface of equipment with the client.**

   Specific types of resistance include body weight, free weights, constant resistance, variable resistance, hydraulics and pneumatics, electronics, isokinetics, and others. Body weight remains the most versatile source of overload and is truly client-centered. Dumbbells and barbells are probably the oldest and most easily understood forms of resistance. Proper instruction and supervision are critical. Generally, machines are safer to use and easier to learn than free weights. Variable resistance equipment is designed around the principle that the force a muscle produces during contraction is not constant. Most often a cam-shaped pulley alters the effective resistance of the weight stack to match the strength curve of the muscle. Alternatives to weight stacks include hydraulics and pneumatics. Isokinetic machines mechanically control the speed of movement. Other types of resistance are possible: elastic bands and tubing, water, and manual resistance.

3. **Select the resistance training methods that will meet your client's needs, time constraints, experience, motivation, and level of condition.**

   The standard set system consists of one (single-set) or more sets (multiple-set) of each exercise. A standard set system can be performed at any resistance, for any number of repetitions or sets, to match the goals of the client. With the pyramid system, the client begins using a relatively light weight and after each set increases the weight so that fewer repetitions can be done, until only one or two repetitions can be performed. The resistance is then progressively decreased each set. The superset system uses several sets of two exercises performed one after the other with little or no rest. A compound set involves two exercises, and a tri-set is a group of three exercises for the same body part, one done after another. A form of training that combines speed of movement with strength is plyometrics. Plyometric training comprises rapid eccentric lengthening of a muscle followed immediately by rapid concentric contraction of that muscle to produce a forceful explosive movement. Circuit weight training consists of a series of resistance exercises in a multiple station system: approximately 10 to 15 repetitions of each exercise, at a resistance of 40% to 60% of maximum (RM), with 15 to 30 s rest between exercises. The split routine system trains various body parts on alternate days. Periodization is a method that can be applied to resistance training and is characterized by systematic cycles of alternating prescription variables such as intensity and volume.

4. **Design a physiologically sound and client-centered exercise prescription for resistance training using the eight-step model of sequenced decisions.**

   Step 1: Assess Needs and Formulate Goals

   Client needs may be related to health (low bone density, low back pain), fitness (strength and endurance), performance (sport-specific power, occupational fitness), education (e.g., regarding diet and supplements), appearance (hypertrophy, weight loss or gain), or rehabilitation (injury, posture).

   Step 2: Select Resistance Equipment

   Sometimes rather simple equipment such as bands or tubing can provide great benefit in return for very low cost.

   Step 3: Select Resistance Training Method

   Your design can become quite distinctive when you manipulate prescription factors within a given system.

   Step 4: Select Exercises and Order of Performance

   Knowing the purpose and benefit of each exercise can help maintain muscle balance and avoid overworking a particular body area.

   Step 5: Assign Resistance Intensity and Weight

   Training intensity is a critical prescription factor providing the stimulus needed for improvement in specific muscular components.

   Step 6: Establish Resistance Volume

   Volume is often described as sets × reps × load. However, the rest between the sets and the speed of the movements all contribute to total "time under tension," which is a more complete measure of volume.

   Step 7: Assign and Monitor Resistance Progression

   The challenge is to shape the overload to suit your client by manipulating the prescription factors according to the principle of specificity—namely, that gains in muscular fitness are specific to the muscle group, training method, and exercise volume.

   Step 8: Design Warm-Up and Cool-Down

   The warm-up and cool-down should reflect the type and magnitude of the work done in the resistance training portion.

Resistance Training Prescription Card

Client Name _____   Trainer Name _____

Client Goals	Special Considerations

Circulatory Warm-Up

Equipment and Mode	Workload	Time	HR/PE Objective

Stretching Warm-Up

Name and brief description	Guidelines

Resistance Workout

Equipment type (e.g., free weights)	Training method

Guidelines

Exercise (brief description)	Muscles	Intensity and weight	Reps	Sets	Rest between sets	Precautions

Progression

Cool-Down

Name and brief description	Guidelines

Note. HR = heart rate; PE = perceived exertion.

From *Client-Centered Exercise Prescription, Second Edition,* by John C. Griffin, 2006, Champaign, IL: Human Kinetics.

Client-Centered Muscle Balance and Flexibility Prescription Model

Chapter Competencies

After completing this chapter, you will be able to demonstrate the following competencies:

1. Describe the factors affecting muscle balance.

2. Describe the causes and results of muscle imbalance.

3. Select and describe assessment items for muscle balance.

4. Describe the factors affecting the quality of a stretch.

5. Describe the advantages and client suitability of various stretching techniques.

6. Select appropriate exercises (stretching or resistance) that target designated muscle groups to improve range of motion or muscle balance.

7. Design a physiologically sound and client-centered exercise prescription for muscle balance and flexibility using the six-step model of sequenced decisions.

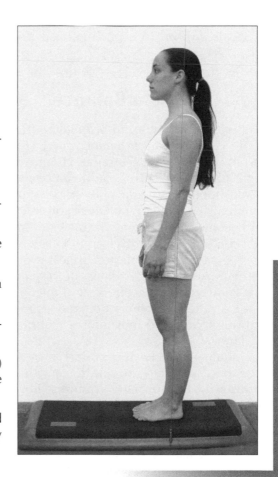

Muscle balance is affected by muscle tightness, flexibility, strength, and endurance, because these factors work together to provide support and movement. Thus, looking at muscle balance is a necessary part of a holistic approach to muscular fitness. Although not a new concept, muscle balance is a new approach to solving problems. It gets right to the heart of your clients' needs, whether they are athletes or fitness enthusiasts or are recovering from injuries.

A muscle must be long enough to allow a normal range of motion and be short and strong enough to provide joint stability. Thus, only after assessing a client's muscle tightness and flexibility, and weakness versus strength and endurance, can we adequately personalize the training program. Setting objectives for muscle balance usually centers around stretching tight muscles, strengthening weak muscles, reducing spasms or inefficient firing, building muscular endurance, or improving posture.

In addition to discussing the preceding issues, this chapter presents the steps involved in the model for muscle balance prescription and two case studies that illustrate the progression from postural analysis to selection of muscle length test items and on to a personalized prescription.

Muscle Balance

Muscle balance is vital to optimal bodily functioning. A loss of muscle balance may be reported as a pain or a general feeling of fatigue or tightness. During screening, you may recognize muscle imbalance from poor posture or poor alignment (chapter 4), and postural deviations will become more common and more exaggerated with aging. Repetitive activity can overuse certain muscles and underuse opposing muscles. This overuse creates a weakness of one group that is overpowered by the strength of the opposing group. A client's job may demand a prolonged position or repeated movements that create an imbalance.

Imbalance may be the underlying cause of headaches, low back discomfort or other joint abnormalities, apparently random aches and pains, or an old injury that keeps emerging. Most clients will approach you with relatively vague initial concerns. Careful questioning about signs, symptoms, or concerns can reveal a potential cause of the muscle imbalance. Such problems are usually multifaceted: They are not limited to strength, flexibility, or endurance but may involve strength of one muscle group and flexibility of an opposing muscle group. Muscle balance also depends on neuromuscular efficiency or the ability of the neuromuscular system to properly recruit movers (agonist), stabilizers, and synergists to produce force or reduce force (antagonists). By considering all these factors, you can best serve your clients.

 Baseball-Related Muscle Imbalance

Your client plays recreational baseball and complains of some discomfort when raising his arm to throw. Because his shoulder felt weak, he had initiated a strengthening program for his shoulders and chest, with no apparent improvement. Your initial observations include a rounded shoulder posture and well-developed chest muscles. This is a classic example of muscle imbalance that needs an integrated approach to prescription. Many of the major upper-body muscles internally (medially) rotate the shoulder. Throwing the ball powerfully uses these muscles. The external (lateral) rotators, however, are relatively small. The stronger and tighter internal rotators involved in throwing are overpowering the weaker external rotators. In baseball, the magnitude and speed of this force are significant. The rounded shoulders are the result of this imbalance and a contributing cause of the shoulder pain. The single-component approach used by the client to strengthen the shoulder actually increased the imbalance. The anterior muscles (internal rotators) need to be lengthened, and the external rotators (posterior) need improved strength and muscular endurance. This is the muscle balance approach.

Causes and Results of Muscle Imbalance

A joint is a pivot point or a fulcrum whose alignment is constantly affected by the pull of the muscles around it. A key to structural balance and posture is equal pull by opposing muscles. Figure 8.1 shows a loss of structural alignment when a short muscle overpowers a longer muscle.

If the muscle is short, it will restrict normal range of motion. Muscles that are too short are usually strong and hold the opposite muscle in a lengthened position. Excessively long muscles are usually weak and allow adaptive shortening of antagonists (Kendall et al. 1993).

To better understand how these imbalances happen, consider the specialized roles played by different sorts of muscles. Muscles can be categorized into two groups (Norris 2000):

1. **Postural stabilizers.** These muscles have a static postural function and primarily stabilize a joint. Their function is more slow-twitch or tonic in nature than that of other muscles. They are often tight and short because of long work periods. Examples include upper trapezius, levator scapulae, transversus abdominis, pelvic floor, quadratus lumborum, iliopsoas, multifidus, erector spinae, and hip adductors.

2. **Phasic mobilizers.** These muscles are primarily responsible for movement. They tend to be more superficial and are often biarticular. They may be weak and fatigue early. Examples include rectus abdominis, gluteus maximus, rectus femoris, peroneals, deltoid, and biceps.

With insufficient variety in muscle use, postural muscles can be activated disproportionately, which inhibits and weakens phasic muscles (Nordin and Frankel 2001). This process can lead to muscle imbalance, poor posture, loss of mobility, and an increase in joint load. Stabilizers and mobilizers react differently to reduced or excessive usage. Most often, we will see tightness in the postural stabilizers and weakness in the phasic mobilizers (table 8.1).

Table 8.1　Postural Stabilizers and Phasic Mobilizers

Tight postural stabilizers	Weak phasic mobilizers
Upper trapezius, levator scapulae	Lower trapezius, rhomboids
Iliopsoas	Rectus abdominis
Erector spinae, multifidus	Gluteus maximus
Hip adductors	Gluteus medius

Causes of Muscle Imbalance

Let's look more closely at the specific causes of imbalance. Muscles can be unbalanced in several ways. They can have unmatched levels of flexibility, strength, or contracture, or a combination of these factors, all of which are discussed subsequently. In addition, muscles can be neurally imbalanced (Blievernicht 2000).

Imbalance Resulting From Tight Muscles

Flexibility is the range of joint motion; **muscle tightness** is the range of muscle length. For muscles that pass over one joint, these two measures are very similar. For muscles that pass over two or more joints (e.g., gastrocnemius, hamstrings, rectus femoris, erector spinae), the range of muscle length will be less than the total range of motion of the joints over which the muscle passes. For example, the knee must be flexed to permit a full range of hip flexion because the hamstrings are too tight if the knee is straight.

Often there is tightness in the most active muscle group, which overpowers the more passive, longer, opposing muscle group. For example, you should always examine the lower leg balance

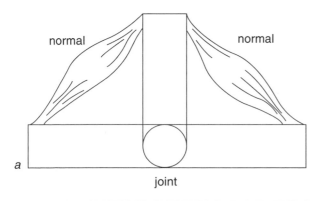 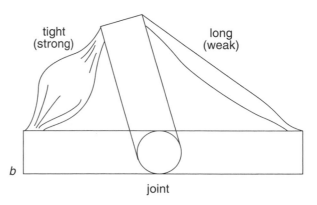

Figure 8.1　Muscle balance: *(a)* joint in structural balance and *(b)* joint misaligned—muscle imbalance.

of clients who are runners. Without proper stretching, constant use of the calf muscles will cause tightness. Calf stretching will help prevent alterations in the running mechanics and subsequent injuries.

Imbalance Resulting From Weak Muscles

Muscle strength testing not only can determine muscles of compromised strength but may also isolate the position of weakness. Muscle weakness has many causes. Even in active people, certain muscles are seldom overloaded. If weakness is attributable to lack of use, prescribe specific exercises for those muscles. With the runner in the previous example, strengthening the anterior shin would prevent problems resulting from unmatched levels of calf strength. If weakness is caused by overwork, fatigue, or strain, prescribe rest—at least in the short term. Relieve the stress before prescribing additional muscular work. Weakness often means an altered proprioceptive input to that muscle, and to improve joint stability, normal proprioception must be restored (Roskopf 2001).

Imbalance Resulting From Muscle Contracture

Commonly known as muscle spasms, muscle contracture also can cause imbalance. Contracture may result from injury, prolonged shortening, or weakness in the opposing muscle. These continued involuntary contractions usually respond to application of heat or cold, progressive static stretching, and, at times, isometric contractions.

A forward-bent position of the trunk and head (spinal flexion), often seen in office workers, requires continuous, prolonged muscle contractions—often at 20% of maximum voluntary contraction (Nordin and Frankel 2001). The pain that results from a lack of oxygen and an accumulation of metabolites can lead to a vicious circle of muscle spasm. In addition, prolonged isometric contractions can cause inflammation and passive shortening of the muscle.

Clients who have chronic low back pain are often diagnosed as having "back spasms." Traditional treatments include rest, ultrasound, various forms of heat, and massage. Although these treatments may relieve symptoms, they do not address the cause of the underlying muscle imbalance.

Imbalance Resulting From Combinations of Strength, Length, and Contracture

You need to prescribe both strengthening and stretching for total body balance. A reduction of tightness is often needed before certain strength exercises can be properly performed. Therapeutic exercises to strengthen weak muscles, stretch tight muscles, and retrain postural awareness and movement patterns are the most effective and lasting means by which muscle balance is restored and maintained.

Low back spasms are often caused by weakness of opposing muscles. In the earlier example of the office worker, the weakness would be in the abdominals around the trunk and the gluteus maximus and hamstrings around the posterior pelvis. Because traditional treatment is passive, it would actually leave the client with **two** weak muscles: the abdominals and the low back muscles! When pain subsides and the traditional treatment has relieved some inflammation and spasm, you would start your client on abdominal strengthening exercises (with precautions for the back—see chapter 11). As in one of the case studies later this chapter, tight hip flexors can place added pressure on the low back. Neuromuscular awareness of postural alignments while standing, sitting, lying, and performing any of the prescribed movement patterns is a critical part of this integrated approach.

Neural Imbalance

Muscles that are strong and shortened are also neurally facilitated, whereas muscles that are weak and lengthened are neurally inhibited. Neurally facilitated muscles contract early and with excessive force during movements. Neurally inhibited muscles respond later and with less force than they would otherwise.

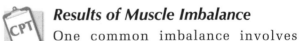

Results of Muscle Imbalance

One common imbalance involves shortened back extensors and hip flexors versus weakened abdominal and buttocks muscles. This imbalance results in an anterior pelvic tilt and excessive lumbar lordosis. In the upper body, there often is tightness of the pectoralis major, upper trapezius, and levator scapulae versus weakness of the rhomboids, lower trapezius, serratus anterior, and the deep flexor muscles of the neck. This is manifested in rounded shoulders, shoulder girdle elevation and abduction, forward head position, and possible cervical lordosis (Nordin and Frankel 2001).

Muscle imbalance may also lead to faulty movements through muscle groups firing in an uncoordinated way. For example, clients with tight rectus femoris and weak abdominals may alter their body mechanics when they perform a hamstring curl. The hips may flex and the back hyperextend near the end of the range of motion. The rectus femoris is stretched under tension as the knee bends, but if the rectus femoris is tight, it will pull on its origin, the anterior superior iliac spine, causing hip flexion. If the abdominals are not strong, they cannot counter the anterior pull on the pelvis, and an anterior tilt results along with a low back hyperextension.

Imbalances may also exist within synergists, that is, a group of muscles that work together to produce a movement. For example, when clients with rounded shoulders perform lateral raises with dumbbells or reach overhead such as lifting a box to a top shelf, substitution patterns may occur. Normally the scapula rotates laterally (upwardly) to allow the shoulder joint to abduct. Clients with rounded shoulders often have an imbalance between the synergists responsible for this movement. They have tight upper trapezius and weaker lower trapezius and serratus anterior. What results is excessive elevation of the shoulder girdle because of the dominant upper trapezius.

Faulty mechanics will usually result when some stabilizers are more passive than others during certain movements. For example, during a strenuous biceps curl, the shoulder girdle may elevate. The middle and lower trapezius should stabilize the shoulder girdle in an adducted and depressed position during elbow flexion. Because the long head of the bicep brachii attaches to the scapula above the shoulder, the levator scapula and upper trapezius overpower their lower antagonists to place the bicep in a stronger prestretched position when fatigue sets in. This also occurs during activities such as shoveling or lifting, when the anterior deltoid or pectoralis major (clavicular) is prestretched by the shoulder girdle elevators. This substitution pattern will often result in a tense neck and upper back.

The human kinetic chain is made up of the muscular, skeletal, and neural systems. If one segment of the kinetic chain is misaligned or not functioning properly, predictable patterns of dysfunction develop, leading to neuromuscular inefficiency and tissue overload (Ninos 2001a). For example, tightness of the gastrocnemius can cause a runner to alter the support phase of her gait. The reduced dorsiflexion and slight turnout may result in increased stress on the plantar fascia and longitudinal arch. As a result, some excess pronation may occur in midstance when the foot is rolling forward but runs out of dorsiflexion range of motion. Further up the chain, this may cause an increased external rotation of the tibia, which in turn adds to the stress being placed on the patellofemoral joint (Ninos 2001b). Tightness of the calf can also affect the mechanics of doing a squat. Without adequate dorsiflexion, lifters will widen their stance and externally (laterally) rotate their feet to compensate for the tight calf. Essentially, the body's kinetic chain seeks the path of least resistance by placing an excessive torque load on the knees, resulting in ever-increasing disability.

The ultimate goal of the kinetic chain is to maintain dynamic postural equilibrium. To accomplish this, it must have adaptive potential. Limited flexibility, muscle weakness, and inappropriate neural firing decrease this adaptive potential. It is your job to detect any existing muscle imbalance and begin the process of restoring balance.

How to Detect Muscle Imbalance

Clients are not going to say that they have muscle imbalance. But you can find out if they do by asking the right questions, as outlined later in this section.

Joint Stress Cycle

As should be clear by now, loss of muscle balance may lead to acute injury or can be the underlying cause of chronic overuse injury. Figure 8.2 is a model of how muscle imbalance can induce injury.

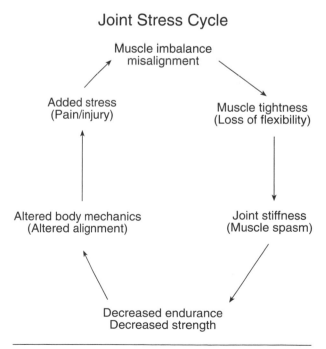

Figure 8.2 The joint stress cycle.

The **joint stress cycle** works like this: If your client has a muscle imbalance, such as tight anterior chest muscles (including shoulder internal rotators), there will often be a malalignment (e.g., rounded shoulders). These muscles lose flexibility, and the joint becomes progressively more stiff until the muscle is in constant partial contracture; it has progressively less endurance and strength. At this point, a person will alter his mechanics—for example, he may throw a ball with a distinct sidearm style. But the adjustments themselves cause additional problems, creating a vicious circle of pain and misalignment.

How do you know if your client is within this joint stress cycle? Most clients, whether active or inactive, are somewhere on the cycle, and you must decide where your client is on the cycle.

Start by obtaining a client history of musculoskeletal problems. Use the *Joint Stress Questionnaire and Observations* on page 221 to gather the client's answers and to record your own observations. This information will tell you where your client is on the joint stress cycle and how to get her out of it.

Muscle Balance Assessment

Faulty body mechanics, as determined by postural screening, should be confirmed by the muscle tests. Select assessment items only after you and your client together have decided on priorities. Chapter 4 describes and interprets the following assessments:

- Postural assessments (including static and dynamic)
- Muscle length and flexibility assessments
  - **Upper body**: pectoralis minor, pectoralis major (sternal), shoulder internal rotators, shoulder external rotators, shoulder abduction range of motion (ROM)
  - **Lower body:** hip flexors (one and two-joint), tensor fascia latae, hamstrings, hip internal rotators, hip external rotators, gastrocnemius, tibialis posterior and soleus (ankle ROM)
  - **Trunk:** lumbar and cervical rotation ROM, sit and reach
- Strength assessments
  - **Upper body:** Push-ups (pectorals, serratus anterior), weightlifting 5RM to 10RM (selected muscles)
  - **Lower body:** Weightlifting 5RM to 10RM (selected muscles)

  - **Trunk:** Biering–Sorenson (erector spinae), five-level sit-up (abdominals), leg lowers (lower abdominals), lateral lift (quadratus lumborum)

Postural analysis will indicate which muscle length and flexibility tests and strength assessments to perform. Interpretation of these tests will tell you what muscles need to be strengthened and which ones need to be lengthened.

Client-Centered Flexibility Prescription

Flexibility is an often neglected component of physical fitness. Enhancing flexibility improves not only joint ROM but also muscle relaxation, muscle balance, and preparation for activity as well. Flexibility should integrate multiplanar soft tissue extensibility with neuromuscular efficiency throughout the full range of motion. Lack of flexibility is often the cause of musculoskeletal injuries, low back pain, and headaches.

Mechanism of Stretch

The effectiveness of a stretch is related to the behavior of the connective tissue and muscle when under stress. Limitation to ROM is attributable 47% to joint structure, 41% to muscle fascia, and 10% to tendons (Brooks 1993). The mechanism of stretch explains why this is so.

The myosin filaments within the sarcomere of the muscle fiber have a strand of very elastic protein called titin extending out to be anchored at the Z line. When a relaxed muscle is stretched passively, its muscle fibers elongate and the actin and myosin filaments slide past each other so that the sarcomeres also lengthen. When the stretch force is removed, the muscle fibers and the sarcomeres spring back to their original resting lengths because of the actions of titin pulling the Z lines closer together (Germann and Stanfield 2002). This elastic mechanism is not dependent on time.

However, muscles are not purely elastic; rather, they are viscoelastic, having both viscous (resistant to flow) and elastic properties. When a muscle lengthens under force it is called **creep.** When a muscle is stretched to a constant length, over time the force (tension) will decrease, and this is called **stress-relaxation.** If the muscle returns to its original length when the force is removed, this is **elastic deformation** (figure 8.3). When connective tissue is stretched, some of the elongation

Joint Stress Questionnaire and Observations

1. Do you currently have any pain? _____

2. If so, in what joint or area do you feel the pain? _____

   In what positions do you feel the pain? _____

   During what movement do you feel the pain? _____

3. Does your occupation or fitness activity overuse one body segment?_____

4. Do you feel you are currently overtraining? _____

5. Do you feel tight anywhere? _____

   Do you feel this tightness during or after activity? _____

6. Do you get tired (muscularly) more easily than you used to?_____

7. Have you experienced a loss of strength? _____

8. Are you compensating in your movements to avoid pain or loss of strength? _____

9. Are things getting worse?_____

10. What do you think is causing this problem? _____

    How could it be alleviated? _____

Watch your client during a workout. Look for altered body mechanics, stiffness, or postural faults, and then answer these questions:

11. Did you notice any altered body mechanics, stiffness, or postural faults when your client walked in?

    _____

12. Did you notice any altered body mechanics, stiffness, or postural faults when your client was active?

    _____

13. Can any altered body mechanics, stiffness, or postural faults be accounted for because of acute symptoms from current or chronic injuries? _____

14. According to these questions and initial observations, where is your client on the joint stress cycle?

    _____

Assessment (chapter 4): Perform a postural screening particularly on the area of greatest concern. Perform muscle length testing to determine whether the muscle length is limited or excessive.

Objectives: Establish specific objectives and a plan for exercise design and monitoring.

From *Client-Centered Exercise Prescription, Second Edition,* by John C. Griffin, 2006, Champaign, IL: Human Kinetics.

is elastic and some may be more permanent when the force is removed **(plastic deformation)** (Hendrick 2000). Connective tissue is the major structure limiting joint range of motion (i.e., sheathing around muscle, tendons, ligaments, and joint capsules).

New evidence suggests that the stretch mechanism has both a direct and an indirect process of decreasing a muscle's "stiffness," which is defined as the force required to change its length. The direct process is via passive viscoelastic changes or deformations. The indirect process is attributable to reflex inhibition and consequent changes in the viscoelasticity from decreased actin-myosin crossbridging (Shrier and Gossal 2000). There is also evidence that we get an increase in range of motion not only because of a decrease in muscle stiffness but also because of an increase in our stretch tolerance (i.e., more force can be applied before we feel pain).

Factors in Stretching Prescription Effectiveness

There has been some controversy about the merits of stretching, particularly as an element of the warm-up, and you must give your clients accurate information in this area. The following section on flexibility prescription begins by examining the factors that can make a stretch program highly successful.

Factors Affecting Stretch Quality

In prescribing any exercise for your client, consider the following factors that directly affect the quality of stretch:

- Duration of the applied force (how long to hold a stretch)

- Intensity of the applied force (how hard to push a stretch)
- Temperature of the tissue (related to pre-stretch warm-up)
- Degree of relaxation of the muscle (amount of tension in a muscle)
- Type of applied force (e.g., ballistic, static, proprioceptive neuromuscular facilitation)
- Alignment of muscle fibers to be stretched (direction of pull on the muscle)

Other prescription factors you should consider in your client's program design include these:

- Number of exercises (within the flexibility program)
- Number of repetitions (number of times the same stretch is performed)
- Other activities within the workout (aerobic, strengthening, sports)
- Frequency of workouts (how often the flexibility program is done per week)

Controlling the Prescription Factors

By prudent selection and control of the prescription factors, you can increase the quality of your client's stretches.

Duration, Force, and Temperature

A stretch of relatively long duration and low force at elevated tissue temperatures will provide an effective permanent stretch **(plastic deformation)** (Sapega et al. 1991). If the duration of stretch is short, the intensity of force is high, and the tissue temperature is normal or cold, the muscle–tendon structure will return quickly to its original length

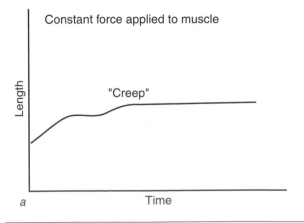
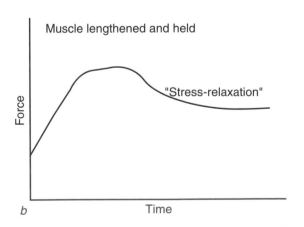

Figure 8.3   If a constant force is applied, (a) the muscle will stretch immediately and then slowly increase in length. If a muscle is stretched to a certain length and held, (b) the force on the muscle gradually reduces.

(elastic deformation) and much of the benefit of the stretch will be lost.

Warming up for stretching has replaced the notion of stretching to warm up. Besides simply raising tissue temperature, warm-up activity stimulates muscle calcium release and motor unit recruitment. However, warm-up without stretching does not increase range of motion (Shrier and Gossal 2000). On the other hand, there has been evidence that high strength and power outputs have been negatively affected after a stretching session (Knudson et al. 2000). However, most clients who have tightness will benefit from a prewarmed, long, static stretch routine done frequently and without the ballistic effect of other activities.

Muscle Relaxation

Attempting to stretch muscles in spasm may cause injury. Connective tissue can be stretched effectively only if the muscle is relaxed. Strain is most often felt around the tendon of a tense muscle. Heat, light aerobics, loosening (see *Active Loosening*), massage, or ROM exercises can provide some relaxation, particularly if your client has come directly from an environment of repeated movements or static posture, such as sitting at a computer terminal. The mode of training can also affect the state of relaxation. For example, proprioceptive neuromuscular facilitation (PNF) involves a phase of isometrically contracting the muscle to be stretched. The proprioceptor is sensitive to the isometric tension, producing a reflex inhibition of the muscle, less resistance to stretch, less discomfort, a possible analgesic effect, and a greater range of motion. But remember—if the muscle–tendon structure is inflamed, rest may be the best prescription.

If the alignment of the muscle–tendon structure is directly in the line of the stretch (or movement), the tensile stretch (or force application) is optimized. Pay special attention to alignment detail when you demonstrate the program to your client.

Program Parameters

A well-rounded flexibility program, or conditioning program, should include at least one exercise for each major muscle group. Your prescription should include the stretch specific to the area of tightness, the proper positioning and execution of the stretch, and the method of stretching best suited to your client. Postural screening and muscle length testing may suggest greater emphasis on, or avoidance of, certain muscle groups.

You can provide the appropriate overload in the form of additional isolation stretches, more repetitions, longer duration, more frequent sessions, or a change of stretching technique. Heyward (2002) suggested 2 to 6 repetitions of each exercise for a minimum of 3 days a week, with the duration of stretch from 10 to 60 s. Bandy et al. (1997) suggested one 30 s stretch per muscle group, but it is likely that longer periods or more repetitions are required in some people, for some muscle groups, or in the presence of injuries.

Teach your clients to read their body's feedback and make their prescription client-centered:

1. Stretch until you feel tension or slight pulling, but no pain.
2. Hold that length of the muscle until there is a noticeable decrease in the tension (stress relaxation).
3. Increase the muscle length until you feel the original tension level.
4. Take a deeper breath and slowly exhale. Repeat Steps 2 and 3 until no further increase.

Flexibility Training Methods

There are two approaches to improve flexibility: decreasing the resistance to the stretch and increasing the strength of the opposing muscle. Decreasing resistance to the stretch can be accomplished by either increasing the connective tissue length or attaining a greater degree of relaxation or analgesic effect in the target muscle. Table 8.2 describes the appropriate stretching techniques for each approach.

You must have thorough knowledge of your clients before you can determine the best approach. A client who participates in competitive sport once or twice a week probably has tight muscle–tendon structures, whereas a previously inactive client may lack the strength of opposing muscles to pull the joint through a larger range of motion. If your client's objective is to attain a ROM that allows ease of daily function or improved posture, static stretching may be the best training method.

Most types of flexibility training fall into three categories: static, dynamic (ballistic), and PNF. Regardless of the method of flexibility selected, always be aware of safety during the demonstration, supervision, and modification (see chapter 5).

Active Loosening

Relaxation, or the minimization of muscular tension, must exist before a stretch is attempted. Reduced tension can assist in stretching out

Table 8.2   Stretching Techniques

Approach	Technique
1. Decrease resistance to the stretch	
a. Lengthen connective tissue. b. Relax stretch reflex of targeted muscle. c. Use an analgesia.	a. Warm-up (including light aerobics), massage, loosening, dynamic stretching b. Static stretch with brief intermittent isometric contractions, relaxation techniques c. Ice or heat applied during a static stretch
2. Increase strength of opposing muscles	
a. Resistance train opposing muscles (muscle balance).	a. Isolation of specific muscles and isometric or concentric contractions
3. Combine approaches	
a. Train for stretch and strength (facilitation).	a. Proprioceptive neuromuscular facilitation

connective tissues. **Active loosening** can relieve muscle tension and promote relaxation (Kuprian 1982). Active loosening exercises include rhythmic swinging of the limbs, active shaking of the limbs, or rotating the torso or limbs.

Many athletes know the effects of shaking the extremities to loosen particular muscles. A sprinter never gets into the starting blocks without thoroughly loosening her legs and arms. She shakes her legs one at a time while in a slight straddle position, and she shakes her arms while standing with the upper body slightly inclined and the arms hanging loosely. Loosening exercises facilitate more rapid recovery from stress through a facilitated blood flow. Failure to loosen up leads to an early loss of strength, slowing of movements, and fatigue (Eitner 1982).

Other examples of effective loosening exercises include these:

- Lifting the shoulders and allowing them to fall
- Lying on the upper back, supporting the waist with the hands, and shaking the legs in the air
- Standing, twisting the trunk to the left and right (avoid excessive momentum, and avoid if any history of back problems)
- Standing, leaning against wall with outstretched arms, swinging each leg back and forth
- Lying supine with knees bent, shaking the legs (especially calves and hamstrings)
- Standing, one arm leaning on a table, letting other arm swing in a circle by rocking body weight in a circular pattern (figure 8.4)

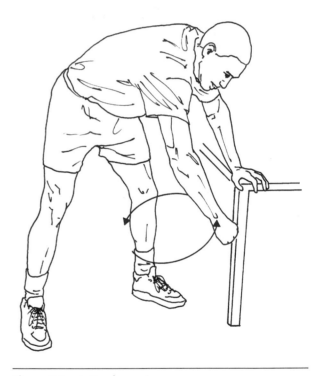

Figure 8.4   Active loosening.

Static Stretching

Static stretching involves controlled elongation of an antagonistic muscle by placing it in a maximal position of stretch and holding it. The Golgi tendon organs (GTOs) in the muscle's tendon are sensitive to the tension of a static stretch. The GTOs' signal to relax overrides the muscle spindles' signal to contract. The muscle spindles need a few seconds to adapt to the lengthened position before they decrease their discharge. The reflex contraction of the muscle to be stretched decreases, and the muscle is more relaxed and prepared to stretch. Recommendations for the optimal time for holding the stretch range from as short as 10 s to as long as 60 s (Heyward 2002). Bandy and colleagues (1997) suggested a 30 s duration, assuming muscle temperature is elevated. If the stretch time is reduced to 15 s, 2 or 3 repetitions should be completed (Sapega et al. 1991). Static stretching can be either active or passive. Shrier and Gossal (2000) found that 30 s static stretches were likely to achieve maximum ROM benefits within 6 to 7 weeks, although results varied with muscle group.

Active Static Stretching

Active static stretching is accomplished by moving the agonist muscle to the end of its ROM and holding it in that position with an isometric contraction of the agonist muscles—without other aid. For example, to stretch the anterior chest and pectoralis minor muscles (figure 8.5), a client would contract the posterior shoulder girdle and shoulder joint muscles. This type of stretch is especially useful for people whose ROM is limited by the strength of the agonist muscles. You will recognize these clients by noting a large difference between their active ROM and assisted (passive) ROM. Active static stretching may also be effective after strength training or heavy eccentric work when a forced stretch may elongate the fibers excessively.

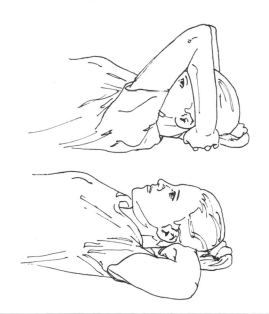

Figure 8.5 Active static stretch.

Passive Static Stretching

In **passive static stretching**, an outside agent applies the force. This form of stretching is effective when the ROM is limited by soft tissue extendibility. Its effect on warmed muscle is to lengthen the connective tissues passively. Pressure or held traction, external leverage, or support of a partner may provide the outside force.

- **Pressure or held traction.** This technique is used in a side-lying quadriceps stretch where the heel is pulled toward the buttock (figure 8.6). The stretch should be gently and gradually increased.

- **External leverage.** This can be seen in figure 8.7, in which the shoulder internal rotators are elongated by the position of leverage in the doorway.

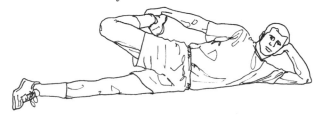

Figure 8.6 Passive static stretch (pressure and traction).

Reprinted, by permission, from V. Heyward, 1998, *Fitness assessment and exercise prescription*, 3rd ed. (Champaign, IL: Human Kinetics), 303.

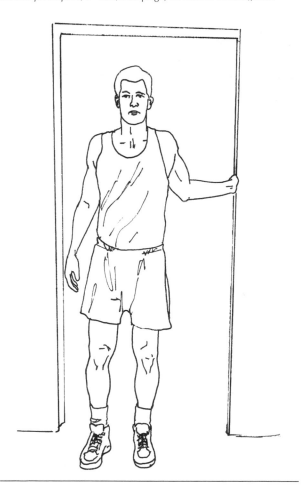

Figure 8.7 Passive static stretch (external leverage).

- **Support of a partner.** The partner assists the stretch beyond an active ROM but must remain in close communication with the client and carefully control the stretch intensity. Figure 8.8 shows a partner hamstring stretch.

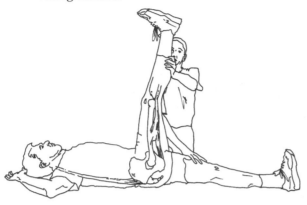

Figure 8.8 Passive static stretch (support of a partner).

Reprinted, by permission, from E.T. Howley and B.D. Franks, 1997, *Health fitness instructors handbook*, 3rd ed. (Champaign, IL: Human Kinetics), 259.

Dynamic Stretching

Active, bouncing movements initiated by contraction of the agonist muscle produce a quick stretch of the antagonist muscle. If uncontrolled momentum becomes a factor in the stretch, it is referred to as a ballistic stretch. Ballistic stretching can cause overstretching, resulting in microtears within the musculotendinous unit. Connective tissue has a safe elastic range, but if stress exceeds a yield point, small tears will occur. Repetition of such microtrauma can cause inflammation (chapter 11). The tearing can also lead to formation of scar tissue, with a gradual loss of elasticity. The risk of injury is higher with this type of stretching than with others and is dependent on the intensity and velocity of the stretch and the temperature of the muscle (Alter 2004).

However, many sports require dynamic or ballistic movements. Because ballistic stretching is functional and does increase ROM (Hendrick 2000), it is reasonable to integrate it into athletic training programs as long as the ballistic stretches correspond to actions required by the sport. If you prescribe this type of stretching for a client, target the specific muscle to be stretched, establish safe alignment, and avoid excessive momentum. Dynamic stretching should follow static stretching and only after the body temperature is sufficiently warm. Dynamic stretching should consist of rhythmic actions similar to those in the client's sport. Start with small movements and gradually increase the range of motion. The exercises can be performed while the client walks 10 to 20 m (11-23 yd). Depending on the sport, common dynamic flexibility exercises include lunge walk (figure 8.9), lunge with a twist, walking knee tuck, high–low walks, and grapevines (with a twist).

Proprioceptive Neuromuscular Facilitation

PNF stretching invokes neurological responses that facilitate stretching. PNF works by generating a force or tension (generally an isometric muscle contraction) in the muscle that stimulates the Golgi tendon organs, which then inhibit the muscle spindles and relax the muscle (autogenic inhibition) (Holcomb 2000). Before the stretch, have your client hold a submaximal isometric contraction against a resistance at the end of the limb's ROM for about 6 s. The static stretch that follows (approximately 15-30 s) also stimulates the Golgi tendon organs to further relax the muscle to be stretched. Your client should repeat

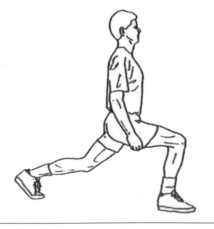
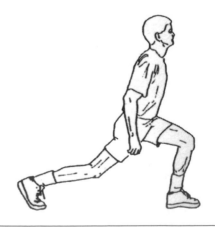

Figure 8.9 Dynamic flexibility: lunge walk.

Reprinted, by permission, from National Strength and Conditioning Association, 1994, *Essentials of strength training and conditioning* (Champaign, IL: Human Kinetics), 328.

the sequence several times, to allow for a greater reflex inhibition and thus a greater stretch.

PNF Methods

McAtee and Charland (1999) summarized the common PNF variations as follows:

• **Hold–relax** uses an isometric contraction of the antagonist at the limit of the initial ROM, followed by a period of relaxation. Then the limb actively moves farther in the same direction against minimal resistance through the new ROM to the new point of limitation. The strong isometric contraction is thought to recruit more muscle fibers and then fire the inverse stretch reflex, relaxing the target muscle and permitting further stretch (Osternig et al. 1990). Hold–relax is effective when ROM has decreased because of muscle tightness on one side of a joint.

• **Contract–relax (CR)** is similar to hold–relax. You provide resistance as the client attempts to move the limb to the initial limit of the ROM of the target muscle. Because your resistance prevents the limb from moving, his muscles contract isometrically. Then your client relaxes, and you again move the limb passively beyond the initial limit. Contract–relax is preferred to hold–relax when ROM is good and when motion is pain-free.

• **Contract–relax, antagonist–contract (CRAC)** is similar to contract–relax, except that after the isometric contraction, the client actively moves his limb into the new ROM (figure 8.10). This active contraction of the agonist is thought to relax the target muscle (called reciprocal inhibition), thereby allowing a better stretch (Voss et al. 1985).

• **Manual isometric stretch** is a modification of a PNF, using the relaxed state of the muscle immediately following an isometric contraction (figure 8.11). Have your client manually resist the contraction of a muscle in the midrange of movement for 6 to 10 s and then move the muscle into a passive static stretch, allowing enough time for connective tissue elongation and neuromuscular relaxation. Figure 8.11 may be performed as a manual isometric stretch of the shoulder.

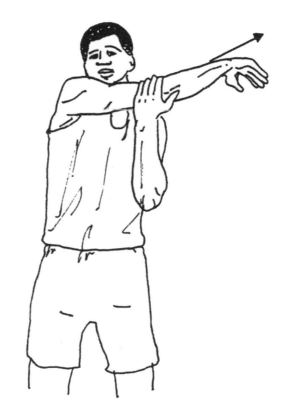

Figure 8.11 Manual isometric stretch.

Reprinted, by permission, from National Strength and Conditioning Association, 1994, *Essentials of strength training and conditioning* (Champaign, IL: Human Kinetics), 302.

Advantages and Client Suitability of PNF Stretching

PNF is considered an advanced method of stretching, both for the client and for personal fitness trainers, who have varying levels of skill in its application. It has a number of advantages and is well suited for certain clients:

• Specific benefits are associated with the PNF method used (see *PNF Methods*).

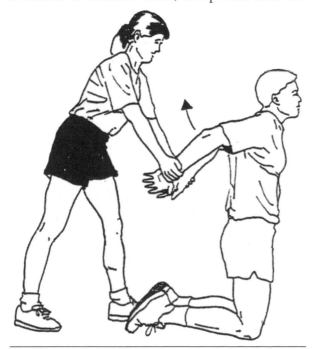

Figure 8.10 Proprioceptive neuromuscular facilitation stretch: pectoralis major (sternal).

Reprinted, by permission, from National Strength and Conditioning Association, 1994, *Essentials of strength training and conditioning* (Champaign, IL: Human Kinetics), 296.

- ROM gains, especially passive mobility, have been equal to or greater than gains with other stretching methods.
- PNF produces strength, muscle balance, and joint stability.
- PNF increases relaxation of the muscle, which allows greater stretch of the connective tissue.
- Because PNF generally requires a partner, it gives you an opportunity to increase rapport with your client.
- PNF can be used to stretch any muscle in the body.
- PNF provides an excellent opportunity to motivate your client.
- PNF is popular with therapists because it approximates "natural" movements.
- PNF can be adapted to be done without a partner.

Despite all these pluses, use PNF with caution. Because it may produce excessive tissue stretch, PNF stretching should be performed only with the supervision of a knowledgeable and experienced personal fitness trainer.

Client-Centered Muscle Balance Prescription

Muscles that are too short are often strong and hold antagonists in a lengthened and weakened position. These muscles need to be lengthened and made more flexible through stretching. Muscles identified as weak and long need to be strengthened. This is best done through simple exercises that isolate and use the muscles in question. For muscle balance to be restored and maintained, therefore, therapeutic exercises to strengthen weak muscles should be combined with stretches for tight muscles.

The steps involved in the model for muscle balance prescription follow this approach. Client goals are established based on counseling con-

cerns and assessment of posture, muscle tightness or joint ROM, and muscle weakness. For each goal, a series of exercises are designed for flexibility of the tight muscles and strength of the weak side. *The Muscle Balance Prescription Model* describes in some detail the six steps of the model. Use the *Muscle Balance Prescription Card* to record program recommendations and guidelines for safety and monitoring for each patient. The card is a useful template to guide this program design process, ensuring that it is client-centered and goal-oriented. The two case studies at the end of the chapter demonstrate the use of the model and prescription card.

Principles of Muscle Balance Prescription

Table 8.3 shows (for the lower body) the progression from postural assessment to the identification of probable areas of muscle imbalance, and it provides guidelines for exercise design. Depending on the exercise movement, every muscle, at some time, is a prime mover (agonist) in a specific action, and each muscle has an opposing muscle (antagonist). Refer to table 8.4 to determine muscle pairs and to aid you in designing exercises based on muscle testing.

Some Precautions

When designing isolated corrective exercises, ensure that the resistance is light enough to prevent the client from compensating by using other muscles. As muscle balance improves, start to replace isolated exercises with more complex movements. However, if the isolated weakness is not corrected, multijoint strengthening exercises will also tend to cause compensation and reinforce the imbalance or create new ones.

When a muscle has excessive tension, the stress should be relieved before you prescribe additional muscular work. There is often reduced neuromuscular input in these muscles. Roskopf (2001) suggested using isometric contractions to restimulate the muscle by increasing sensory input to the brain. Corrective isometrics can act as precursors

The Muscle Balance Prescription Model

Step 1: Assess Needs and Formulate Goals

Clients' needs may be related to health or injury, fitness, or performance improvement. Their needs can also be identified by fitness assessments (posture, tightness, ROM, weakness) or an observed compensation in some movement patterns.

Step 2: Select the Training Method for the Fitness Component

You must select the training method that best meets your client's needs, time constraints, experience, and level of condition. Your design can become quite distinctive when you manipulate prescription factors within a given system. Training methods such as standard sets or a specific circuit may be appropriate for strengthening, whereas static stretching or PNF may be selected for tightness or ROM.

Step 3: Select Exercises and Order of Performance

To restore and maintain muscle balance, combine therapeutic exercises to strengthen weak muscles with stretches for tight muscles. You must know the purpose and benefit of each exercise and choose those that maintain muscle balance and retrain muscles that have been over- or underworked. Modifications may be necessary because of physical limitations and current or past injuries. Order your selection of specific exercises using the following guidelines:

- Deal with each identified goal sequentially, as a unit of exercises.

- Work areas of weakness or imbalance while your client is still fresh.

- Have the client do a light warm-up and then stretch, followed by strengthening exercises and then any functional neuromuscular exercises.

- Select exercises for each related muscle group maintaining agonist–antagonist and bilateral symmetry, which promotes a balanced development.

- Choose exercises that are functional for the demands on the client; these often include exercises in more than one plane.

- Include stabilizers (e.g., lower spine muscles) later in the session.

Step 4: Provide Prescriptive Recommendations

Program recommendations may include equipment selection, exercise load, or volume. Often there is no need for specialized equipment. Some simple equipment that can be useful may include bands and tubing, pulleys, or other small equipment such as medicine balls and plyo balls, body bars, dumbbells, wobble boards, Theraballs, balance discs, Bosu trainers, and mats.

Exercise volume is one of the most important prescription factors. Volume is often described as sets × reps × load. The intensity or load must be heavy enough to cause temporary fatigue. If your client is using weights, strength and endurance improvements will come with 8 to 12 repetitions and a 75% load. Two sets are usually sufficient to produce excellent benefits. Frequency is sometimes more than 3 days per week when retraining an imbalance.

Step 5: Provide Progression, Monitoring, and Safety Guidelines

The universal principle of conditioning is progressive overload, that is, periodically raising the workload to increasingly challenge the muscle group. The object is to shape the overload to suit your client by manipulating the prescription factors according to the principle of specificity—namely, that gains in muscular fitness are specific to the muscle group, training method, and exercise volume.

To ensure safe and effective progression, modify only one volume factor at a time (e.g., increase reps up to about 15, then increase the load and drop the reps back down). Program cards that allow quick recording of these factors can save time and encourage regular recording. Visually monitor primary safety precautions and execution mechanics.

Step 6: Design Warm-Up and Cool-Down

The warm-up and cool-down should reflect the type and magnitude of the work done in the training portion. After some warming, have the client statically stretch the muscle groups to be used in the workout. In the cool-down, relieve anticipated muscle tightness and have the client stretch tight postural muscles (e.g., anterior chest, hip flexors, hamstrings).

Muscle Balance Prescription Card

Client name:	Trainer name:
Client goals:	**Assessment rationale:**
1.	1.
2.	2.
3.	3.
Flexibility prescription for goal 1: *Exercise name and description*	**Strengthening prescription for goal 1:** *Exercise name and description*
Exercise name and description	*Exercise name and description*
Exercise name and description	*Exercise name and description*
Flexibility prescription for goal 2: *Exercise name and description*	**Strengthening prescription for goal 2:** *Exercise name and description*
Exercise name and description	*Exercise name and description*
Exercise name and description	*Exercise name and description*
Flexibility prescription for goal 3: *Exercise name and description*	**Strengthening prescription for goal 3:** *Exercise name and description*
Exercise name and description	*Exercise name and description*
Exercise name and description	*Exercise name and description*
Program recommendations:	**Safety and monitoring guidelines:**

From *Client-Centered Exercise Prescription, Second Edition,* by John C. Griffin, 2006, Champaign, IL: Human Kinetics.

Table 8.3 Exercise Design From Muscle Testing: Lower Body

Postural fault	Muscles in shortened position	Muscles in lengthened position	Exercise implication
Flexed knee	Popliteus Hamstrings at knee	Quadriceps Sartorius	• Stretch knee flexors • Stretch hip flexors if tight; may contribute
Medially rotated femur (often associated with pronation of foot or toeing in)	Hip medial rotators	Hip lateral flexors	• Stretch hip medial rotators • Strengthen hip lateral rotators
Knock-knee	Tensor fascia latae Lateral knee joint structures	Medial knee joint structures	• Stretch tensor fascia latae
Postural bowlegs	Hip lateral rotators Quadriceps Foot everters	Hip medial rotators, popliteus, tibialis posterior, and long toe flexors	• Strengthen hip medial rotators
Ankle pronation	Peroneals and toe extensors	Tibialis posterior and long toe flexors	• Strengthen inverters and muscles supporting the arch
Ankle supination	Tibialis (especially posterior)	Peroneals	• Strengthen peroneals

Table 8.4 Opposing Muscles

Movement direction	Agonists	Antagonists
Foot and ankle		
Anteroposterior	Dorsiflexors (tibialis anterior, peroneus tertius)	Plantar flexors (gastrocnemius, soleus)
Lateral and rotary	Tibials (tibialis anterior and posterior)	Peroneals (peroneus longus and brevis)
Knee		
Anteroposterior	Flexors (hamstrings, gastrocnemius)	Extensors (quadriceps)
Hip		
Anteroposterior	Flexors (iliopsoas, rectus femoris, pectineus, tensor fascia latae, sartorius)	Extensors (gluteus maximus, hamstrings)
Lateral	Abductors (gluteus medius, tensor fascia latae)	Adductors (adductor longus, brevis, magnus, gracilis, pectineus)
Rotary	Internal rotators (gluteus minimus, tensor fascia latae)	External rotators (gluteus maximus, six external rotators)
Trunk		
Anteroposterior	Flexors (rectus abdominis, external oblique)	Extensors (erector spinae, deep posterior spinal group)
Lateral	Lateral flexors—left oppose right (quadratus lumborum, external and internal obliques, erector spinae group)	Same
Rotary	Rotators to the same side (internal oblique, erector spinae group)	Rotators to the opposite side (external oblique, deep posterior group)

(continued)

Table 8.4   *(continued)*

Movement direction	Agonists	Antagonists
Pelvis		
Anteroposterior	Forward tilt (hip flexors, trunk extensors)	Backward tilt (trunk flexors, hip extensors)
Lateral	(Gluteus medius and minimus)	(Quadratus lumborum, external oblique)
Shoulder joint		
Anteroposterior	Flexors and horizontal adductors (anterior deltoid, pectoralis major)	Extensors and horizontal abductors (posterior deltoid, latissimus dorsi, teres major)
Lateral	Abductors (deltoids, supraspinatus)	Adductors (latissimus dorsi, teres major, pectoralis major)
Rotary	Internal rotators (subscapularis, teres major)	External rotators (infraspinatus, teres minor)
Shoulder girdle		
Vertical	Elevators (trapezius 1 and 2, levator scapula, rhomboids)	Depressors (trapezius 4, pectoralis minor)
Lateral	Abductors (serratus anterior, pectoralis minor)	Adductors (trapezius 2, 3, and 4, rhomboids)
Rotary	Lateral rotators (trapezius 2 and 4, serratus anterior)	Medial rotators (pectoralis minor, rhomboids)
Elbow		
Anteroposterior	Flexors (biceps brachii, brachialis, brachioradialis)	Extensors (triceps brachii, anconeus)
Radioulnar		
Rotary	Pronators (pronator quadratus, pronator teres, brachioradialis)	Supinators (supinator, brachioradialis, biceps brachii)
Wrist		
Anteroposterior	Wrist flexors	Wrist extensors
Lateral	Abductors (radial side)	Adductors (ulnar side)

to designing exercises to strengthen concentric contractions. Roskopf suggested a protocol using 6 repetitions of 6 s contractions progressing from 50% intensity to 70%, 100%, and maximal force on the last three contractions.

The previous chapter discussed in detail the prescription factors for resistance exercises. For a client dealing with the weakness underlying muscular imbalance, refer to the detailed guidelines in chapter 7.

Strengthen Movement Patterns . . . Not Just Muscles

After constantly repeating a particular faulty movement pattern, clients need to be reprogrammed to perform the movement correctly. This can be difficult, because the faulty movement is by now ingrained in the central nervous system and has contributed to the muscle imbalance and poor posture. To address this condition, put your client's kinesthetic and postural awareness to use. Have clients perform the exercises with little or no load initially. Once they can do the unloaded movement properly, add a Theraband or tubing and continue to monitor the movement mechanics. There are several good examples where this has proven to be very effective:

• Clients with weak lower trapezius and overactive upper trapezius: Excessive scapular elevation can occur with dumbbell lateral raises. Start with light tubing and teach the client to pull outward, not upward, avoiding any shoulder shrugging.

• Clients who need to be aware of a neutral spine position: Promote postural awareness in a seated position on a stability ball. Establish awareness of what muscles are contracting to stabilize and then begin small movements in all directions while maintaining a good kinesthetic sense of the lumbar–pelvic position.

• Clients with winged scapulae that need to be stabilized against the rib cage: Teach clients to "set" their scapulae in proper alignment with your tactile feedback. Progress to a modified push-up and emphasize the involvement of the serratus anterior with fully protracted scapulae at the top of the exercise. Similarly, emphasize the rhomboids by pinching the scapulae in the lowered position.

Check your clients for alignment and compliment good form during their resistance exercises. Balance the number of push–pull movements in the maintenance prescription. Progress to more functional total-body exercises and identify the things clients do in everyday life that need the same degree of attention as their workout. Few of us are immune from these daily risks: the new mother who undergoes repeated spinal flexion with caring for her child, the career driver with a poor seat or poor core stability who has constant intervertebral compression, the office worker with his telephone wedged between his ear and shoulder, and the personal trainer who constantly stoops to pick up weights and leans over to spot clients.

Case Studies

Inherent in musculoskeletal fitness are alignment and muscle balance. Screening for common postural faults provides a direction for follow-up muscle testing. The goals of training for performance, rehabilitation, or fitness may differ, but the need to maintain muscle balance is important for all. Setting objectives for muscle balance usually centers around stretching tight muscles, strengthening weak muscles, reducing spasm, building muscular endurance, or improving posture. Remain vigilant for those clients whose postural assessment or other screening indicates that they should be referred to another health care professional.

Two case studies will illustrate the progression from postural analysis to selection of muscle length test items and on to a personalized pre-scription. The case studies detail a number of muscle tests presented in chapter 4.

Case Study 1: 37-Year-Old Working Mother

Rose was a 37-year-old bank teller with two children, ages 3 years and 18 months. She did not exercise regularly. Rose had headaches caused by neck tension and pain. She wanted to exercise at home and could devote 25 to 30 min, 4 or 5 days per week, to her program. Her primary objectives were to improve upper-body endurance and eliminate neck pain.

Assessment

A cursory check of Rose's posture, with particular attention to upper torso alignment, revealed some areas that warranted further examination. I believed that an apparent lack of balance could be confirmed with some muscle tightness assessment.

The postural assessment helped to fine-tune the priorities. I observed no significant problems with Rose's feet, knees, or pelvis, but I did note the following misalignments: depressed chest, increased cervical curve, forward shoulders, palms rotated medially, scapulae abducted, and a forward head (tables 8.5 and 8.6).

Interpretation

The combination of postural faults just described often creates neck and shoulder tension and discomfort, because the weight of the head is supported by the posterior muscles rather than the skeletal system. Strengthening of the anterior neck muscles (deep neck flexors and sternocleidomastoid) can help restore balance.

The shoulder girdle and neck musculature are linked. It was clear to me that muscle length testing could help determine the underlying cause of Rose's rounded-shouldered posture. The pectoralis minor exerts a forward and downward pull on the front of the scapula and may alone cause the roundness. Tightness of the pectoralis major will contribute to the forward pull of the shoulders and may cause an internal rotation of the shoulder, as seen by the palms facing backwards. Because Rose was relatively untrained, I suspected weak and overstretched posterior scapular adductors (trapezius and rhomboids) and a depressed chest (which often accompanies rounded shoulders).

Chapter 4 described procedures for muscle length assessments for the pectoralis minor, pectoralis major (sternal-S), shoulder internal rotators, and shoulder external rotators. The "normal"

Table 8.5 Assessment of Segmental Posture: Upper Body (Case 1)

Alignment scale: 5 (Good) 4 3 (Faulty) 2 1 (Very faulty)

Joint	View	Good alignment	Faulty alignment	Score	Left (L)/ Right (R)	Comments
Head	L P	Erect and balanced	Protruding, chin forward Tilted and rotated	3		Head and chin forward
Arms and shoulders	A	Arms relaxed; palms facing body	Arms stiff, away from body Palms facing backward	3		Palms rotated medially
	L	Shoulders back	Shoulders rounded and forward	2		Shoulders rounded
	A/P	Shoulders level	One or both shoulders up, down, or rotated	5		
	P	Scapulae: flat on ribcage; 4-6 in. (10-15 cm) apart	Scapulae: prominent-winged, far apart	3		Scapulae abducted: 6 in. (15 cm) apart

Score: 16 /25

Note. A = anterior; P = posterior; L = lateral.

Table 8.6 Assessment of Segmental Posture: Spine (Case 1)

Alignment scale: 5 (Good) 4 3 (Faulty) 2 1 (Very faulty)

Joint	View	Good alignment	Faulty alignment	Score	Left (L)/ Right (R)	Comments
Spine and pelvis	A/P	Hips level, weight even on both feet	One hip higher (lateral tilt), hips rotated (forward one side)	5		
	P	No lateral curve to spine (posterior view)	C- or S-curve scoliosis Ribs prominent one side	5		
	L	Natural lumbar curve	Lordosis: forward tilt of pelvis and flat back: pelvis tilts backward	5		
	L	Natural thoracic curve	Kyphosis: thoracic rounding	4		Some thoracic rounding
	L	Natural cervical curve	Cervical lordosis: forward head	3		Increased cervical curve and forward head
Trunk	L	Flat or slightly rounded abdomen	Protruding lower or entire abdomen	5		
	L	Chest slightly raised	Hollow chest and rounded back	3		Depressed chest
Head	L P	Erect and balanced	Protruding, chin forward Tilted and rotated	3		As noted in table 8.5

Score: 33/40

Note. A = anterior; P = posterior; L = lateral.

values quoted for the tests are conservative: Any deviation from them deserves attention. Here is what I found for Rose (table 8.7):

- Pectoralis minor: moderate tightness, left and right
- Pectoralis major (sternal): left and right arms 5° off table
- Shoulder internal rotators: left and right forearms 10° off table
- Shoulder external rotators: normal ROM
- Early and excessive elevation of scapulae when shoulder joint abducted

Prescribing for Rose

It seemed clear that Rose's forward chin, cervical lordosis, and a tight neck would benefit from exercises designed to stretch the neck extensors and strengthen the neck flexors. Her rounded shoulders should respond to stretches for tight pectoralis minor and major and to strengthening exercises for shoulder extensors, external rotators, and scapular adductors (see table 8.4).

Several exercises are beneficial for both areas, with simple training methods appropriate for the home environment. Static stretching is the suggested method for lengthening the tight muscles. Isometric exercises, tubing, and calisthenics are the appropriate strength training techniques. I prescribed these exercises for Rose, as described in table 8.8.

Follow-Up

Weekly phone conversations with Rose seemed very promising. She managed to devote nearly an hour every day to her prescription. She liked the convenience of working out at home and the easy-to-follow program. I joined her for a workout in the third week and was amazed at her rapid increase in muscular endurance, especially in the posterior shoulder area. However, the dull ache in her neck had not disappeared. My concern at this point was that Rose might be overtraining and perpetuating the symptoms.

I didn't want to discourage Rose from her exercise habit, but some modifications were necessary. We designed a workout log to track the volume of work and any symptoms. She agreed to exercise only 3 days per week for 30 min. To maintain an adequate overload, I moved her up to heavier tubing and substituted bent-over flys with some newly acquired dumbbells for the supine scapular retraction exercise. We selected a starting weight that brought Rose to fatigue by the eighth to tenth repetition on the first set.

I scheduled a reassessment in 5 weeks to judge the effectiveness of the prescription for Rose's posture and muscle balance. Continued weekly phone calls confirmed a reduction in neck pain and tension headaches.

Prescriptions are rarely a straight highway to success. But with regular monitoring and follow-up modifications, the journey can resume in the right direction.

Note: If your clients are seeking gains in strength and endurance, select a starting weight that brings them to fatigue by the eighth to tenth repetition on the first set. Adjust the weight, if necessary, and have them do as many repetitions as possible on the second set. Refer to table 8.8 for progressions and other guidelines.

Table 8.7   Assessment of Shoulder and Chest Tightness (Case 1)

Assessment	Results (observations)	Normal range of motion	Pain
Shoulder internal (medial) rotation: tightness of infraspinatus, teres minor	L: 70°_____ R: 70°_____	70°	No
Shoulder external (lateral) rotation: tightness of subscapularis	L: 80°_____ R: 80°_____	90°	No
Pectoralis major (sternal) length	5° off table	Table level	No
Pectoralis minor length	L: Moderately tight R: Moderately tight		No
Shoulder joint abduction (dynamic shoulder alignment)	Early and excessive elevation of scapulae	180°	Neck tightness

Table 8.8   Muscle Balance Prescription—Case 1

Client name: Rose	Trainer name: John
Client goals: 1. Relieve neck pain by stretching neck extensors and strengthen neck flexors 2. Correct rounded shoulders by stretching chest and front shoulder and strengthen back shoulder and scapular muscles	**Assessment rationale:** 1. Forward chin and head lean—cervical lordosis, tension in neck 2. Rounded shoulders, internal rotation of shoulder, abducted scapulae, tight anterior muscles
Flexibility prescription for Goal 1: **Chin tuck** Pull head straight back, keeping jaw and eyes level.	Strengthening prescription for Goal 1: **Resisted neck flexion** Facing forward with finger tips on forehead, bend head forward through a full range. Give moderate resistance. (20 s × 2)
Lateral neck stretch Grasp arm and pull downward and across body while gently tilting head.	
Flexibility prescription for Goal 2: **Shoulder internal rotator stretch** Keep palm of hand against door frame, elbow bent at 90°. Turn body from fixed hand until stretch is felt.	Strengthening prescription for Goal 2: **Resisted diagonal shoulder extension** Grasp tubing with arm reaching above shoulder and across body. Gently pull downward and away from your body. Return slowly to starting position.
Supine wand thrust Hold wand with involved side palm up, push with uninvolved side (palm down) out from body, keeping elbow at side until you feel a stretch. Then pull back across body, leading with uninvolved side.	**Resisted shoulder external rotation** Using tubing, and keeping elbow in at side, rotate arm outward away from body. Keep forearm parallel to floor.
Door frame pec stretch Keep palm of outstretched horizontal arm against door frame. Turn body until a stretch is felt. Vary the level of the arm.	**Supine scapular retraction** With fingers clasped behind head, pull elbows back while pinching shoulder blades together.
Program recommendations: • For clients who prefer dumbbells, upper back strengthening exercises may be replaced with bent-over flys or reverse flys. • For stack-weight users, rowing and pull-downs could be substituted. • For clients seeking gains in strength endurance, select a starting weight that brings them to fatigue by the eighth to tenth repetition on the first set.	**Safety and monitoring guidelines:** • Hold stretches for 15-30 s, longer but not harder if tension is more significant. • Repeat stretches 2 or 3 times. • Do a circulatory warm-up before muscle balance workout.

Case Study 2: 45-Year-Old Weekend Warrior

Kevin was a divorced 45-year-old broker who worked long hours. He played old-timers hockey once a week for 6 months of the year. He had moderate low back discomfort. He had just joined a local fitness club and was willing to commit to three 50 min workouts per week. He wanted to lose fat from the trunk area and improve the condition of his back.

Assessment

Kevin was concerned about his back and trunk region. An overview of his posture revealed some areas to examine further. His prolonged stress and sitting posture at work were obvious concerns. To confirm an apparent lack of balance, I assessed the strength and tightness of the muscles that attach to the spine and pelvis. The postural assessment (table 8.9) helped to fine-tune the priorities.

Kevin's postural chart showed nothing significant at the feet, knees, shoulder, scapulae, or head. I did note the following misalignments: an anterior tilt to the pelvis, a protruding abdomen, and an increased curvature to the low back with accompanying discomfort.

Muscle testing showed tightness in the one-joint hip flexors (the iliopsoas crosses only the hip) and two-joint hip flexors (the rectus femoris crosses both hip and knee). Further assessment revealed some tightness of the hamstrings; five-level sit-up test (chapter 4) revealed weak abdominals, and a modified trunk forward flexion assessment disclosed low back tightness (tables 8.10 and 8.11).

Chapter 4 describes procedures for muscle length assessments for hip flexors, hamstrings, and forward trunk flexion. As was true with the previous example, any deviation from the "normal" values given for these tests should lead to further investigation. The observations I made for Kevin are as follows:

- Hip flexors: one-joint and two-joint hip flexors tight, tensor fascia latae also tight

Table 8.9   Assessment of Segmental Posture: Spine (Case 2)

Alignment scale:

	5 (Good)	4	3 (Faulty)	2	1 (Very faulty)

Joint	View	Good alignment	Faulty alignment	Score	Left (L)/ Right (R)	Comments
Spine and pelvis	A/P	Hips level—weight even on both feet	One hip higher (lateral tilt); hips rotated (forward one side)	5		
	P	No lateral curve to spine (posterior view)	C- or S-curve scoliosis Ribs prominent one side	5		
	L	Natural lumbar curve	Lordosis: forward tilt of pelvis and flat back: pelvis tilts backward	3		Increased curve in low back—anterior pelvic tilt
	L	Natural thoracic curve	Kyphosis: thoracic rounding	5		
	L	Natural cervical curve	Cervical lordosis: forward head	5		
Trunk	L	Flat and slightly rounded abdomen	Lower or entire abdomen protrudes	3		Protruding abdomen (entire trunk)
	L	Chest slightly raised	Hollow chest and rounded back	5		
Head	L P	Erect and balanced	Protruding, chin forward Tilted and rotated	5		

Score: 36/40

Note. A = anterior; P = posterior; L = lateral.

Table 8.10   Assessment of Hip, Knee, and Back Tightness (Case 2)

Hip/Knee Assessment	Results (observations)	Normal ROM	Pain Y/N
Hamstring length	L: 80°_____ R: 75°_____	80° (males) 90° (females)	N
Hip flexors: 1 joint (tightness of iliopsoas)	L: 10° off table R: 10° off table	Thigh table level	N
Hip flexors: 2 joint (tightness of rectus femoris)	L: 60°_____ R: 60°_____	Knee: 80°	N
Tensor fascia latae tightness	L: abduction and rotation_____ R: abduction and rotation_____		N
Hip internal (medial) rotation (tightness of gluteus maximus, piriformis)	L: _____ R: _____	35°	
Hip external (lateral) rotation (tightness of gluteus minimus, anterior gluteus medius)	L: _____ R: _____	45°	
Back Assessment	Results (observations)	Normal ROM	Pain Y/N
Spinal rotation: Lumbar Cervical	L: 40°; R: 45°_ L: _____; R: _____	45° 65-70°	N
Sit and reach test: actual visual	24 cm Short muscles in low back—no roundness in low back	"good": 28-33 cm (males), 32-37 cm (females)	felt tight

- Hamstrings: 75° to 80º (low normal)
- Forward trunk flexion: hamstrings normal, short muscles in low back (no roundness)
- Lumbar rotation: 40° to 45° (low normal)

Interpretation

The increased lumbar lordosis had caused the weight of the upper body to settle on the low back, aggravating any low back problems. Although it is common in such cases to see exaggerated curves in the thoracic and cervical regions (to compensate for the lumbar curve), Kevin did not exhibit such symptoms. The anterior tilt to his pelvis, in conjunction with the lumbar lordosis, is very common and likely resulted from one or several muscle imbalances. Tight hip flexors pulled his pelvis forward and down—a condition often associated with short spinal extensors, which also contribute to anterior pelvic tilt. Weak and perhaps overstretched abdominals are not sufficient to withstand such forces. I decided that strengthening the hip extensors (gluteus maximus and hamstrings) would resist the pull of the very strong hip flexors.

Prescribing for Kevin

Because Kevin had lumbar lordosis and anterior pelvic tilt and tested positive for tight erector spinae and hip flexors, he could alleviate his low back stress with exercises that stretched the back extensors and hip flexors and that strengthened the abdominals and hip extensors. Table 8.4 is a useful reference for muscle pairs.

The exercise design began with therapeutic exercises for the lumbar lordosis, followed by exercises for the related anterior pelvic tilt (see table 8.12). The methods of training included static stretching for muscle tightness. To strengthen the abdominals, Kevin started with

Table 8.11 Strength and Endurance Testing (Case 2)

Muscle	Test	Rating system (circle one)	Comments
1) 2) 3) 4)	Weightlifting	1. Exercise: _____ 5-10RM _____ ; 1RM _____ 2. Exercise: _____ 5-10RM _____ ; 1RM _____ 3. Exercise: _____ 5-10RM _____ ; 1RM _____ 4. Exercise: _____ 5-10RM _____ ; 1RM _____	
Erector spinae	Biering–Sorenson	E.g., ages 20-29 male (m) and female (f) [s] Needs improvement • Fair • Good • Very good • Excellent (m) ≤ 85 • 86-98 • 99-132 • 133-175 • 176-180 (f) ≤ 65 • 66-101 • 102-135 • 136-179 • 179-180	
Rectus abdominis	Five-level sit-ups	1) 2) × 3) 4) 5) No. of reps: 8 at level 1	Terminated because of loss of form and partial fatigue
Lower abdominals	Leg lowers	75° = poor, 60° = fair, 30° = good, 5° = excellent ° = Degrees when back arches while lowering legs	
Quadratus lumborum	Lateral lift	**Right shoulder** Grade 1: Shoulder 1 in. off floor without difficulty Grade 2: Shoulder 12 in. off floor with difficulty Grade 3: Shoulder 2-6 in. off floor Grade 4: Unable to raise shoulder off floor **Left shoulder** Grade 1: Shoulder 12 in. off floor without difficulty Grade 2: Shoulder 12 in. off floor with difficulty Grade 3: Shoulder 2-6 in. off floor Grade 4: Unable to raise shoulder off floor	
Serratus anterior	Push-up	Strong = Scapula flat in down phase Weak = Scapular "winging" in down phase	

only the resistance of gravity and body weight. For the hip extensors, I suggested that he add resistance from tubing or from the appropriate machines at the fitness club.

Follow-Up

I had an opportunity to talk with Kevin during most of his club visits. The first 4 weeks of his program preceded the start of his hockey season. After a guided demonstration and three workouts on his own, I introduced some aerobic intervals that simulated the shift changes for his hockey. I explained that the aerobic activity would have an added benefit for his back.

Because he enjoyed the aerobic intervals, we continued them throughout the hockey season using different equipment for a cross-training effect (see chapter 6). A month into the season, Kevin began coming in only twice a week as opposed to three times as prescribed. This would

not have been a concern had not Kevin indicated that his home workouts had pretty much dropped off.

Kevin was in an "action stage" (see chapter 1), and his risk of relapse was high. I could tell he felt guilty about the transgression, but I reassured him that this was a normal state of affairs and our job now was to deal with the lapse. With his two club aerobic workouts and weekly hockey, he was pleased with the cardiovascular improvements he was feeling. However, he was taking two days of rest after his hockey because his back felt tight and fatigued. Although he agreed that he needed to do the muscle balance exercises more frequently, Kevin admitted that he had little motivation to follow his home program. We came up with two modifications. First, I linked Kevin up with one of our apprenticing personal trainers for an additional 15 min per visit of guided strengthening and stretching

Table 8.12 Muscle Balance Prescription—Case 2

Client name: Kevin	Trainer name: John
Client goals: 1. Alleviate low back discomfort and reduce lumbar lordosis by stretching back extensor muscles and strengthening abdominals 2. Relieve back discomfort symptoms and pelvic tilt by stretching hip flexors and rotators and strengthen hip extensors	**Assessment rationale:** 1. Increased curve in low back; tight low back during sit-and-reach; protruding abdomen; only 8 reps at level 1 2. Anterior pelvic tilt, tight one- and two-joint hip flexors, tight tensor fascia latae, deep buttock ache

Flexibility prescription for Goal 1: **Supine knees to chest** Pull both knees in to chest until a comfortable stretch is felt in low back. Keep back relaxed.	**Strengthening prescription for Goal 1:** **Curl-up—Level 1** With arms at side, tilt pelvis to flatten back. Raise shoulders and head from floor. Return in a controlled fashion.
Seated back stretch Sit on the edge of a chair with legs spread apart. Tuck your chin and slowly bend downward. Relax in a comfortable stretch. Return slowly.	**Abdominal crunch** With legs over footstool or chair and arms positioned at side of head, tilt pelvis to flatten back. Raise head and shoulders from the floor.
Flexibility prescription for Goal 2: **One-joint hip flexor lunge** Slowly push pelvis downward from a front lunge until stretch felt in front of hip.	**Strengthening prescription for Goal 2:** **Supine hip thrusts** Start in a supine position with lower legs vertical and pillow under head. Slowly raise buttocks, keeping stomach tight.
Side-lying quad stretch Pull heel toward buttocks until comfortable stretch in front thigh. Tilt pelvis backward.	**Resisted hip extension** With tubing around involved ankle and opposite end secured, bring leg backward, keeping knee secure.
Wall lean stretch With arm against wall, slowly lean hips toward wall. Cross inside leg behind for increased stretch.	
Supine piriformis stretch Cross legs with involved leg on top. Gently pull opposite knee toward chest. Stretch should be felt in buttock and hip area.	
Program recommendations: • Stack weight leg extensions or other machines may be substituted to strengthen hip extensors. • For clients seeking gains in strength endurance, select a starting weight that brings them to fatigue by the eighth to tenth repetition on the first set.	**Safety and monitoring guidelines:** • Hold stretches for 15-30 s, longer but not harder if tension is more significant. • Repeat stretches 2 or 3 times. • Do a circulatory warm-up before muscle balance workout. • Monitor discomfort in buttocks and low back; if symptoms worsen, seek medical attention.

similar to his prescribed exercises. To deal with the tightness created by the hockey, I gave him five stretches—specifically adapted to the bench in his locker room—that he agreed to do before and after each game.

Client-centered prescription involves carefully listening to your client's feedback and modifying the path as necessary in response. It often involves side trips and doubling back, but it always moves in the direction of better health for your client.

Highlights

1. **Describe the factors affecting muscle balance.**

   Muscle balance is affected by muscle tightness, flexibility, strength, and endurance, as these factors work together to provide support and movement. A muscle must be long enough to allow a normal range of motion and short and strong enough to provide joint stability. Muscle balance also depends on neuromuscular efficiency or the ability of the neuromuscular system to properly recruit movers, stabilizers, and synergists to produce force or reduce force (antagonists).

2. **Describe the causes and results of muscle imbalance.**

   A joint is a pivot point or a fulcrum whose position is constantly affected by the pull of the muscles around it. Joint alignment and posture are affected by these forces. If the muscle is short, it will restrict normal range of motion. Muscles that are too short are usually strong and hold the opposite muscle in a lengthened position. Excessively long muscles are usually weak and allow adaptive shortening of antagonists. Muscles can be unbalanced in several ways: unmatched levels of flexibility, strength, contracture, or a combination of these factors.

   One common imbalance involves shortened back extensors and hip flexors versus weakened abdominal and buttock muscles. This imbalance results in an anterior pelvic tilt and excessive lumbar lordosis. The ultimate goal of the human kinetic chain is to maintain both a static and dynamic postural equilibrium. Muscle imbalance may also lead to faulty movements through muscle groups firing in an uncoordinated way.

3. **Select and describe assessment items for muscle balance.**

   If your client has a muscle imbalance, there will often be a malalignment. In a cyclic fashion, when muscles lose flexibility, the joint becomes progressively more stiff until the muscle is in constant partial contracture exhibiting progressively less endurance and strength. At this point, a person will alter his mechanics. Faulty body mechanics, as determined by postural screening, should be confirmed by the muscle tests for tightness, range of motion, and weakness.

4. **Describe the factors affecting the quality of a stretch.**

   Muscles are not purely elastic; rather, they are viscoelastic. That is, they have both viscous (resistant to flow) and elastic properties. When a muscle lengthens under force it is called **creep.** The stretch mechanism has both a direct and indirect process of decreasing a muscle's **stiffness,** which is defined as the force required to change the muscle's length. The direct process is via passive viscoelastic changes or deformations. Indirectly, the stretch mechanism is attributable to reflex inhibition and consequent changes in the viscoelasticity from decreased actin–myosin cross-bridging.

   When you are prescribing flexibility exercises, the following factors directly affect the quality of stretch:

   - Duration of the applied force
   - Intensity of the applied force
   - Temperature of the tissue
   - Degree of relaxation of the muscle
   - Type of applied force (e.g., ballistic, static)
   - Alignment of muscle fibers to be stretched

5. **Describe the advantages and client suitability of various stretching techniques.**

   Active loosening exercises such as rhythmic swinging of the limbs can relieve muscle tension and promote relaxation. **Static stretching** (actively or passively) involves controlled elongation of an antagonistic muscle by placing it in a maximal position of stretch and holding it. The Golgi tendon organ's signal to relax overrides the muscle spindles' signal to contract and the muscle is more relaxed and prepared to stretch. **Dynamic stretching** through bouncing movements produces a quick stretch of the antagonist muscle. If momentum is uncontrolled, the stretch becomes a ballistic stretch and can cause overstretching and microtears. However, many sports require dynamic movements and it is reasonable to integrate these functional movements into athletic training programs. **Proprioceptive neuromuscular facilitation (PNF)** (e.g., contract–relax, antagonist–contract) involves the client actively moving the limb into the new ROM after an isometric contraction. This active contraction of the agonist is thought to relax the target muscle (called reciprocal inhibition), thereby allowing a better stretch. PNF stretching requires an experienced trainer but produces excellent ROM gains, strength, muscle balance, and joint stability.

6. **Select appropriate exercises (stretching or resistance) that target designated muscle groups to improve range of motion or muscle balance.**

   Setting objectives for muscle balance usually centers around stretching tight muscles, strengthening weak muscles, reducing spasm, building muscular endurance, or improving posture. As muscle balance improves, start to replace isolated exercises with more complex movements. After constantly repeating a particular faulty movement pattern, clients often need to be kinesthetically reprogrammed to perform the movement correctly.

7. **Design a physiologically sound and client-centered exercise prescription for muscle balance and flexibility using the six-step model of sequenced decisions.**

   For muscle balance to be restored and maintained, therapeutic exercises to strengthen weak muscles should be combined with stretches for tight muscles. The steps involved in the *Muscle Balance Prescription Model* includes:

   1. Assess needs and formulate goals

   2. Select the training method for the fitness component

   3. Select exercises and order of performance

   4. Provide prescriptive recommendations

   5. Provide progression, monitoring, and safety guidelines

   6. Design warm-up and cool-down

   The *Muscle Balance Prescription Card* records specific program recommendations and guidelines for safety and monitoring. Remain vigilant for those clients whose postural assessment or other screening indicates that they should be referred to another health care professional.

Client-Centered Weight Management Prescription Model

Chapter Competencies

After completing this chapter, you will be able to demonstrate the following competencies:

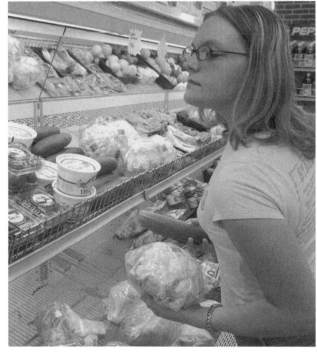

1. Take a two-pronged approach to improving a client's "shape" and helping him lose weight by (a) modifying eating behaviors and (b) integrating activity (not merely fitness prescription).

2. Identify behaviors most often identified as the reasons for a client's weight problem, that is, what is eaten (e.g., overeating or eating the wrong foods) and why it is eaten (e.g., emotional eating).

3. Describe several ways to expend energy: resting metabolism, metabolizing food (thermic effect of food), and physical activity (thermic effect of exercise).

4. Provide information to clients about counting calories and the merits of diet versus exercise.

5. Use the Energy Deficit Point System to encourage clients to become more active and to estimate the weight loss value of these lifestyle changes.

6. Use a 10-step model to design a physiologically sound and client-centered exercise prescription for weight management.

We must help our clients accept a large range of healthy weights and variations in body size, and we also need to educate them about the merits of diet versus exercise and the issue of counting calories. The Energy Deficit Point System is presented in this chapter to encourage clients to become more active and to estimate the weight loss value of these lifestyle changes. We must recognize the importance of integrating a resistance training segment into a weight management prescription that will prevent loss of lean body mass while increasing resting energy expenditure, and often increasing energy expenditure per pound.

In the case study in this chapter, you will learn how to apply the model for weight management prescription with physiological justifications and client-centered (behavioral) justifications for each choice made.

What to Tell Your Clients

A large and growing number of clients ask for assistance to "get into shape." By "getting into shape," most clients mean that they want to shed extra pounds. It is a formidable task to create behavioral change in the midst of overwhelming cultural pressures to succumb to the junk-food diets and sedentary living that have led to epidemic weight gain and ill health. So how can we most effectively help those who wish to transform their physical shape?

Improving a client's shape and helping him lose weight require a two-pronged approach: (a) modifying eating behaviors and (b) integrating activity (not merely fitness prescription). The most effective weight loss programs focus on these two components. Inadequate attention to either one of these decreases the likelihood of long-term, healthy weight management.

Eating Behaviors

The human body is a remarkable machine. It can consume nearly a ton of food in a year and not change its weight. However, overeating, eating the wrong foods, and emotional eating are the behaviors most often identified as the reasons for weight problems. A number of nutrition essentials and resources should be among your tools of the trade, although you cannot replace the services of a qualified nutritionist (see *Nutrition for CPTs*).

Nutrition for CPTs

Nutrition Essentials

1. The U.S. My Pyramid or Canada's Food Guide to Healthy Eating

The U.S. My Pyramid model helps with daily food choices by dividing food into five groupings. For a 2,000 calorie intake, it supports a foundation of wholesome breads, cereals, and grains at each meal (6 oz). It recommends at least 2.5 cups of vegetables, 2 cups of fruit, 5.5 oz of beans and animal proteins, and 3 cups of dairy foods. The Dietary Guidelines for Americans (2005) recommends consuming a variety of nutrient-dense foods within the basic food groups while limiting the intake of saturated and trans fats, cholesterol, added sugars, salt, and alcohol. The tip of the pyramid lists refined sugars and saturated fats, which are foods to be used sparingly. In a similar way, Canada's Food Guide encourages selecting a variety of foods from each of four food groups. The number of servings depends on age, body size, activity level, gender, and pregnancy or breast-feeding status. Canada's Food Guide suggests 5 to 12 servings of grain products, 5 to 10 servings of vegetables and fruit, 2 to 3 servings of meat and alternatives, and 2 to 4 servings of dairy products.

2. Portion Sizes and Servings

Portion sizes may not be as large as most clients think. With the emphasis on getting more for your money, many people have lost sight of standard portion sizes. Eating large portion sizes can lead to overeating, resulting in overweight. To keep your eye on portion size, use the visual images presented in table 9.1 to help you (Dietitians of Canada 2005).

3. Food-Label Savvy

A good place to start to keep track of the foods you eat is at the grocery store. Nutritional labeling posts the nutritional values on most packaged foods. The marketing claims often placed on the front of

Table 9.1   Visualizing Portion Sizes

Food group	Specific foods	Portion size	Looks like
Grain products 5-12 servings	Pasta, rice Bagel	125 ml (1/2 cup) 1/2 small	1/2 baseball 1 hockey puck
Vegetables and fruits 5-10 servings	Fresh (e.g., apple, orange) Dried fruit Baked potato	1 medium piece 60 ml (1/4 cup) 1 medium	1 baseball 1 golf ball Computer mouse
Meats and alternatives 2-3 servings	Meat, poultry, fish Cooked kidney beans Nuts (e.g., peanuts, almonds)	50-100 g cooked 125-250 ml (1/2-1 cup) 75 ml (1/3 cup)	Deck of cards 1/2-1 baseball Cupped palm of hand
Milk products 2-4 servings	Yogurt Cheese	175 ml (3/4 cup) 50 g (2 oz)	Yogurt container (6 oz) 3 dominoes

Data from Fleck and Kraemer 2004; Heyward 2002.

What to Look for in a Cereal

If your favorite cereal doesn't meet these criteria, combine it with others to achieve a healthy mix.

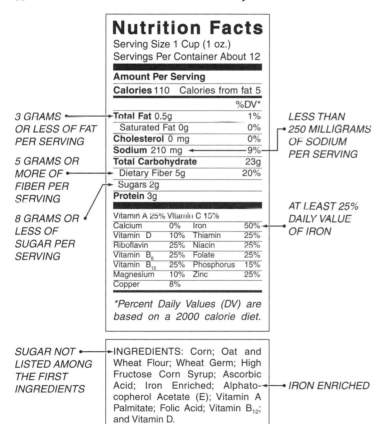

the package can be misleading. Claims of fat free, low sodium, or high fiber are recorded accurately on the nutrition label. Nancy Clark (2003) showed how to use the nutritional facts on the label to evaluate the value of a cereal (figure 9.1).

Packaged programs, self-inflicted diets, and gym gurus are often unsuccessful because one approach does not fit everyone. Clients seeking professional advice on weight loss programs that are individually tailored to their lifestyle and food needs are best referred to a registered dietitian. Use *Healthy Eating Resources* to locate a local registered dietitian or to find reliable information.

Figure 9.1   What to look for in a cereal.

Reprinted, by permission, from N. Clark, 2003, *Nancy Clark's Sports Nutrition Guidebook*, 3rd ed. (Champaign, IL: Human Kinetics), 62.

Healthy Eating Resources

American Web Sites and Journals

> American Dietetic Association: www.eatright.org
>
> Food and Nutrition Information Center: www.nal.usda.gov/fnic
>
> American Journal of Clinical Nutrition: www.ajcn.org
>
> Nutritional Reviews: www.ilsi.org
>
> USDA-Center for Nutrition Policy and Promotion: www.mypyramid.gov

Canadian Web Sites

> Dietitians of Canada: www.dietitians.ca
>
> Canada's Food Guide for Healthy Living: www.hc-sc.gc.ca/hppb
>
> Canadian Institute for Food Science and Technology: www.cifst.ca

One of the best nutrition resources for active people is Nancy Clark's third edition (2003) of *Sports Nutrition Guidebook*. Human Kinetics. ISBN: 0-7360-4602-X.

What You Eat

It is unfair, and for the most part unproven, to suggest that all people with weight problems overeat. Even if the cause of increased fat deposit is not overeating, treatment for overweight clients usually involves a reduction in daily energy intake. Yet dieting can reduce the resting metabolic rate, shift the energy balance back in the direction of energy storage, and counteract caloric reduction (Williams 1995). Repeated diets may have decreased your client's ability to lose weight and increased his ability to gain weight (Blackburn et al. 1989).

The average American consumes nearly 40% of calories from fat (25-30% is recommended). This amount of dietary fat can itself be a cause of obesity. It has been shown that naturally lean people have a difficult time gaining weight on a low-fat diet but gain easily on high-fat diets (Tremblay et al. 1989). Eating a high-fat diet promotes body fat formation. The body uses one fourth to one third less energy to process dietary fat than it does to convert protein or carbohydrate to body fat (Dattilio 1992). In other words, a given caloric quantity of excess dietary fat is more fattening than a calorically similar quantity of excess carbohydrate. This means that what you eat (diet composition) may be as important as total calories in the promotion of obesity.

Miller (1991) demonstrated that middle-aged obesity is characterized by reduced carbohydrate intake. His data suggested that consumption of natural or complex carbohydrates (such as whole grains) assists in weight loss, whereas obesity correlates with excess consumption of "added" or refined sugars. He also found that a high fiber intake assists in weight loss because of the increased consumption of natural carbohydrates (vegetables, fruits, grains).

Clients are more likely to follow eating recommendations if you can integrate their food preferences assuming moderation and include all food groups. Even the most knowledgeable clients need encouragement to make the best choices on a daily basis. The National Heart, Lung, and Blood Institute (2000) provided recommended elements of a basic low-calorie diet for healthy adults (table 9.2).

Fast Food Fat

I have a friend who often found himself on the road at mealtime. He usually picked up a cinnamon bun with butter in the late afternoon, to hold him till dinner. His wife prepared wonderful nutritious dinners such as chicken breast, baked potato, salad, and juice. What changed his habit was his shock in learning that the afternoon snack had more calories than his dinner! He was also surprised that not all hamburgers are created equal. For example, McDonald's Big Mac has almost 600 kcal with its high-fat sauce, whereas a regular hamburger contains only 150 kcal (from carbohydrate, fat, and protein). Fast food snacks may be high-fat meals—choose carefully!

Why You Eat

Helping clients discover why they eat is as important as knowing what they eat. Clients who were rewarded with food as children may confuse being fed with being loved. Some people eat when they are bored. With the boom in television watching, many are not aware of the amount they consume each night after their "last" meal!

These clients need extra help to become more aware of when and why they eat. A daily log of the food, quantity, time, place, and emotional state may provide insights for you and your client and help you devise strategies to counteract her personal triggers for overeating or for eating the wrong things. Many clients may need guidance

Table 9.2   Recommended Daily Intake

Component	Recommended daily intake
Calories	500-1,000 kcal/day reduction
Protein	About 15% of total calories
Carbohydrate	≥55% of total calories
Fat (saturated and unsaturated)	≤30% of total calories
Cholesterol	<300 mg/day
Sodium chloride	<2,400 mg/day
Calcium	1,000-15,000 mg/day
Fiber	20-30 g/day

National Heart, Lung, and Blood Institute: Clinical Guidelines on the Identification, Evaluation and treatment of Overweight and Obesity in Adults: Executive Summary. National Institutes of Health publication no. 00-4084, Rockville, MD, October 2000.

in preparing food, packing a nutritious lunch, or judging food serving sizes. To avoid temptations to give into excuses, instruct your clients to do the following:

- Plan alternatives ahead of time. Have some prepared meals in the freezer that can be thawed faster than a pizza delivery.
- Use stick-on notes to post inspirational messages on the refrigerator, for example, "Contrary to popular belief, chocolate is not one of the food groups."

- Share goals and temptations with a friend or spouse and ask for their help when the going gets tough.
- Use smaller plates and bowls so food portions seem larger.

Integrating Activity

The late Jean Mayer, an international authority on weight control, reported that no single factor is more frequently responsible for obesity than lack of physical activity. If inactivity is not a major cause for obesity in some cases, it is the consequence of obesity and plays a definite role in maintaining it.

We live busy lives, and lack of time is the most frequently quoted barrier to becoming more active. Combine this with a dislike for strenuous exercise and often a sense of physical embarrassment and you have the formula for sedentary living. We need a new strategy to help overweight clients. Recent research (Andersen and Jakicic 2003) and public health guidelines (ACSM 2000; CSEP 2003; HHS 2005) suggest that sedentary individuals can derive significant health benefits from accumulating 30 min or more of moderately intense activity on most days (see figure 9.2).

Although some clients will follow a structured aerobic-based exercise prescription for weight loss, many will not. With these clients, your challenge is to help them buy into the concept and practice of activity "integration." We need to direct these clients toward activities that could be part of their current lifestyle. Thoughtful counseling should

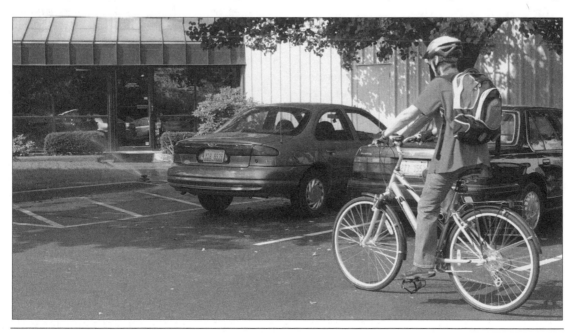

Figure 9.2   Many clients can fit aerobic work into their daily routines by biking or walking to work.

identify daily opportunities to walk, such as delivering a message in person, three floors up, or perform manual tasks, such as washing the car, gardening, or doing repair jobs around the house. Andersen and Jakicic (2003) compared the effects of performing several 10 min bouts of home exercise throughout the day with a single, longer bout. Overweight patients were more likely to adhere to the shorter prescription than those who exercised in longer bouts.

A compelling argument against exercise as a means of weight loss is that it expends so few calories: "One piece of cake and I've blown my whole aerobics class!" In the short term this is true. But compare mild exercise with the return we expect when we invest money at interest. The immediate payback usually is not large; but if we are patient and stay with the investment, it will grow substantially over time. For example, if you walk briskly for about 2 miles a day, it would expend enough calories in a month to 6 weeks to account for a loss of nearly 2 lb. When we combine mild diet reduction with increased activity, it is reasonable to expect a 10% reduction in body weight in 6 months (Bartlett 2003).

Sources of Energy Expenditure

There are three ways to expend energy: resting metabolism, metabolizing food (thermic effect of food), and physical activity (thermic effect of exercise).

Resting Metabolic Rate

The resting metabolic rate (RMR) is the energy expended to maintain normal body functions if we are simply lying in bed. It is usually the primary source of energy expenditure (60-75%) and would be about 1,600 kcal/day for someone weighing 70 kg (154 lb)—the equivalent of jogging 16 miles!

Obese people have daily RMRs approximately 500 kcal higher than nonobese people. This may seem like good news. However, when an obese person loses excess weight, the RMR may drop to 15% to 20% below that of a normal-weight person of similar height and weight (Nieman 1990). This is because fat is less metabolically active than muscle, and dramatic dieting can decrease lean body tissue so that the proportion of fat to lean tissue actually increases, slowing the "internal furnace"! This makes it even more difficult to lose weight at the same levels of energy expenditure than before the dieting. You can estimate RMR by multiplying the body weight in pounds by a factor of 10 for women and 11 for men (Heyward 2002). For example, if our 70 kg client was a female, her RMR would be approximately 1,540 kcal (154 lb × 10 kcal/lb or 70 kg × 22 kcal/kg). Given the higher energy expenditure of muscle, of course, individuals with more muscle have a higher RMR than those of the same weight with less muscle.

Thermic Effect of Food

The thermic effect of food (TEF) is the increase in energy expenditure above the RMR that can be measured for several hours after a meal. The average client's TEF is 7% to 10% of the total ingested calories and may last more than 3 hr. The TEF is higher after carbohydrate and protein meals than after fat meals (Miller 1991). With appropriate adjustments in meal plans, you could eat more and still lose weight!

Thermic Effect of Exercise

Any physical activity will raise the baseline rate of metabolism (RMR). The energy expended for physical activity is the thermic effect of exercise (TEE). The most significant factor affecting this TEE is the intensity of the exercise. For example, a briskly walking average-sized adult male may expend 5 kcal/min (compared with 1 kcal/min while lying). The same man jogging easily may burn 10 kcal/min. And if the intensity is up to a level barely sustainable by the best athletes for a full workout (10-12 mph), the rate of caloric expenditure may be more than 20 kcal/min (Williams 1995). On the other hand, Klesges and colleagues (1993) indicated that the resting energy expenditure decreases while watching television in approximately inverse proportion to the temptation to consume high-calorie snacks!

Energy expenditure is affected not only by the intensity but also by the efficiency of movement. A more awkward swimmer or runner will burn more calories going the same distance at the same speed as an expert swimmer. Heavier people also burn more calories for any given amount of work, because it takes more energy to move a heavier load.

Exercise may also facilitate weight loss by increasing postexercise energy expenditure (Brehm 1996). Cycling at 70% $\dot{V}O_2$max for 20 to 80 min is reported to produce a 5% to 14% elevation in RMR for 12 hr after exercise. Present this bonus to your clients as their physical condition improves and their enjoyment of activity increases.

What Effect Does Exercise Have on Fat Metabolism?

The two major sources of energy during exercise are fats (in the form of fatty acids) and carbohydrates (in the form of muscle glycogen).

A mixture of fats and carbohydrates is usually used during exercise, the ratio depending on the intensity and duration of the exercise and on the diet and physical condition of the individual.

Fat cells are specialized for the synthesis and storage of triglycerides. Before energy release from fat, triglycerides are broken down into free fatty acids (FFAs). Although some fat is stored in all cells (some in the muscle cells and a small amount in the blood), the most active sources of FFAs are the fat cells within adipose tissue. Once FFAs diffuse into the blood stream, they are delivered to active tissues where they can be used for energy (figure 9.3). As blood flow increases with exercise, more FFAs are removed from fat cells and delivered to active muscle (figure 9.3(1)). During exercise, the muscle cells first use fatty acids from the blood and from the muscles' own stores of triglycerides. As exercise continues or increases in intensity, the blood FFAs begin to be in short supply and must be replenished by the vast stores of triglycerides in the adipose tissue.

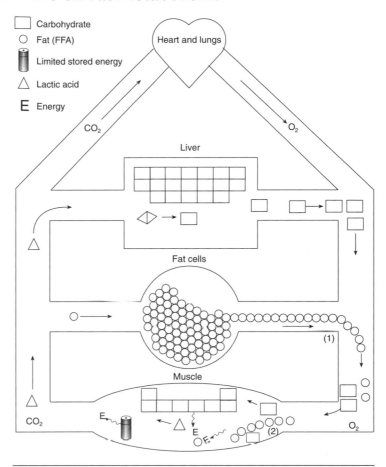

Figure 9.3 Schematic of energy production during light exercise.

During rest, the body metabolizes only about 30% of the FFAs that are released from adipose tissue. The other 70% are converted back into fat (i.e., triglycerides) (figure 9.3). During exercise, only about 25% of these FFAs are reconverted into triglycerides, providing much more FFA to the muscle cells (figure 9.3(2)).

During light exercise (25-50% of $\dot{V}O_2$max), about 30% to 50% of the total energy cost is derived from carbohydrate whereas the other 50% to 70% comes from FFAs. As the exercise intensity increases toward 60% to 65% $\dot{V}O_2$max, the muscle triglycerides become increasingly important as the source of fatty acids (Romijn et al. 1993) (figure 9.4).

Carbohydrate is the preferred energy source during high-intensity exercise, such as 65% to 70% of $\dot{V}O_2$max and above (figure 9.4). FFAs alone cannot sustain exercise at this intensity, and their contribution diminishes. Hodgetts and colleagues (1991) suggested that an increase in blood lactic acid levels may block release of FFAs from the adipose tissue (figure 9.4(3)).

Although carbohydrate becomes more important as an energy source during high-intensity exercise, trained endurance athletes may be able to use fats more efficiently at higher exercise intensities. Even regular exercisers who increase their anaerobic thresholds will be able to burn more fat during intensity levels of 65% to 70% of their $\dot{V}O_2$max.

Common Client Concerns

Clients usually come to you with a mix of information and disinformation about weight management. Two of the most common areas of confusion are counting calories and the relationship of diet, exercise, and weight control.

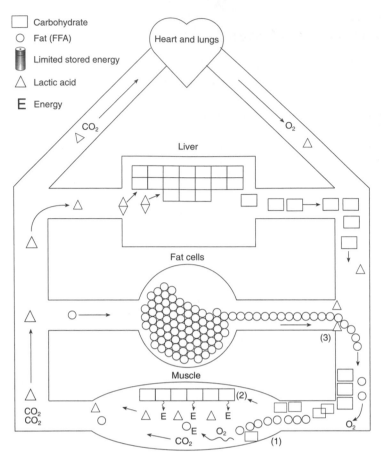

Figure 9.4   Schematic of energy production during high-intensity exercise.

Should Clients Count Calories?

If a person routinely consumes more calories than he expends, he will gain weight regardless of the composition of his diet. Conversely, if your client uses more calories than he ingests, he will lose weight. A 3,500 kcal deficit will result in a loss of 1 lb (0.45 kg) of body tissues; a 3,500 kcal excess will result in the gain of 1 lb of body tissue. If your client needs to count the calories he expends and the calories he consumes to ensure the balance (for weight maintenance) or deficit (for weight loss) between them, counting calories is important. Clients often will need to start out counting calories but will eventually reach the point where they develop a feel for their caloric balance. When making food choices, they should keep in mind that protein and carbohydrate contain only 4 kcal/g, whereas fat contains 9 kcal/g and water contains no calories (McArdle et al. 1991).

Because the body has different components (water, fat, fat-free mass), changes in these components may bring about weight fluctuations that

appear to contradict the caloric balance concept. For instance, early weight loss may be primarily loss of water. Also, exercise increases the fat-free mass (which is heavier, although more compact than fat) while it is decreasing fat, so weight loss on the scales may be slower than might be expected (figure 9.5).

Counting Calories for the Blue Jeans

Gwen is a good example of someone who benefited from counting calories. Gwen entered our employee fitness program weighing 150 lb (68 kg) and set realistic goals of losing 10 lb (4.5 kg) and fitting into her blue jeans. She had been maintaining her weight for the last year and believed that she could achieve a daily 500 kcal deficit (3,500 kcal/week) by reducing her diet by 250 kcal and increasing her activity by 250 kcal, on average. Gwen joined our noon aerobics class 3 days a week (3 × 300 kcal) and started walking to work 5 days a week (5 × 150). A weekend golf game or tennis match burned an extra 500 kcal. At the end of each day, Gwen recorded food deficit calories and the caloric worth of her activities. Each day did not add up to 500 kcal, but the week's total gave her a 3,500 kcal deficit. After a greater than 1 lb (0.45 kg) loss in the first 2 weeks (probably water loss), it looked like things were starting to plateau. However, by the end of 10 weeks, she had lost the 10 lb. More important for Gwen, she arrived at work that Friday casually dressed in blue jeans.

Which Is More Effective: Diet or Exercise?

There are pros and cons to using exercise alone or dieting alone, but either can be effective in reducing weight. You must consider each client individually when establishing an appropriate treatment strategy. Overweight clients are somewhat less likely to stay with an exercise program. Inactivity may be the cause of the problem, or it may be the result of the excess weight. Clients should include exercise because if they only follow a calorie-restricted diet, they risk losing lean body tissue. Walberg (1989) showed that diet-only programs lead to decreased resting energy expenditure and ongoing weight management dif-

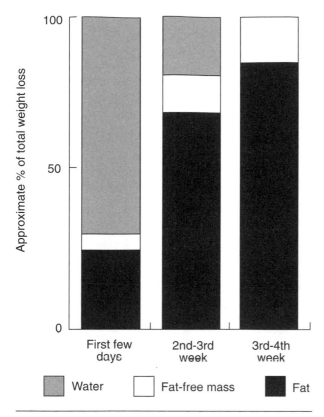

Figure 9.5 Percent composition of weight loss.

ficulties. The slower metabolism helps conserve a dwindling energy reserve from lack of food. But the restrictive dieting also makes it progressively harder to lose weight. It may be only a matter of time before the weight is gained back and another crash diet starts a "yo-yo" effect. Many clients have already tried diet restriction alone for some time and are among the 95% of all people who lose weight only to gain it back within 2 years.

Compared with exercise alone, dieting alone can produce more rapid weight reduction early in a program. Although exercise may provide slower results, it can help maintain lean body mass and prevent any decrease in resting energy

expenditure. Weight lost by dieting is about 75% fat and 25% protein. Combining exercise and diet can reduce that protein loss to only 5% (Garfinkel and Coscina 1990). Exercise counterbalances the disadvantages of dieting alone, and once excess body fat has been lost, continued exercise is important to maintaining a stable, healthy body weight. Marks and colleagues (1995) showed that aerobic cycle exercise and resistance training are equally effective in maintaining fat-free mass while encouraging weight loss.

Every client is different in terms of her degree of motivation to change diet or exercise. Keeping in mind that a 3,500 kcal deficit will result in a loss of 1 lb (0.45 kg) of body tissue, table 9.3 identifies four "routes" that a client may take, each resulting in the loss of about 1 lb/week.

Is Resistance Training for Weight Loss or Weight Gain?

Most clients want resistance training programs to build muscle strength, endurance, power, or size. However, resistance training can also be a valuable adjunct to a weight management prescription. It can contribute to both weight loss and weight maintenance.

Here are some facts about weight management and resistance training that will encourage your clients who are interested in weight loss or maintenance:

- A weight reduction program can cause loss of protein tissue (primarily muscle) along with body fat. Weight training can prevent significant loss of lean body mass.

- Weight training can also prevent decreases in resting energy expenditure, keeping the furnace stoked! In fact, each additional pound of muscle tissue can raise the RMR by 35 kcal/day (Campbell et al. 1994). If

Table 9.3   Diet and Exercise Plans to Lose 1 lb (0.45 kg) per Week

Exercise	Intensity	Duration	Frequency	Required kcal exercise expenditure per week	Required diet kcal deficit per week	Required diet kcal deficit per day	Total kcal deficit per week
None	—	—	—	—	3,500	500	3,500
Yes	Moderate	30 min	3 × /week	1,050	2,400	350	3,500
Yes	Moderate	30 min	5 × /week	1,750	1,700	250	3,500
Yes	Moderate	60 min	5 × /week	3,500	None	None	3,500

your client adds 2 lb (0.90 kg) of muscle tissue as the result of resistance training, it could raise her RMR by 70 kcal/day (35 × 2), which equals 25,550 kcal/year (70 × 365) or the equivalent of 7.3 lb (3.3 kg) of fat (25,550/3,500).

- Andersen and Jakicic (2003) reported that acute strenuous resistance exercise is associated with modest but prolonged elevations in postexercise metabolic rate and possibly fat oxidation.

- Lifting lighter weights for more repetitions (e.g., 15-25) and 1 or 2 sets can maintain muscle endurance and tone with little chance of significantly altering muscle size.

- Clients need not worry that new muscle cells will turn into fat in the future: It is physiologically impossible.

- Although resistance training does burn calories, the effect is relatively small compared with that of aerobic exercise. Thus, the optimal prescription for many is a combination of aerobic exercise and moderate resistance training.

Unique Role of Exercise in Weight Management

Recent American and European surveys (Bartlett 2003, Simopoulos 1992, Williams 1995) have shown that approximately 35% to 40% of adult women and 25% to 30% of adult men are currently attempting to lose weight. What all of these people must understand is that every calorie they eat must be expended or conserved in the body, so weight gain has usually resulted from a long period in which energy intake has exceeded energy expenditure. Calorie intake and calorie outgo must be balanced if clients are to maintain weight and "unbalanced" in the appropriate direction if clients are to gain or lose weight.

We have at our disposal a positive and powerful tool for manipulating this energy balance: physical activity. We have seen the unique role that this tool has on fat metabolism, metabolic rate, and energy expenditure. In this section we examine how to integrate everyday activity and exercise into our prescriptions and ensure that each combination is suited both to the goals of weight control and to the individual client.

Aerobic Training and Body Composition

Heyward (2002) described four changes relating to fat loss and the conservation of lean body tissues that results from aerobic training:

- The percentage of the energy used during submaximal exercise that is derived from the metabolism of FFA is larger than the percentage used during rest or intense exercise.

- Endurance training raises the point at which lactic acid levels sharply increase (called the anaerobic threshold). Because lactic acid inhibits fatty acid metabolism, conditioned people burn more fat during exercise than do unconditioned people.

- Resting energy expenditure (REE) may not decrease during calorie-restricted diets if regular exercise is maintained.

- Increased levels of epinephrine and norepinephrine released during exercise stimulate the mobilization of fat from storage and activate the enzyme lipase, which breaks down triglycerides into free fatty acids.

Creating the Deficit

To manage their weight, clients need to understand the following principles:

- Weight loss should not exceed 1 kg (2 lb) per week.

- Caloric deficit should not exceed 1,000 kcal/day.

- Aerobic activity should be performed daily, in one or several sessions.

- Aerobic activity, if sustained for at least 10 min, may include home or occupational activities in addition to fitness, recreation, and sport activities (table 9.4).

- Total energy expenditure is higher with longer-duration, lower-intensity exercise; however, RMR can remain elevated for 30 min or longer after high-intensity exercise (Heyward 2002).

- Resistance training effectively maintains FFM, which uses more calories at rest.

Inactive, sedentary individuals may only expend 15% additional energy beyond their RMR. At the other extreme, laborers and very active athletes may expend double their RMR. For most clients, our goal is to help them move into light activity, which may provide 35% to 40% of additional expenditure beyond their RMR. Larger deficits will come by encouraging moderate activity, adding 50% or more to their total daily caloric expenditure.

If at rest the average-sized adult burns 60 to 70 kcal/hr, with even light activity this can be tripled. As conditioning increases to allow a moderate level of activity such as tennis, brisk power walking, or moderate aerobics, the furnace can be stoked to about eight times its normal burning capacity, increasing our potential to burn more calories in the same period of time.

Many resources (including table 9.4) list the energy costs of a wide variety of physical activities. When using these lists, remember that

- they refer only to the time that your client is actually moving, which may be only 35 to 40 min of an hour-long basketball game; and

- actual energy expenditure may vary because of skill level, air resistance, and terrain, and body weight and gender can affect the data (body weight adjustment is listed below the table).

Energy Deficit Point System

Table 9.4 provides the energy requirements for many home, occupational, and fitness activities. You can calculate the total caloric expenditure for each activity by multiplying the $kcal \cdot kg^{-1} \cdot min^{-1}$ by the client's body weight (kg). By multiplying this by the number of minutes of that activity, you have the client's energy expenditure for that session. Doing the detailed calculations and keeping a physical activity log can be very helpful for some clients; however, it is time-consuming and, of course, is still an estimate. To simplify the use of this information, the first column lists "energy points" associated with each group of activities. These points are a conservative estimate of the number of calories burned per minute of activity.

How to Use the Energy Deficit Point System

The Energy Deficit Point System is based on the calculations and the accumulated research represented in table 9.4, yet it is as easy as 1–2–3. Simply perform the following steps:

1. **Prescribe and record the fitness activity** of your client's choice. In addition, identify or credit home or occupational activities that are performed during the week. Record the "energy points" associated with the activities. For example

Activity A: _____ Energy points

Activity B: _____ Energy points

2. **Prescribe and record the length of time** in minutes that your client will devote to those activities (minimum continuous time is 10 min). This provides the energy points for that session of activity. For example

Activity A: _____ Energy points × _____ min
= _____

Activity B: _____ Energy points × _____ min
= _____

3. **Prescribe and record the number of times** in a week that this will be repeated. This provides the energy points for that activity for the week. For example

Activity A: _____ Energy points × _____ min
× _____ /week = _____

Activity B: _____ Energy points × _____ min
× _____ /week = _____

Total weekly energy points: _____

Energy Deficit Point System Example

Let's apply this technique to a plausible situation you might encounter with a client. You recommend that your client take her dog for a 20 min brisk walk every day. To create an additional energy deficit, you design a 30 min calisthenic circuit including Therabands that she will do 3 times a week. She also recognized that if she helps with the weekly Saturday cleaning of the apartment, she deserves some credit!

To apply the Energy Deficit Point System:

Step 1: Prescribe the activities

Activity A: Walking the dog (3.0 mph) =
5 Energy points

Activity B: Calisthenic circuit = 6 Energy points

Activity C: Cleaning = 5 Energy points

Step 2: Prescribe the durations

Activity A: 5 Energy points × 20 min = 100

Table 9.4 Point System for Energy Requirements

Energy points	Energy range	Home or occupational activity	Fitness or recreational activity
2	1.5-2.0 METs 2.0-2.5 kcal/min 0.013-0.016 kcal·lb^{-1}·min^{-1} 0.029-0.035 kcal·kg^{-1}·min^{-1}	Desk work Word processing Playing cards	Strolling (1 mph)
4	2.0-3.0 METs 2.5-4.0 kcal/min 0.016-0.026 kcal·lb^{-1}·min^{-1} 0.035-0.057 kcal·kg^{-1}·min^{-1}	Dressing Driving a car Riding a lawn mower Making a bed Washing Playing a musical instrument	Walking (2.0 mph) Cycling (5 mph) Stretching Hatha yoga Bird-watching Bowling Playing catch, baseball, Frisbee
5	3.0-4.0 METs 4.0-5.0 kcal/min 0.026-0.032 kcal·lb^{-1}·min^{-1} 0.057-0.070 kcal·kg^{-1}·min^{-1}	Showering House painting Sweeping floors Cleaning windows Pushing light power mower Vacuuming Active child care and play	Walking (3.0 mph) Golf, using power cart Cycling (6 mph) Bicycle ergometer (300 kg·m^{-1}·min^{-1}) Light calisthenics Tai chi Curling Volleyball, noncompetitive
6	4.0-5.0 METs 5.0-6.0 kcal/min 0.032-0.039 kcal·lb^{-1}·min^{-1} 0.070-0.086 kcal·kg^{-1}·min^{-1}	Gardening, weeding, raking Mopping floors Light carpentry Washing and waxing the car	Walking (3.5 mph) Golfing: walking and carrying clubs Cycling (8 mph) Bicycle ergometer (450 kg·m^{-1}·min^{-1}) Stepping: stair height (18/min) Jogging on minitrampoline Water aerobics and calisthenics Weightlifting (moderate) Many calisthenics Baseball, general Basketball, shooting baskets Badminton, social singles or doubles Dancing: line, polka, fast pace Skiing, downhill, light effort
7	5.0-6.0 METs 6.0-7.0 kcal/min 0.039-0.045 kcal·lb^{-1}·min^{-1} 0.086-0.099 kcal·kg^{-1}·min^{-1}	Gardening, digging Walking downstairs Scrubbing floors Carrying objects (15-30 lb, 7-14 kg) Manual labor (moderate)	Walking (4.0 mph) Walk and jog combination Jogging in place (60-70 steps/min) Hiking, cross-country Cycling (10 mph) Bicycle ergometer (600 kg·m^{-1}·min^{-1}) Aerobic dance (low impact) Stepping: stair height (24/min) Softball, fast or slow pitch Skiing, downhill, moderate effort Tennis, doubles

Energy points	Energy range	Home or occupational activity	Fitness or recreational activity
8	6.0-7.0 METs 7.0-8.0 kcal/min 0.045-0.052 kcal·lb⁻¹·min⁻¹ 0.099-0.114 kcal·kg⁻¹·min⁻¹	Chopping wood Climbing stairs (slowly)	Walking (5.0 mph) Cycling (11 mph) Stepping: stair height (30/min) Aerobic dance (moderate) Water aerobics (vigorous) Rowing machine (moderate) Weightlifting (vigorous) Racquetball, casual, general Soccer, casual, general Skiing, cross-country, light effort
10	7.0-8.0 METs 8.0-10.0 kcal/min 0.052-0.065 kcal·lb⁻¹·min⁻¹ 0.114-0.143 kcal·kg⁻¹·min⁻¹	Sawing hardwood Snow shoveling	Jogging (5.0 mph) Jogging in place (120 steps/min) Cycling (12 mph) Bicycle ergometer (750 kg·m⁻¹·min⁻¹) Swimming laps (slow to moderate) Circuit resistance training Heavy calisthenics (e.g., push-ups, sit-ups, jumping jacks) Skating, roller or ice Skiing, cross-country, moderate effort Tennis, singles
11	8.0-9.0 METs 10.0-11.0 kcal/min 0.065-0.071 kcal·lb⁻¹·min⁻¹ 0.143-0.156 kcal·kg⁻¹·min⁻¹	Climbing stairs (moderate speed) Shoveling 10 shovels/min (30 lb or 14 kg load)	Running (5.5 mph) Cycling (13 mph) Bicycle ergometer (900 kg·m⁻¹·min⁻¹) Rowing machine (vigorous) Aerobic dance (vigorous/step: 6-8 in.) Water jogging Rope skipping (<75 rpm) Hockey, recreational
11+	≥10.0 METs ≥11.0 kcal/min ≥0.071 kcal·lb⁻¹·min⁻¹ ≥0.156 kcal·kg⁻¹·min⁻¹	Climbing stairs (quickly)	Running (6.0 mph = 10 METs 7.0 mph = 11.5 METs 8.0 mph = 13.5 METs 9.0 mph = 15 METs) Deep-water running Cycling (>13 mph) Bicycle ergometer (≥1,050 kg·m⁻¹·min⁻¹) Swimming, laps (vigorous) Rope jumping (120-140 beats/min = 11-12 METs) Martial arts

Note. 1 MET = energy expenditure at rest; approximately 3.5 ml·kg⁻¹·min⁻¹.

Energy range depends on efficiency, rest pauses, and body size. Values are based on client of 154 lb or 70 kg. Add 10% for each 15 lb or 7 kg above 154 lb or 70 kg.

Ainsworth et al. 2000, Heyward 2002, Hoeger and Hoeger 1999, Sharkey 1978.

Activity B: 6 Energy points × 30 min = 180

Activity C: 5 Energy points × 100 min = 500

Step 3: Prescribe frequency

Activity A: 5 Energy points × 20 min × 7 /week = 700

Activity B: 6 Energy points × 30 min × 3 /week = 540

Activity C: 5 Energy points × 100 min × 1 /week = 500

Total weekly energy points: 1,740

This represents a conservative estimate of 1,740 kcal/week and should represent 1 lb of weight lost every 2 weeks.

Final Word on Changing Shape

Fitness professionals often take a purely physiological approach to weight management, examining weight and health in terms of metabolic normality, body composition (leanness and fat), and functional capacity. This approach tends to focus on health enhancement, on an acceptable standard, on performance, or on aesthetics. Such a focus, however, may not connect with your client's needs.

Our eyes see what our brains tell them to see. Body image is the mental image we have of our own physical appearance. More than 50% of adult women are dissatisfied with their weight. The concern with weight often starts in high school, but the handicap is felt long after in terms of personal and professional fulfillment. For such clients, the mental image of the ideal weight is often distorted. You need to help them realize that an acceptable and realistic standard may be a "tolerable" weight that is within a healthy standard (chapter 4).

Once your clients realize that you are considering the psychological and social pressures they face, and that you don't simply see their weight as a risk factor, the doors will be open to talk about weight in relation to well-being, body image, and social acceptance. Deemphasize any absolute measure of weight or body composition in the counseling, and encourage your client to find her own desirable and healthy weight. Ask her if she is happy with her weight. To really enjoy a high quality of life, she needs to be happy with herself. Then ask her if she wants to change enough to implement exercise and dietary changes. These simple questions will help establish a degree of commitment to define a "tolerable" weight for her.

For clients with a body image goal, I like to use a "mirror" analogy: I challenge them to change the reflection they see. It becomes an attitude challenge. Our goal is to promote a personal acceptance of a large range of healthy weights and variations in body size. Searching through magazines to find appropriate images of body shape can be helpful. Less frequent use of scales and a few new pieces of clothing can also help toward a more positive self-attitude. Be realistic about your "reflection" but recognize the continuing benefits of appropriate eating and physical activity habits.

The Weight Management Prescription Model

The model for weight management prescription is similar to that used in chapter 6 for cardiovascular prescription. Resistance exercise is incorporated into this weight loss prescription to minimize the reduction of lean body mass and to increase the resting metabolic rate, so you will need to consult chapter 7 for the model recommended for the design of resistance training programs.

Table 9.5 outlines a 10-step model for the design of a physiologically sound and client-centered exercise prescription for weight management. Each step involves a sequenced decision that you must make. Many of the choices available for each decision are listed for each step. Following a brief background to each of the steps, a sample case study is presented including the choices that were made for the client and a justification for those choices.

Step 1: Assess Client's Needs and Formulate Goals

Client needs may be related to medical or high-risk (elevated blood lipids, hypertension), educational (eating habits), or motivational factors. Client needs also can be defined by results of fitness assessments (skinfolds), by lack of self-esteem, or by special designs necessitated by physical limitations caused by weight or orthopedics. Careful screening procedures can identify when medical intervention is warranted. Often the client is unaware of emerging needs such as borderline hypertension or lack of core strength. Recording an activity profile can establish current levels of energy expenditure (see table 9.4).

Table 9.5 Model: Exercise Prescription for Weight Management (Aerobic and Resistance Exercise)

Decisions	Choices
1. Assess client's needs and formulate goals	• Screening: medical history, intervention needed (e.g., meds) • Limitations (e.g., CV risk, orthopedic, injury, test results) • Activity profile and history (review current energy expenditure) • Design considerations (e.g., time and equipment availability) • Priorities: health, fitness, appearance • Motivational strategy, personality, learning style • Stress management issues • Food management habits and strategies (review current diet) • Weight loss goal (kcal deficit goal)
2. Select aerobic equipment and exercise	• Treadmill, run, walk • Bicycle, ergometer • Elliptical trainer • Rower • Stepper • Swim • In-line • ACSM Group I and II—aerobic (less weight-bearing)
3. Choose aerobic training method	• Continuous • Interval • Circuit • Cross-training, sports • Active living
4. Select aerobic intensity and workload	Recommended training zone: • % $\dot{V}O_2$ reserve, % maximum METs, % HRR, perceived exertion (e.g., 50-70% $\dot{V}O_2$ reserve or HRR; sufficient to complete duration and tolerate the exercise without risk) • Calculate corresponding workload (e.g., ACSM metabolic formulas) or client selects a workload that elicits an appropriate HR (e.g., 50-70% HRR); verify selection during demo-client trial • Calculate kcal/min (e.g., chart or L/min × 5 kcal) • Recreational sport and active living (kcal chart) • Manipulate balance with duration (kcal/session) and frequency (kcal/week) to promote high kcal expenditure • Confirm consistency with goals and needs
5. Select aerobic volume (duration and frequency)	• Total work per session (intensity and duration) • 20-30 min, progressing to 45+ min • 250-500 kcal/session • Minimum 3 ×/week; work toward 5-6 ×/week • Total kcal deficit per week (intensity, duration, and frequency): 1,000-2,000 kcal/week • Supplement with active living recommendations • Kcal deficit from diet modifications

(continued)

Table 9.5 *continued*

Decisions	Choices
6. Assign and monitor aerobic progression	• Stage of progression (ACSM: initial, improvement, maintenance) • Methods of progression—FITT (e.g., increase time initially) • Rate of progression (build kcal deficit, e.g., 10%/week) • Monitoring to cue progression timing • Monitoring to suit client's objectives but avoid overtraining • Monitoring to motivate
7. Assign resistance exercise type and equipment	• Choice suits goals, needs, preferences • Simple, complex, multijoint, single joint • Equipment (and brand) pros and cons • Constant, variable, accommodating resistance • Free weight, machine • Bands, tubes, balls, boards • Equipment features (e.g., ROM limited, pivot locations) • Exercise order
8. Choose resistance training method	• Standard (simple) sets • Circuit • Supersets • Compound set • Pyramids (ascending, descending) • Split routine • Negatives (forced repetition) • Plyometrics

9. Assign and monitor resistance progression	• Volume first, intensity second
	• One volume factor modified at a time
	  (e.g., 1: Increase reps: $2 \times 12\text{-}15$; then 3×10)
	  (e.g., 2: [Strength]: 2×12 at 100; then 3×8 at 110; then 4×6 at 120)
	• 5% increase in load is very tolerable (when upper limit of reps met)
	• Increase reps when tolerated in second set
	• Progress (e.g., machines to free weights) when good strength base
	• Monitoring, follow-up checks should cue progression timing
	• Related to client's objectives (motivation)
	• Primary safety precautions listed

10. Design warm-up and cool-down	• CV warm-up and cool-down transitions (e.g., after aerobic segment) • Specific joint and muscle stretching • Suits nature of the prescription and client specifics (e.g., mode, time, intensity, monitoring)

Note. CV = cardiovascular; MET = metabolic equivalent; HR = heart rate; HRR = heart rate reserve; FITT = frequency, intensity, time, and type; ROM = range of motion.

As discussed in chapter 1, goal setting is the process of specifying what needs to be done, when and how to do it, and what the anticipated outcomes will be. Integrating needs, wants, and lifestyle will increase the probability of compliance with any prescription. It is often easier to begin with long-term goals that are more global and then formulate several shorter-term goals that could be accomplished before there are major changes in assessment measures such as target weight loss, skinfolds, or body mass index. You play a vital role by helping your clients set realistic, measurable goals and recording them in clinical notes and for the clients. As mentioned earlier, there should be a two-pronged approach to goal setting: "eating behavior" goals may include food management habits and strategies for stress management, whereas "activity integration" goals may require flexibility in the program design, purchase of home equipment, or time management.

Step 2: Select Aerobic Equipment and Exercise

The client's own preferences and availability of equipment will often narrow the choices very quickly. We must be informed about equipment, including specific functions and brand differences, because a client's selection to use or to purchase should be based on comparisons of pros and cons. Even for equipment of the same type (i.e., treadmills, bicycles, or elliptical trainers), there are frequently different features on the information displays or in the braking mechanism that would be better suited to your client.

Aerobic exercise is the best type of program for losing body fat. It also provides significant other health and cardiovascular benefits. Aerobic exercise involves large muscle groups, so you can look beyond walking, jogging, stair climbing, and bicycling to activities that also incorporate shoulder and trunk muscles such as cross-country skiing, swimming, skipping, rowing, elliptical training, and aerobic dance. Weight-supported activities such as swimming and water aerobics are excellent choices, especially for deconditioned or restricted clients; however, complementary weight-bearing activities should be added when tolerated. A circuit involving a number of aerobic modes of exercise can add some variety and cross training. Other activities such as tennis, squash, basketball, baseball, hockey, and occupational and home maintenance activities have an aerobic component to them, but skill levels and competitiveness can place these activities at excessively high intensity levels. The action should be continuous, maintaining the energy expenditure level. It appears that aerobic exercise modes are equally effective in altering body composition (Heyward 2002).

Even with all these choices, there remains a single mode of exercise that consistently maintains adherence, suits the overweight client, and has a proven track record for weight management. I refer to walking or its progressive extensions, walk–jog–run. Walking with hand weights can increase energy expenditure by 5% to 10%, nearly 1 kcal/min (Williams 1995). For hypertensive clients, carrying weights in the hands tends to increase blood pressure more than weights strapped to the wrist. Walking faster or on an incline may be an alternative.

Flexibility exercises targeted at the muscles used in the aerobic activity may be integrated within the session depending on the design (e.g., interval or circuit). Resistance exercises focused on large muscle groups are often part of a complete weight loss prescription for lower-risk clients.

Step 3: Choose Aerobic Training Method

A variety of training methods allow us to match specific benefits to the appropriate client. Continuous training methods are well suited to low to moderate intensities and for clients initiating a weight loss program. Pacing and reduced injuries are advantages over interval training. However, the ACSM (2000) recommended interval training for higher-risk clients who can tolerate only low-intensity exercise for short periods of time (1-2 min). Shorter, more intense intervals with intermittent recoveries may be better suited to the temperaments of your former athletes . . . . just monitor carefully. Recently, Peterson and colleagues (2004) demonstrated that caloric expenditure was similar with 30 min of intermittent exercise compared with 30 min of continuous exercise as long as both occur at a moderate intensity level (70% $\dot{V}O_2$max) and the intermittent sessions are at least 10 min in length.

An active lifestyle can effectively complement a more formal exercise prescription and make a significant difference in the speed of weight loss or the ease of weight maintenance. Active living may not produce profound cardiovascular benefits, but for energy expenditure, "every little bit counts." Every time your client is about to relapse from her exercise program, remind her that washing the car, mowing the lawn, vacuuming the carpet, gardening, or doing house repairs are bonus calorie-burners that are every bit as valid as a trip to the gym.

The Zen of Walking

My 63-year-old neighbor was approaching retirement and knew he wanted to play golf every day. His weight and blood pressure had been creeping up, and he was concerned about his future quality of life. He bought a portable music player and set aside his "walking time" after work each day. Gradually adding loops to his walking route to progressively extend his time, my neighbor had lost almost a pound a week in the first 3 months. The walking time became a cherished time of sanctuary and rejuvenation. It would never replace golf, he told me, but it became more than just a means of losing weight. Surely there is a Zen of walking.

Step 4: Select Aerobic Intensity and Workload

Every client has an optimal intensity, depending on her condition and the length of the exercise. At very low intensities, our bodies rely predominantly on fat metabolism. At higher intensities, carbohydrates are the predominant energy source. This has led some people to conclude that to lose fat weight, low-intensity exercise is preferable. The fact is that higher-intensity exercise burns more calories per minute. Even though the proportion of fat calories used is smaller during high-intensity exercise, the total number of fat calories used in high-intensity exercise greatly exceeds those used in low-intensity workouts of equal duration.

Other physiological factors also support higher-intensity activity. First, the RMR can stay elevated for hours after a bout of intense exercise. Second, the cardiovascular training effect created by higher-intensity training increases the activity of certain muscle enzymes involved in burning fat. These enzymes favor the burning of fat rather than glycogen (Bean 1996).

However, for an unfit client, higher intensities cannot be tolerated for long enough duration to produce significant caloric expenditure. Nonetheless, there are many health benefits to regular lower-intensity exercise that may normalize metabolic disorders common in obese clients. We must always turn back to our clients in making prescriptive decisions—in many cases, lower-intensity (longer duration and frequent) exercise may be most suitable. Showing obese clients how to live more actively on a daily basis may prove more successful than regimented programs (see table 9.4). Many overweight clients have orthopedic limitations, and they will sustain fewer injuries with a lower intensity. If previously inactive clients can get into the habit of exercise, their fitness may gradually improve to the point that we can prescribe higher-intensity levels of activity (e.g., 70-75% HRR) without driving them away. As our clients' cardiovascular fitness improves, so does their anaerobic threshold. This increases their ability to work at higher absolute intensities (e.g., speed on the treadmill) for longer and still burn fat and not just carbohydrate.

Step 5: Select Aerobic Volume (Duration and Frequency)

If losing weight is your client's priority, your prescription should stress duration or total energy expenditure (intensity × duration). One of your initial challenges is to bring your clients to a point of sufficient aerobic fitness that they can sustain moderate intensity for enough time to burn a lot of calories. If a client is jogging at an 8 min/mile pace and fatigues after 3 miles (4.8 km), she has burned approximately 336 kcal (24 min × 14 kcal/min). If she reduces her speed to a 9 min/mile pace, she can complete 4 miles (6.4 km) and burn 450 kcal (36 × 12.5 kcal/min). Duration and total distance are more important than speed (intensity) alone. The slower pace also avoids the inhibiting effect of lactic acid on fat mobilization.

Similarly, a jogger, because his activity is continuous, uses considerably more calories in an hour than a hockey player, who may be moving for only 40% of the game. Be aware of this principle if you base your prescription on a chart of caloric expenditures per minute for various activities. Skill levels, such as in racket sports, can significantly change the energy expenditure per hour.

The benefits of avoiding labor-saving devices—taking the stairs, walking to work, and generally living more actively—accumulate during the day and effectively extend the daily energy expenditure. This approach may be well suited to your client's lifestyle and level of commitment and may firmly place him in the action stage of change. It is possible to use frequent short bouts of moderate day-to-day activities to lose the equivalent of 2 lb (0.90 kg) of body fat per month (table 9.6).

It is quite evident that the more a person exercises, the greater his weekly caloric expenditure. Exercise frequency complements duration and intensity, and the combination of these three factors yields the *volume* of activity, often measured in kcal/week. Four sessions per week are satisfactory, provided duration and intensity are adequate. A frequency of three times per week usually requires such high intensities or very long sessions to reach sufficient weekly caloric expenditures that clients often get discouraged or injured. A daily program is most likely to establish a behavioral habit and promote adherence.

Step 6: Assign and Monitor Aerobic Progression

The perpetual challenge is to find a rate of progression that builds the caloric deficit without overtraining or reducing compliance. Duration is usually the first factor to increase. Volume is the goal, but often frequency is limited by other commitments and intensity should only increase

Table 9.6   Health-Related Fitness Prescription

Day	Activity (150 lb [68 kg] person)	Kcal
Monday	30 min at fitness club—aerobic	250-300
Tuesday	Brisk walk to work—30 min Stairs—5 min	200-250
Wednesday	30 min at fitness club—aerobic	250-300
Thursday	Brisk walk to work—30 min Stairs—5 min	200-250
Friday	Brisk walk to work—30 min Stairs—5 min Wash and wax car—30 min	300-350
Saturday	Gardening—30 min Housecleaning—30 min	300
Sunday	Mowing lawn—30 min Raking and yard work—30 min	400-450
	Total	1,900-2,200

when the cardiovascular or orthopedic condition permits. An increase of 10% in the weekly caloric expenditure (e.g., duration increased from 40 min to 44 min) is usually well tolerated.

Peak exercise heart rates or perceived exertion scores that begin to decrease in successive workouts should signal a time to progress. Slower recoveries and increased signs of fatigue may indicate that the current level should be reduced or the progression was too rapid.

Monitoring progress at follow-up sessions should begin by reviewing the steps taken toward goals. "You were going to try to get out for a walk on your lunch time last week. Were you able to get away?" If the goals were specific and measurable, it is easy to focus on the projected outcomes, being careful to create a natural link between the client's behavior and his body composition and health goals.

Feedback should go beyond recognition and encouragement. Clients need to take ownership of their program by anticipating and strategizing for difficult situations, such as holidays, stressful work periods, or missed appointments. When clients feel discouraged, they need to focus on daily behaviors and short-term successes.

Step 7: Assign Resistance Exercise Type and Equipment

The choice of resistance equipment or the type of exercise must suit the clients' goals, needs, preferences, and availability. Complex, multijoint exercises with large muscle groups allow a client to get a full-body workout with maximum caloric expenditure. Look also to maintain balance in your exercise selection: agonist–antagonist and bilateral symmetry. The order of the exercises may be somewhat predetermined by the training method.

In selecting equipment, consider the best method of resistance, the type of equipment, and the interface of that equipment with your client (ergonomics). Machines offer various types of resistance (e.g., gravity, variable resistance, hydraulics, pneumatics, isokinetics) that may or may not suit your client. Equipment features such as range of motion limits and adjustable seating are particularly important for large and small-sized clients. When equipment is limited, a lot can be accomplished at home with bands, tubes, balls, boards, and gravity. For more detail see chapter 7.

Step 8: Choose Resistance Training Method

Resistance training methods combine the selection of load, reps, sets, and rest (see chapter 7) with the sequence of exercises to produce specific muscular fitness outcomes. Depending on the type and availability of equipment, the time devoted to resistance training will limit the number of reps and sets and the number of exercises selected. For example, in a 50 min lunchtime workout, your client may only have 20 min for resistance work. Cullinen and Caldwell (1998) reported that moderate to intense resistance training 2 days a week for 12 weeks significantly increased fat-free mass and decreased percent body fat.

For the purposes of weight management and body composition, exercises are usually arranged to provide maximum work with sufficient recovery. Alternating push–pull exercises in a circuit or in standard sets allows good balance (agonist–antagonist) and recovery.

Step 9: Assign and Monitor Resistance Progression

It is advisable to increase volume first and then intensity. Only modify one volume factor at a time. For example: increase reps 2 × 12-15 and then 3 × 10. Begin to increase the reps when they are tolerated in the second set. A 5% to 10% increase in load is very tolerable when the upper limit of reps has been met. Progressions with training methods or equipment (e.g., machines to free weights) should occur only when there is a good strength base.

Regular monitoring or follow-up checks should cue the best time for progression. The rate and method of progression are related to the client's objectives and level of motivation. Techniques such as periodization are discussed in chapter 7.

Step 10: Design Warm-Up and Cool-Down

The warm-up should include a gradual increase in the aerobic activity sufficient to raise the body temperature and approach the low end of the target heart rate. Selected stretching of active muscle groups is facilitated with the warmth and elasticity of the muscle and connective tissue. The length of the warm-up should be longer if the fitness level of the client is low, cardiovascular risk level is high, or there is a possibility of sporadic higher exertion (e.g., competitive sports).

The cool-down is important for overweight clients to avoid blood pooling, rapid changes in blood pressure, and postexercise muscle stiffness. If 10 min are devoted to the cool-down within a 45 to 50 min exercise session, this can include a 3 to 5 min gradual tapering after the aerobic portion of the workout with 5 to 7 min of specific muscle stretching afterwards. Ensure that your client's heart rate is below 100 beats/min or within 20 beats/min of the original heart rate and that your client looks and feels recovered.

Case Study

A 42-year-old insurance broker, Fred, was a prime example of creeping obesity. He had coached basketball for 17 years but had done nothing for the last 5 years. He claimed that a busy insurance practice and a new cottage had left him little time for regular exercise. He had noticed the weight problem, but it was his last medical check-up (elevated cholesterol and borderline hypertension) that motivated him to seek help with an exercise program.

Our first task was to focus on his priorities—to determine what he wanted to achieve, not just what his doctor wanted. His objectives were to

- lose 12 lb (5.4 kg) in the first 6 months and a total of 24 lb (10.8 kg) in the first year by exercise alone,
- reduce his elevated cholesterol level to a normal range, and
- reduce the fat around his waist (if possible) and strengthen that area.

Assessment, Discussion, and Action

The assessment provided me with the following data (table 9.7):

After I explained the assessment results and the implications of his doctors' findings, Fred was committed to making some immediate changes. He decided to walk the 20 min to work each day and to set aside three 10 min sessions in his office

Table 9.7   Fred's Assessment Data

Risk factors	
	Weight, cholesterol, borderline hypertension, and lifestyle (physician approval to continue was obtained—PARmed -X)
Body composition	
Weight	84.1 kg (185 lb)
Height	172.5 cm (5 ft 8 in)
Body mass index	28 (overweight)
Body fat	24.5%
Abdominal girth	96.5 cm (38 in)
Cardiovascular	
Resting heart rate	80 bpm
Blood pressure	Resting: 135/88 (high normal), recovery: 135/84
Oxygen uptake	33 ml/kg/min = fair, with early leg fatigue and slow recovery
Musculoskeletal	
Strength	Weak abdominals but average upper-body strength on push-ups and grip strength
Posture	Lumbar lordosis and rounded shoulders

each week to do muscle strengthening exercises. He planned to coach a basketball team and to be physically active in their 1-1/2 hr practice once a week. We discussed the possibilities for cross-country skiing at his cottage during the winter. After Fred's wife attended the follow-up session, she agreed to eliminate her own high-cholesterol, high-fat snacks at night and reduce between-meal "junk" eating. This was important for Fred, because he feared that if these foods were available in the house, he wouldn't be able to resist them. The rest of their menu appeared reasonable except for the number of times they ate at fast food outlets.

Prescription Summary

To see how I filled out Fred's prescription card, see figure 9.6.

Brisk walk to work (10 trips at 20 min each) at 7 kcal/min	1,400 kcal/week
Basketball practice (approximately 40 min active) at 10 kcal/min (Substitute cross-country skiing at the cottage as suits schedule)	400 kcal/week
Diet modification (reduce snacks and fast food)	1,700 kcal/week
Deficit:	3,500 kcal/week

Strength and endurance work on trunk: Three core exercises for various abdominal and back muscles, 2 sets of 10-15 each (progress with third set)

Strength and endurance work on upper back: Three tubing exercises (attached to office door) for posterior shoulder joint and shoulder girdle muscles

The prescription card will guide Fred or another personal trainer when I am not there. Specific workloads, times, and monitoring levels are listed for the warm-up and again for the aerobic workout. Upper and lower limits that include perceived exertions are useful with intermittent training methods such as basketball or the uneven terrain of cross-country skiing. After a brief aerobic cool-down, on the days that he has time, Fred can add his resistance exercises, checking his card periodically for descriptions, weight, reps, sets, and precautions. I would prefer to be there for decisions about progression.

Results

For the first month of the program, Fred followed the program and eating habits very closely and lost 4 lb (1.8 kg) (3,500 kcal/week). He set up a corner of his office with a mat, tubing, some music, and a monitoring chart. His wife continued to be a good support, and besides a few meal celebrations, by the sixth month both had significantly modified their eating habits. Weather and work pressures permitted Fred to walk to work an average of 3 days per week for the remainder of the 6 months. By this time the weight loss was almost 15 lb (6.8 kg), his waist girth was down 2 in. (5 cm), his blood pressure was consistently 130/84, and the basketball was a lot of fun! Although the cardiovascular results showed no significant improvement (perhaps the intensity was too low), he felt less fatigued and generally more energized. Even if Fred's absolute aerobic capacity remained the same, his relative capacity improved with his loss of weight. He certainly "carried" himself better and avoided any injuries in the 6 months. His physician was pleased with the lowered weight and blood pressure and was confident that his blood cholesterol would soon follow. Fred's wife was the gatekeeper in the kitchen and she would often join Fred on a walk or ski. Not only was she instrumental in motivating Fred, she too lost about half the weight that Fred shed!

 ## Justification of the Weight Management Prescription Case Study

Each personal fitness trainer will have a slightly different approach to the case study prescription. However, as you make choices, be sure you have a strong rationale for each one. Take another look at the choices made in the previous prescription. Provide physiological justifications and client-centered (behavioral) justifications for each choice made. This exercise has been started in table 9.8.

Prescription Card for Weight Management
(Aerobic and resistance exercise)

Client name   Trainer name

Client goal	Special considerations

Circulatory Warm-Up

Equipment and mode	Workload	Time	HR/PE objective

Stretching Warm-Up (Name and brief description)

Name and brief description	Guidelines

Aerobic Workout

Intensity and training range

Lower limit: _____%HRR _____beats/min _____RPE   Upper limit: _____%HRR _____beats/min _____RPE

	Equipment	Training method	Frequency	Kcal/session
1				
2				

Phase	Workload	Time	Phase	Workload	Time
Warm-up			Warm-up		
Peak			Peak		
Cool-down			Cool-down		

Progression and Monitoring

Resistance Workout

Equipment type (e.g., free weights)	Training method

Goals	Guidelines

Exercise (brief description)	Muscles	Weight	Reps	Sets	Precautions

Progression

Cool-Down

Name and brief description	Guidelines

Note. HR = heart rate; PE = perceived exertion; RPE = rating of perceived exertion.

From Client-Centered Exercise Prescription, Second Edition, by John Griffin, 2006, Champaign, IL: Human Kinetics.

Fred's Prescription Card

Client name:	Trainer name:
Fred	John

Client goals	Special considerations
• Lose 12 lb in the first 6 months and a total of 24 lb in the first year • Reduce elevated cholesterol level and BP to a normal range • Reduce fat around waist and strengthen that area	• Basketball and cottage motivators • Spouse support with meals

Circulatory Warm-Up

Equipment and mode	Workload	Time	HR/PE Objective
• Good walking and basketball shoes	Light to moderate	First 2-3 min of walk or ski	HR: 120-130 RPE: 11-12

Stretching Warm-Up

Name and brief description	Guidelines
Walking: stretch lower body (including hip flexors) Skiing: chest stretches plus walking stretches or 15 easy lunges with arm action Basketball: do along with team	• Walking: WU, gradually • Increase speed • Skiing: WU, start skiing slowly • Basketball: WU, ease into drills

Aerobic Workout

Intensity/training range

Lower limit: 50% HRR, 129 beats/min, 12 RPE   Upper limit: 65% HRR, 144 beats/min, 14 RPE

	Equipment	Training method	Frequency	Kcal/session
1	Walking shoes	• Continuous for walking	10 trips/week	10 × 20 min × 7 kcal/min = 1,400 kcal/week
2	Cross-country ski equipment Basketball shoes	• Continuous for cross-country • Intermittent for basketball practices	1×/week	40 min × 10 kcal/min = 400 kcal/week

Phase	Workload	Time	Phase	Workload	Time
Warm-up	See above		Warm-up	See above	
Peak	Walking: 7 kcal/min (7 energy points); 50-55% HRR (129-134 beats/min); RPE: 12-13	20 min each	Peak	Skiing and basketball: 10 kcal/min (10 energy points); 55-65% HRR (134-144 beats/min); RPE: 13-14	50 min
Cool-down	Keep moving at work		Cool-down	Gradually decrease intensity Allow HR recovery before resistance work	

Progression and monitoring

- Walking: increase the route length or vigour of the arm action (power walk) or speed
- Skiing and basketball: increase duration of active time
- Skiing and basketball: check heart rate (or RPE) at peak times and modify or active recovery
- Monitoring chart (modified calendar) recorded completed activities, weight, blood pressure, and waist girth on a weekly basis

Resistance Workout

Equipment type (e.g., free weights)	Training method
Tubing, mat, music, monitoring chart	Standard sets for resistance work: three specific shoulder strengthening exercises and three core exercises

(continued)

Figure 9.6 Fred's prescription card.

- Reduce fat around waist (if possible) and strengthen that area
- Work shoulders for skiing

Guidelines

- WU: do an easy set of 5-10 (50% 1RM)
- Two sets of 10-15 reps

Exercise (brief description)	Muscles	Weight	Reps	Sets	Precautions
Shoulder strengthening 1 Lat pull-down (machine)	Latissimus dorsi	65-75% 1RM	10-15	2	
Shoulder strengthening 2 Bench press (machine)	Pectoralis major	65-75% 1RM	10-15	2	
Shoulder strengthening 3 Triceps pull-down (Theraband)	Triceps brachii	65-75% 1RM	10-15	2	
Specific core exercise 1 Twisting curl-up, knees bent	Abdominal obliques		10-15	2	Stop if loss of form Maintain neutral spine
Specific core exercise 2 Four-point alternate arm–leg extensions	Erector spinae		10-15	2	Stop if loss of form Maintain neutral spine
Specific core exercise 3 Reverse curl-up	Rectus abdominis		10-15	2	Stop if loss of form Maintain neutral spine

Progression and monitoring

Increase to 3 sets once 15 reps are reached consistently.
Use monitoring chart (modified calendar) to record completed activities, weights, reps, and sets weekly.

Cool-Down

Name and brief description	Guidelines
Walking: stretch lower body (including hip flexors) Basketball: do along with team Skiing: do chest stretches plus walking stretches All exercises: gradually decrease speed Resistance: stretch back, chest, and hip flexors	Feel recovered before ending cool-down Monitor BP periodically

Note. BP = blood pressure; HR = heart rate; PE = perceived exertion; RPE = rating of perceived exertion; WU = warm-up; HRR = heart rate reserve; BP = blood pressure.

Figure 9.6 *(continued)*

Table 9.8 Exercise Prescription for Weight Management: Justification (Aerobic and Resistance Exercise)

Decisions	Physiological and client-centered (behavioral) justification
1. Assess client's needs and goals	• Two pounds per month is safe and was projected from energy deficit. • Physician reported elevated cholesterol and borderline hypertension. • Waist girth and abdominal visceral fat are high risk and affecting posture. • Client's highest priority was creeping obesity. • Change was motivated by doctor and check-up results. • Client was concerned about appearance.
2. Select aerobic equipment	• Walking is safe, well tolerated, and convenient. • Client can walk long enough to burn calories. • Walking is transportation and time efficient. • Skiing and basketball are enjoyable, so the client is motivated.
3. Choose aerobic training method	• Continuous exercise provides for sufficient fitness and exercise tolerance. • Interval exercise includes active recoveries that are self-selected, allowing higher intensity. • Exercises provide high energy expenditure. • Client finds the exercises fun.
4. Select aerobic intensity and workload	• In walking, intensity and workload match, and monitoring is easy. • HR is easily maintained in appropriate range for objectives. • Skiing is self-regulated; RPE is helpful. • Intensity and workload suit lifestyle.
5. Select aerobic volume (duration and frequency)	• Total weekly caloric expenditure is good. • Recreation is a bonus and in time can be expanded. • Walking is an active lifestyle integration.
6. Assign and monitor aerobic progression	• Progressive overload will improve CV and ability to increase kcal/min at same RPE. • Exercise provides preparation for jogging (i.e., walk volume and basketball). • Power walking increases energy expenditure. • Increasing time and pace will increase weight loss and decrease CV risk factors. • Monitoring will guide time and extent of CV overload. • Monitoring chart (calendar) is motivational.
7. Assign resistance exercise type and equipment	• Equipment works multijoint large muscles of chest, back, and trunk. • There is a minimum of equipment, which is easily substituted if no equipment. • Program is simple and short, which provides motivation.
Exercise 1	• Assists ski poling and balances pecs; improve rounded shoulders
Exercise 2	• Assists basketball and skiing and balances lats
Exercise 3	• Provides third exercise isolation and assists basketball shooting and passing and ski poling
Exercise 4	• Provides core stability, back support, and strong flexion + rotation; improve lumbar lordosis
Exercise 5	• Balances abdominals, stabilizes back, and assists lifting activities
Exercise 6	• Strengthens flexion and improves appearance; stabilizers fatigued last; improve lumbar lordosis
Exercise 7	
Exercise 8	
8. Choose resistance training method	• Standard sets allow recovery of muscle groups. • Method is suited to recreational activities of interest. • Two sets of 10-15 reps are sufficient for strength and body composition changes.
9. Assign and monitor resistance progression	• Three sets are well tolerated and build volume. • Monitoring will guide time and extent of resistance overload. • Monitoring chart (calendar) is motivational.
10. Design warm-up and cool-down	• Increases venous return • Provides gradual return to preexercise state • Carries less chance of dizziness, light-headedness • Increases myocardial perfusion • Clears metabolic wastes and lactic acid • Stretches target previously active muscles

Note: HR = heart rate; RPE = rating of perceived exertion; CV = cardiovascular.

Highlights

1. **Take a two-pronged approach to improving a client's shape and helping him losing weight: (a) modify eating behaviors and (b) integrate activity (not merely fitness prescription).**

   The U.S. My Pyramid and Canada's Food Guide to Healthy Eating help with daily food choices and encourage selecting a variety of foods from each major food group. Make your client aware of portion size; eating large portion sizes can lead to overeating resulting in overweight. A good place to start to keep track of the foods one eats is by reading nutritional labeling at the grocery store.

   No single factor is more frequently responsible for obesity than lack of physical activity. Direct clients toward activities that could be part of their current lifestyle like walking and performing manual tasks.

2. **Identify behaviors most often identified as the reasons for a client's weight problem, that is, what is eaten (e.g., overeating or eating the wrong foods) and why it is eaten (e.g., emotional eating).**

   A given caloric quantity of excess dietary fat is more fattening than a calorically similar quantity of excess carbohydrate. This means that what you eat (diet composition) may be as important as total calories in the promotion of obesity. Helping clients discover why they eat is as important as knowing what they eat. Many clients may need guidance making choices about food preparation, how to pack a nutritious lunch, how to judge food serving sizes, or how to avoid temptations. Help clients accept a large range of healthy weights and variations in body size.

3. **Describe several ways to expend energy: resting metabolism, metabolizing food (thermic effect of food), and physical activity (thermic effect of exercise).**

   The resting metabolic rate (RMR) is the energy expended to maintain normal body and is usually the primary source of energy expenditure (60-75%). When an obese person loses excess weight, the RMR may drop to 15% to 20% below that of a normal-weight person because fat is less metabolically active than muscle. There is a thermic effect of food (TEF) above the RMR for several hours after a meal. Any physical activity will also raise the baseline rate of metabolism and is called the thermic effect of exercise (TEE). Exercise may also facilitate weight loss by causing an increase in postexercise energy expenditure.

4. **Provide information to clients about counting calories and about the merits of diet versus exercise.**

   Clients often will need to start out counting calories but will eventually reach the point where they develop a feel for their caloric balance. Calories don't account for the early weight loss attributable to water loss or the increases in fat-free mass with exercise. Compared with exercise alone, dieting can produce more rapid weight reduction early in a program. Once excess body fat has been lost, continued exercise is important to maintaining a stable, healthy body weight. As conditioning increases to allow a moderate level of activity, it increases our potential to burn more calories in the same period of time.

5. **Use the Energy Deficit Point System to encourage clients to become more active and to estimate the weight loss value of these lifestyle changes.**

   Table 9.4 provides the energy requirements for many home, occupational, and fitness activities. You can calculate the total caloric expenditure for each activity by multiplying the kcal$\cdot$kg$^{-1}\cdot$min^{-1} by the client's body weight (kg). By multiplying this by the number of minutes of that activity, you have the client's energy expenditure for that session.

6. **Use a 10-step model for the design of a physiologically sound and client-centered exercise prescription for weight management.**

   Each step of this model involves a sequenced decision that you must make. Many of the choices available for these decisions are listed for each step in table 9.5.

   - Step 1: Assess client's needs and goals
   - Step 2: Select aerobic equipment and exercise
   - Step 3: Choose aerobic training method

- Step 4: Select aerobic intensity and workload
- Step 5: Select aerobic volume (duration and frequency)
- Step 6: Assign and monitor aerobic progression
- Step 7: Assign resistance exercise type and equipment
- Step 8: Choose resistance training method
- Step 9: Assign and monitor resistance progression
- Step 10: Design warm-up and cool-down

Each personal fitness trainer will have a slightly different approach to prescription; however, it is important that you have a strong rationale for each choice that you make.

PART III

Design Issues for Injury Recovery and Prevention

Our understanding of the effects of physical activity on human health has advanced in recent years, not only among fitness professionals but also in the general population. Consequently, fitness consumers increasingly want specific results, more choices, and more guidance about how to exercise, particularly when recovering from injury. Many of us—whether clinical kinesiologists, personal trainers, physical therapists, athletic trainers, chiropractors, physical educators, or fitness specialists in private or community settings—have noted the lack of resources for guiding these informed consumers.

Part III examines the intrinsic and extrinsic biomechanical causes of soft tissue injuries. Each type of tissue has different biological properties that influence its mechanism of injury and adaptation to training. The most common types of fitness injuries are caused by repetitive microtrauma in which soft tissue becomes inflamed or degenerates

with damage that can be cumulative, resulting in ligament strains, joint synovitis, muscle myositis, or tendinitis. All inflamed tissues follow the same basic pattern of healing involving: inflammation, proliferation or repair, and remodeling. Specific objectives for range of motion, strength, and activity demands must be set to progress from one phase of healing to the next.

Part III also focuses on exercise prescription for clients recovering from or having a history of orthopedic injury. You will find a brief description and background information on functional anatomy for plantar fasciitis, Achilles tendinitis, shin splints (medial tibial stress syndrome), patellofemoral syndrome, hamstring strain, low back pain, and rotator cuff tendinitis (impingement syndrome). You will also find probable causes and strategies for prevention as well as specific exercise designs for stretching and strengthening damaged tissues for each of these injuries.

Preventing and Treating Injuries

10

Chapter Competencies

After completing this chapter, you will be able to demonstrate the following competencies:

1. Describe the causes of soft tissue injury to ligaments, tendons, cartilage, and muscles.

2. Describe the biomechanical characteristics of each kind of soft tissue that determine its vulnerabilities to injury.

3. Describe the phases of injury healing.

4. Prescribe exercise appropriately for each healing stage.

5. Describe how to minimize risk of injury or reinjury.

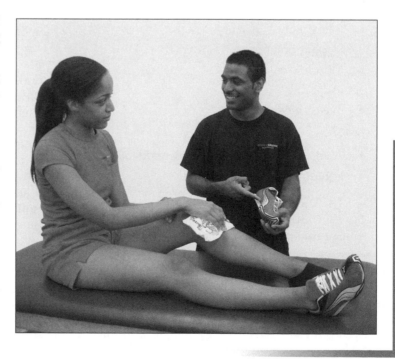

Injuries to ligaments, tendons, cartilage, and muscles are called soft tissue injuries. To help your clients deal with such injuries, you must be familiar with the causes of soft tissue injury, the biomechanical characteristics of each kind of soft tissue that determine its vulnerabilities to injury, the phases of injury healing, how to prescribe exercise appropriately for each healing stage, and how to minimize risk of injury or reinjury.

Causes of Soft Tissue Injury

The biomechanical causes of soft tissue injuries can be classified as intrinsic risk factors, extrinsic risk factors, or some combination of the two. The biological causes of overuse soft tissue injuries can be explained as repeated microinsult to the tissues.

Biomechanical Roots of Injury

The following list of intrinsic and extrinsic risk factors identifies issues that can contribute to overuse injuries either alone on in combination. The cycle of overuse injury, healing, and reinjury will not be broken until the contributing intrinsic or extrinsic factors have been addressed.

Intrinsic and Extrinsic Risk Factors

Intrinsic

- Malalignment
- Muscle imbalance
- Inflexibility
- Hypermobility
- Muscle weakness
- Instability
- Excess weight

Extrinsic

- Training errors (excessive or repeated forces)
- Equipment
- Environment
- Technique
- Sport-imposed deficiencies

Often but not always with overuse injuries, there will be a final event in which the loading pattern exceeds the tissue strength and injury becomes apparent, but the circumstances leading up to the injury may be just as important as the final mechanism (figure 10.1).

$$I + E > Injury$$

| Intrinsic risk (Predispose the client) | Extrinsic risk (expose the client) | (Combination and interaction of I and E leave client vulnerable) |

Figure 10.1 Risk and cause of injury.

Reprinted, by permission, from L. Jozsa and P. Kannus, 1997, *Human tendons* (Champaign, IL: Human Kinetics), 47.

Intrinsic Factors

Intrinsic risk factors are biomechanical characteristics unique to an individual. Each client has a specific structure, alignment, movement mechanics, and injury history that constitute an "intrinsic" risk. Poor muscle strength or muscle imbalance, hypo- or hypermobility, excess weight, and malalignment all prevent the optimal distribution of loading. Subsequent exposure to extrinsic risk factors, such as type of training, equipment, or the environment, will affect those with a higher intrinsic risk more readily.

For example, overpronation of the ankle produces a whipping action on the Achilles attributable to the excessive range of motion. These torsion forces may be related to degenerative changes to the tendon (Achilles tendinitis). Clement and colleagues (1984) reported that almost 60% of injured runners overpronated. Excessive pronation has also been linked to higher incidence of shin splints attributable to the increased stretch of the tibialis anterior. In fact, torsion of the tibia that comes with pronation makes it difficult for the patella to track evenly during gait. Patellofemoral syndrome can result (see chapter 11). Careful observation of the Achilles and subtalar joint while your client is standing and walking should reveal a pronation problem. A medial wearing pattern on the heel of your client's shoe is additional evidence.

Always screen clients as discussed in chapters 3 and 4, and carefully follow up after your prescription to monitor any potential risk. It also can be useful to do some sleuthing on your client's history of injuries—you may uncover an intrinsic predisposing factor that has not been corrected. Careful supervision and appropriate intervention can minimize the effects of a client's intrinsic risk factors.

Extrinsic Factors

Training errors are the primary extrinsic factor associated with overuse injuries. Clement and colleagues (1984) identified training errors in 75% of tendon injuries and overuse syndromes. Changes in duration, intensity, or frequency of activity are common mechanisms of extrinsic overload: too soon, too much, too often, or with too little rest. But risk increases with any kind of change in the loading pattern, for example, during transitions from preseason to competition, with a change of technique, or with something as simple as a new pair of shoes.

The risk factors most commonly introduced by these training errors are

- excessive force in the development of momentum,
- eccentric overload, and
- work volume overload.

Depending on the extent and frequency of the overload or excessive force, any of these three biomechanical risk factors can cause either

- repetitive submaximal tissue overload that leads to microtrauma with incomplete cellular repair and subsequent deterioration of connective tissue, or
- abusive tissue overload that causes acute injury attributable to macrotrauma and may initiate tendinitis or other injury that is resistant to healing and continues as an overuse injury.

Fitness activities often follow patterns of repetitive submaximal tissue overload. Initial studies of high-impact aerobic dance revealed a high incidence of lower-extremity injuries (Griffin 1987): The inherent repetitive overload causes fatigue, loss of strength, and microtrauma to the tibialis posterior, soleus, and gastrocnemius. Without continuing rest and ice treatment, tissue repair is inadequate and subsequent performance is painful, weak, and restrictive. People in this situation suffer from shin splints or Achilles tendinitis. Overuse injuries to the muscle–tendon are so common in fitness activities used for conditioning in specific sports that some of the injuries have taken on common names, such as tennis elbow, swimmer's shoulder, and jumper's knee. Table 10.1 lists the common sites of overuse tendon injuries (Hess et al. 1989).

Figure 10.2 shows how repetitive submaximal tissue overload injuries can be percolating before any symptoms emerge. If training loads exceed the tissue's ability to repair itself between activity sessions, injuries will eventually result. Common

Table 10.1 Common Sites of Overuse Tendon Injuries

Tendon	Common name
Adductor brevis, gracilis, pectineus, iliopsoas	Groin pull
Achilles	Achilles tendinitis
Patellar	Jumper's knee
Common wrist extensor tendon	Tennis elbow (lateral epicondylitis)
Common wrist flexor	Golfer's elbow (medial epicondylitis)
Supraspinatus	Swimmer's shoulder (impingement)
Other rotator cuff tendons (infraspinatus, teres minor, subscapularis)	Rotator cuff tendinitis
Tibialis posterior	Shin splints

situations when this occurs are at the beginning of a program, at a point of progression, or at training camp when the duration, intensity, and frequency of training increase at the same time. Generally there are two kinds of fitness and sports activities that lead to repetitive submaximal tissue overload damage: endurance activities and those associated with repetitive actions.

Momentum

Excessive or uncontrolled momentum is a common technique error in sport, recreational activities, and occupational tasks. You should develop the ability to spot high-momentum movements that place clients at risk. Because momentum is the product of velocity × mass, momentum is high when a large part of the body moves rapidly. A joint experiences even greater forces as

- the mass of the moving part is farther away from the joint (longer lever) or
- the movement goes to the end of the range of motion.

At risk during actions such as these are the joint capsule, musculotendinous unit, and other soft tissue structures. The following design illustrates progressive increases in exercise momentum.

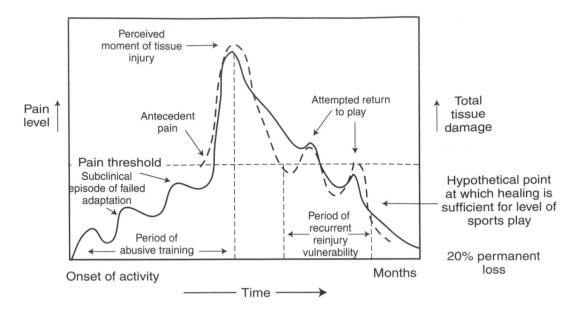

Figure 10.2 Chronic microtrauma.

Reprinted from *Clinics in Sports Medicine*, vol. 11(3), W.B. Leadbetter, "Cell-matrix response in tendon injury," pgs. 533-578, Copyright 1992, with permission of Elsevier.

Example: Triceps Kickbacks (dumbbells)

Level A. Upper arm stays by side of body; elbow extends and returns. (Small body part, short lever, momentum low but depends on weight used.)

Level B. At the end of elbow extension, the entire arm extends at the shoulder; return. (Additional arm weight provides greater momentum, greater range of motion, and longer lever.)

Level C. Same as level B with a rotation of the spine as the weight is lifted higher. (As shoulder reaches end of its range of motion, momentum forces trunk to rotate; addition of any speed to force a heavy weight up would create dangerous torque strain on the back.)

Level C takes the range of motion of the shoulder and elbow beyond a safe point. The high-momentum actions described introduce a repeated tensile stretch to the muscle–tendon unit, including the low back.

Momentum Quiz

The buildup of momentum is very common in fitness activities, and many movements are contraindicated. To test your skill of recognizing momentum and the risk it may present, try the following quiz.

For each of the following exercises identify

A. how the momentum is produced (mass × velocity) and

B. possible adverse effects.

Example

Full neck circles

A. The head is quite heavy; if done quickly, momentum will affect the neck.

B. Facet joints of the cervical spine will be jammed during the hyperextension phase; may affect the neck arteries.

Quiz

1. Straight-leg speed sit-ups

    A.

    B.

2. Stepping down and up quickly from a high aerobic step (bench)

    A.

    B.

3. Full squat with barbell

    A.

    B.

4. Throwing a plyoball with one hand

    A.

    B.

5. Changing directions quickly in a squash game

    A.

    B.

Answers

1A. All mass above the hips is being raised and lowered rapidly.

1B. Hip flexors are exerting a strong anterior pull on the pelvis and low back.

2A. Body weight and gravity combine on the down phase.

2B. The ankle (Achilles), knee, and possibly the back may be injured if client has a forward bend posture.

3A. Body and barbell weight and gravity combine on the down phase.

3B. Knees and possibly back can be injured if form is poor.

4A. Weight of ball, trunk, and arm at the angular velocity is created by the torque of the summed kinetic chain of joints.

4B. Eccentric strain is placed on the shoulder rotator cuff, both preparatory and follow-through phases.

5A. Weight and speed of the body move in the initial direction.

5B. Muscles and joints of the lateral or posterior lower leg must counter with high eccentric forces.

Always stress quality of motion. Every individual has a unique **stop point** for each joint, linked to muscle tightness and muscle strength. This is the point in a joint's range of motion (ROM) that, for motion to continue, would require involvement of another joint. Identifying the stop point requires a learned "intuitive inhibition"; you can help your clients discover these stop points by carefully observing excessive movement as they exercise.

Eccentric Contraction Patterns

You should also evaluate your clients' **eccentric contraction patterns.** Eccentric contractions generate the greatest muscular forces. Extreme strain is placed on connective tissue when it is elongated under tension, creating considerable potential for microtearing. Eccentric contractions occur when

- muscles attempt to counter the force of momentum by slowing down the action—examples include ballistic arm action, especially with hand weights, and the follow-through action during racket sports;
- muscles attempt to counter the force of gravity—examples include any lowering of a limb or of the body, such as the lower body's strain during the support phase of running (figure 10.3).

Sports can overload musculoskeletal systems in predictable patterns. For example, sports involving throwing may leave the external rotators of the shoulder fatigued from continual eccentric deceleration of the arm. This chronic fatigue leads to a loss of flexibility, weakness, and eventual injury (figure 10.4). Eccentric overload is evident in the high incidence of lower leg injuries during many aerobic weight-bearing activities (Houglum 2001, Styf 1988). Eccentric patterns also appear in dynamic front lunges, which require many eccentric contractions to counteract the force of gravity—gastrocnemius, soleus, and tibialis anterior to control the speed of ankle dorsiflexion, quadriceps to control knee flexion, gluteus maximus and hamstrings to control hip flexion, and probably the erector spinae, which controls the downward tendency of spinal flexion. Furthermore, eccentric overload seems to be particularly associated with delayed-onset muscle soreness.

Delayed-Onset Muscle Soreness

Aside from the pain of a muscle or connective tissue injury, vigorous exercise can produce delayed-onset muscle soreness (DOMS). DOMS can emerge 8 to 12 hr after certain exercise, is generally at its worst within the first 2 days following the activity, and subsides over the next few days.

DOMS is thought to be a result of microscopic tearing of the muscle fibers (Ross 1999). Others (Szymanski 2001) believe that the symptoms of DOMS are associated with damage to the connective tissue around the muscle, accumulation of calcium, release of intracellular proteins, and inflammation. In addition to microscopic tearing, swelling may take place in and around the muscle. This swelling increases pressure on nerves and other structures, resulting in pain and stiffness. The amount of damage depends on the intensity, duration, and type of exercise. As noted previously, activities in which muscles forcefully contract while they are lengthening tend to cause the most soreness. These eccentric contractions occur in activities involving a braking action such as running downhill, lowering weights, descending stairs, performing plyometrics, and performing the downward phases of push-ups and squats. Unaccustomed activities involving sudden major changes in the type or length of exercise may also cause delayed soreness.

Understanding Soft Tissue Injuries

Each type of tissue has different biological properties that influence its mechanism of injury and adaptation to training. The phases of recovery

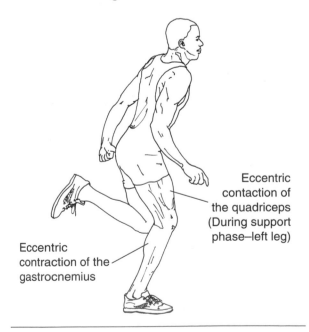

Eccentric contaction of the quadriceps (During support phase—left leg)

Eccentric contraction of the gastrocnemius

Figure 10.3   Eccentric contractions in running.

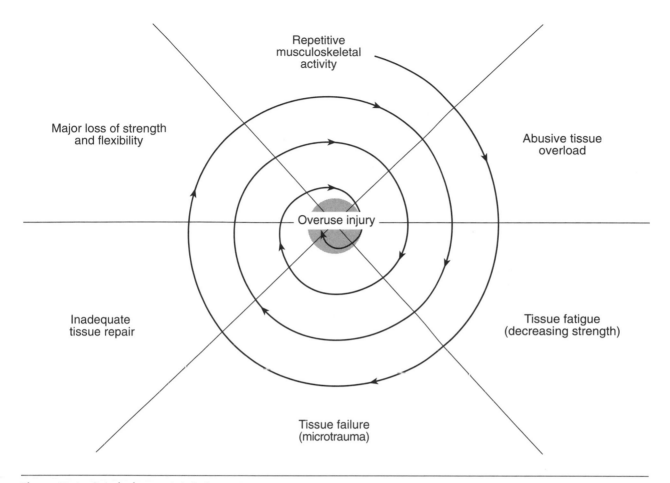

Figure 10.4   Spiral of overuse injuries.

from injury involving inflammation are the same, however, no matter what tissue is involved. Understanding tissue type characteristics and the phases of healing will better equip you to prevent tissue degeneration and to promote proper healing.

Types of Soft Tissue

Soft tissue, such as ligaments, tendons, and cartilage, is susceptible to injury. Its structure is suited to its function, but the external forces often exceed its structural integrity.

Ligaments

Ligaments run from bone to bone, holding the bones together. Ligaments are like a flat mesh that reinforce the joint or joint capsule.

The organization of the tough collagenous fibers in the ligament can be parallel, oblique, or even spiral (as in the anterior cruciate ligament). The fibers are arranged to provide the best stabilization for the joint. Ligaments contain slightly more elastic fibers than do tendons.

Overuse injuries to ligaments are less common than the acute injury from a sudden overload or stretch in an extreme position. However, throwers (e.g., baseball players) may stretch their shoulder capsular ligaments and powerlifters their cruciate ligaments, reducing the joint's stability and leaving it susceptible to injury.

Providing more than passive stabilization, ligaments also contain proprioceptors that, when injured, reduce our ability to sense position or movements of the joint. Therefore, progressive kinesthetic activities are beneficial before returning to full functional training.

Tendons

Tendons attach muscle to bone. They vary in length and can be round, or, if the muscle is broad and flat, the specialized tendon (aponeuroses) is also this shape.

Structurally, tendons closely resemble ligaments. The main difference is the tendon's parallel collagen arrangement in successively larger bundles. Progressing from interior to exterior as well as smaller to larger, these layers are tropocollagen,

collagen, subfibril, fibril, fascicle with an outer endotendineum, and finally the tendon with an outer epitendineum (figure 10.5).

Tendons consist primarily of collagenous fibers (70%) embedded in a gel. The endotendineum, which is the connective tissue sheath surrounding fibrils of collagen, carries blood vessels and nerves. The epitendineum (the outermost layer) is like an elastic sleeve allowing free movement of the tendon against surrounding structures.

Muscle and tendon function as one unit. Injury may occur at any point along this muscle–tendon unit: in the muscle belly, in the tendon, at the musculotendinous junction, or at the tendon–bone attachment. The connective tissue surrounding similar bundles of muscle fibers infolds and attaches to the tendon's collagenous projections within the myotendinous junction. At the other end, the tendon attaches to the periosteum and the bone's fibrocartilage, with a few fibers penetrating the bone itself.

Tendons are the soft tissues most likely to incur overuse injury. Advances in the understanding of tendon pathology indicate that Achilles, patellar, epicondylar, and rotator cuff tendinosis is often misdiagnosed as tendinitis. Because tendinosis is the sequel to unsuccessfully treated tendinitis, and (unlike tendinitis) does not involve inflammation, treating tendinosis as if it were tendinitis will not help it (Kahn et al. 2000). Because these tendinosis conditions involve degenerative changes including loss of collagen, altered fiber organization, and vascular disruption, a treatment must be devised that will address these degenerative problems. As the implications of this paradigm change are further understood, the current recommendations for treatment may also change somewhat, enhancing our clients' recovery.

Cartilage

Bones contact one another, forming a joint, but are separated by a layer of smooth, resilient hyaline cartilage. Some joints contain fibrocartilage structures that, together with the shape of the bone surfaces, influence movement.

Hyaline cartilage covers the articular surface of joints. Although 70% water, it has a meshwork of collagen fibers aligned horizontally on the surface, crisscrossed in the middle, and vertically near the bone. Hyaline cartilage is not supplied with blood vessels or nerves, so the cartilage cells obtain oxygen and nutrients by diffusion. Regular loading maintains a cycle of nutrients in and around the cartilage. Injuries can be from acute joint trauma in which underlying bone is also injured (osteochondral). Degenerative changes can also occur because of cartilage failure or increased loading (osteoarthritis).

Fibrocartilage is found in the knee's meniscus, the wrist, labrum around the shoulder and hip, and the intervertebral disc. Fibrocartilage is strong yet resilient, helping to absorb shock and facilitate fit

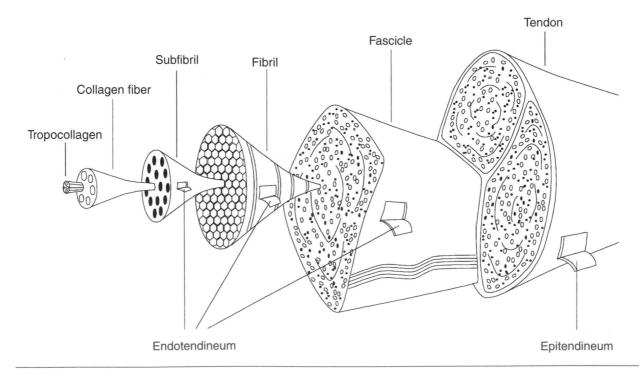

Figure 10.5   The structure of a tendon.

and stability. Although some fibrocartilage has blood supply, it shares the same limited ability to heal itself as the nonvascularized hyaline cartilage.

Structural Strength of Tissues

Terms of Structural Biomechanics shows how tissues such as ligaments, tendons, and muscles react to stresses such as stretching (tensile stress). Initially, the wavy configuration of the collagenous fibers in the connective tissue straightens out. Relatively little force is needed to elongate the tissue, and the relationship between the load (force) and the deformation (stretch) is linear. In this "elastic zone," the tissue can act like a spring, and once the load is removed, the tissue returns to near its original length. If the change in length exceeds a "yield point" (which is about 4% for a ligament), there is more permanent deformation

(lengthening) with some slippage of collagen cross-links. Eventually collagen fibers start to rupture, and the tissue becomes injured.

The relationship between stress and deformation of tendons is similar to that of ligaments. Some activities and sports, such as soccer, basketball, and rugby, require repetitive loading up to 8% change in length (Bahr and Maehlum 2004), potentially causing collagen fibers to rupture. Tendinitis is an inflammatory response within the tendon as a result of microstructural damage to the collagen fibers. The tendon is particularly vulnerable because the force of a contracting muscle is transmitted through the tendon.

To understand the relationship between loading and deformation of hyaline cartilage, remember that the collagen fibers are organized as a meshwork. Deformation increases linearly, straightening the fibers until tearing occurs rather abruptly.

 ## Terms of Structural Biomechanics

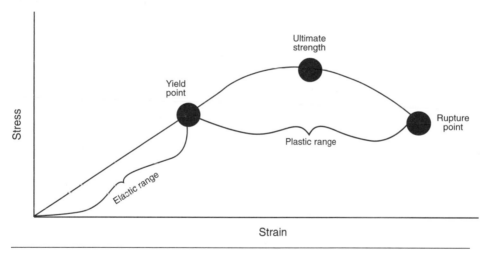

Stress–strain graph.

stress–strain curve (load deformation)—The deformation (strain) increases proportionally to the stress resisting the load. The muscle–tendon complex has properties of elasticity up to a point (elastic range), after which permanent deformation (plastic range) and ultimately a rupture will occur.

stress—Reaction forces to external loads set up within the tissues (e.g., stress created in bone, ligament, and tendon within the arch of the foot to support body weight)

strain—Deformation; changes in tissue size, shape, length

tensile—Pulling apart (e.g., tendon, ligament, muscle)

shear—Sliding apart (e.g., joint surfaces, L5-S1, epiphyseal plates)

compression—Pressure (e.g., intervertebral disc, cartilage)

elasticity—Ability to return to original dimension immediately

plasticity—Ability to retain changes in size or length when load is removed

resilience—Ability of tissue to vigorously return to its original size when unloaded

damping—Characteristic of tissue to return to its original size less vigorously than it was deformed (i.e., loss of energy)

absorbed strain—Process that occurs if loading goes into the plastic range, when a considerable amount of energy may be lost (dissipated during permanent deformation)

Phases of Inflammatory Injury Healing and Reconditioning

The most common types of fitness injuries—and as many as 50% of all sports injuries—are caused by repetitive microtrauma in which soft tissue becomes inflamed or degenerates. The damage can be cumulative, resulting in ligament strains, joint synovitis, muscle myositis, or tendinitis. Injury occurs most often when a tissue like the tendon has been stressed repeatedly until it is unable to endure further tension. All inflamed tissues (ligament, tendon, muscle, cartilage, and bone) follow the same basic pattern of healing (table 10.2). Injuries need inflammation to heal, but inflammation does not always result in healing.

You must recognize the phase and characteristics of the healing phases of injury involving inflammation. The process of returning to regular activity or competition involves this natural phased healing, preparation of the tissues for return to function, and the use of proper techniques to maximize reconditioning. Specific objectives for range of motion, strength, and activity demands must be set to progress from one phase of healing to the next. The three phases of healing are inflammation, proliferation or repair, and remodeling. These stages are described next, and the appropriate exercise strategies for each phase are described in detail in the section on *Exercise Prescription for Injured Clients* (p. 286). Because not much is known about either the process of or treatment for tendinosis, discussion will be limited to healing involving inflammation (figure 10.6).

• Phase 1 (Inflammation): During inflammation, which generally lasts only a few days, the injury is stabilized and contained and debris is removed. The phase begins with bleeding and the release of blood products such as platelets into the injured area. Both vasodilation and increased capillary permeability are induced by histamine that is released by damaged cells (Germann and Stanfield 2002). These vascular changes cause the redness, warmth, swelling, and pain of inflammation. Platelets help stimulate the clotting mechanism, forming a meshwork of fibrin and collagen (Bahr and Maehlum 2004). Neutrophils move through the capillary walls to the injury, where they release enzymes that dissolve the damaged extracellular matrix. Later, macrophages remove debris and excess fluid partially caused by the rupture of cell walls. The damaged lymph vessels are unable to drain the excess fluid (edema) until the area becomes stable and the vessel repaired (Houglum 2001). With a loss of blood flow and oxygen to other healthy cells, the area may experience hypoxia, cell damage, and further edema. The inflammatory substances and edema may cause function-inhibiting pain. Phase 1 inflammation needs to occur but should be minimized by applying ice, compression, elevation, and rest.

• Phase 2 (Proliferation or Repair): Once the macrophages remove most of the debris from the area, the next step is the growth of new blood vessels (angiogenesis) and other tissue. Growth factors enter the area and are responsible for the local migration and proliferation of fibroblasts and endothelial cells. Fibroblasts are important for the development of new capillaries and the extracellular matrix (Houglum 2001), which has both a fibrous component (collagen and elastin) and a gel-like ground substance. The ground substance fills the spaces between the fibrous elements and reduces friction when stress is applied. At the same time, there is a continuous breakdown and removal of extracellular matrix and cellular debris (Bahr and Maehlum 2004). Also, the new matrix draws water into the area, increasing edema. As the injured tissue is repaired, its tensile strength increases.

Table 10.2   Healing Phases of Inflammatory Injury

Phase	Characteristic	Duration
Inflammation	Localized redness, swelling (edema), increased temperature (warmth), pain (tender), loss of normal function	Up to 5 days
Proliferation or repair	Scar tissue red and larger than normal because of edema; increased collagen fiber production	3-21 days
Remodeling	Redness (vascularity) reduced, water content of scar reduced, and scar tissue density increased; collagen fiber alignment and increased tissue strength	7 days to ≥1 year

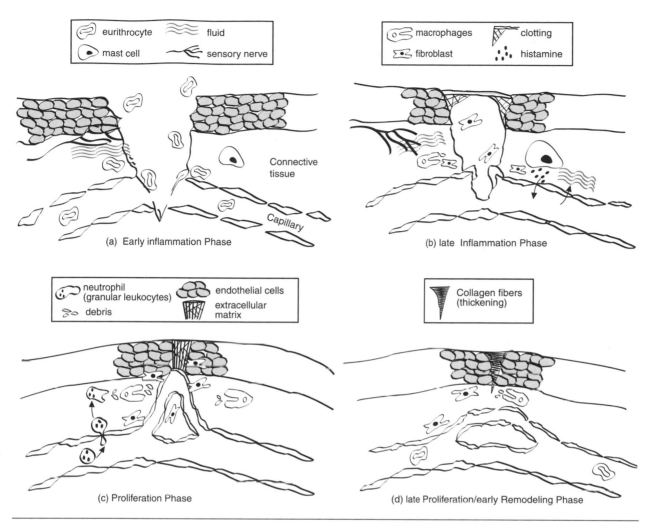

Figure 10.6 Phases of healing: *(a)* inflammation phase, *(b)* late inflammation phase, *(c)* proliferation phase, and *(d)* late proliferation and early remodeling phase.

• Phase 3 (Remodeling): With some overlap of phases, remodeling begins as some of the fibroblasts become myofibroblasts to shrink the wound (Houglum 2001). This scar tissue contraction and adhesion formation can cause a loss of motion at a joint. The number of macrophages reduces and mature blood supply is established by selective removal of capillaries with low blood flow. Swelling and wound sensitivity are reduced with the loss of extracellular matrix substances. Remodeling of the scar tissue involves the formation of thicker collagen fibers in the direction of tissue tension. As fluid is reduced in the area, the collagen fibers can produce more cross-links with each other. When the fibers are aligned in a parallel fashion, collagen can form the greatest number of cross-links to increase tensile strength, and the form and function of this scar tissue depend significantly on the degree to which the tissue is loaded by stretching and contractile exercises while the tissue is remodeling. Proprioceptors such as the muscle spindles and Golgi tendon organs, which monitor muscle length, tension, and rate of change, may be damaged and will start to repair in this stage.

Treating and Preventing Overuse Injuries

If your clients are to maintain long-term fitness, you must be able to treat whatever injuries they already have and minimize the occurrence of new ones. To do this, you must be able to recognize the signs and symptoms of overuse; prescribe appropriately for injured clients, taking the phases of recovery into account; and control risks of further injury.

Defining the Boundaries

Rehabilitation and reconditioning are a team-oriented process requiring all members of the sports medicine team to work together. You must recognize the responsibilities of different health care providers who may be needed throughout the healing and strengthening phases. Although you will need to understand the mechanism of injury, the different types of injury, and the physiological healing process, in addition you must establish a communication network of health care practitioners to facilitate referral and dialogue. Because of your unique knowledge and insight into exercise design, modification, demonstration, monitoring, and health promotion, you can serve a vital role during the final stages of an advanced rehabilitation and reconditioning program (Earle and Baechle 2004).

During the initial counseling session you should determine past injuries, current pains, and potential causes of injury. In many cases, your clients will approach you after they have started their program and experienced some discomfort. At this stage, effective questioning and probing are critical to determine your client's needs. With your client, fill out the *Pain Questionnaire* on page 285 to establish a history and possible causes of her pain.

Recognizing Overuse

Defining the Boundaries helps to identify the areas of expertise of personal fitness trainers and ensure that overstepping these areas is avoided. In addition, most certification programs for personal trainers such as ACSM, NSCA, or CSEP have published competencies and a scope of practice in the area of injury prevention and treatment.

Some clients do not take pain seriously and will mask it until it becomes acute. Ask clients about pain and be alert for signs of pain while they are exercising. Urge them to seek help when they first experience pain. During movement, your client may show signs of feeling pain or warmth, or you may notice swelling or crepitus. Crepitus is a crackling sound similar to the sound of rolling hair between the fingers by the ear. To ensure early intervention so that problems will not become serious, watch carefully for any of these symptoms of overuse.

The series of events that lead to overuse injury are remarkably predictable (O'Connor et al. 1992). When a movement is performed repeatedly and the tissue becomes irritated and inflamed, overuse injury occurs. Although inflammation from tissue damage is required for proper healing, an excessive or prolonged inflammatory response can become self-destructive. To prevent tissue degeneration and promote proper healing, you must interrupt the spiral of overuse discussed earlier (figure 10.4). The following situations often lead to tissue damage:

- A change in execution (e.g., joint alignment)
- A change in the client's interface with equipment (e.g., set-up or starting position, change of shoes)
- Failure of execution with no spotting
- Increase in load or intensity
- Omission of warm-up or cool-down
- Resumption of training after a period of inactivity
- Addition or deletion of exercises from the original prescription
- Change in location of workouts (e.g., surface) or environment (e.g., temperature)
- Addition of supplemental activity such as a sport

Be aware of your client's comments or behaviors, as they may reveal an emerging overuse injury:

- Has she changed her gait or running pattern?
- Does she regularly take painkillers before exercise?
- Does her pain increase even after a good warm-up?
- Does her pain continue even after the intensity has been reduced?

Nirschl (1988) described a pain phase scale for overuse injuries. This scale is useful for initial assessment and as a way to monitor a program's rate of progress (see *Pain Scale for Overuse Injuries*).

Pain Questionnaire

1. Do you have any current pain? _____

2. What are the symptoms? _____

_____

3. How long have you had these symptoms? _____

4. Have you had any related conditions in the past, and what treatment was provided? _____

_____

5. In what joint or area do you feel the pain? _____

6. In what positions do you feel the pain? _____

_____

7. During what movement do you feel the pain? _____

_____

8. Do you feel the pain more or less before activity? _____

9. Do you feel the pain more or less after activity? _____

10. How long does the pain last? _____

11. Do you get tired (muscularly) more easily than you used to? _____

12. Have you experienced a loss of strength? _____

13. Are you compensating in your movements to avoid pain or loss of strength? _____

_____

14. Do you feel tight anywhere? _____

15. Have you changed your prescription? _____

16. Have you recently increased your exercise volume or intensity? _____

_____

17. Have you changed your location of exercise, type of equipment, or other conditions? _____

_____

18. Have you recently changed shoes or are your shoes worn? _____

19. Is the injury or pain getting worse? _____

20. What do you think is causing this problem? _____

_____

21. How could it be alleviated? _____

_____

From *Client-Centered Exercise Prescription, Second Edition,* by John C. Griffin, 2006, Champaign, IL: Human Kinetics.

Pain Scale for Overuse Injuries

Phase 1: Stiffness or mild soreness after activity. Pain usually gone within 24 hr.

Phase 2: Stiffness or mild soreness before activity that is relieved by warm-up. Symptoms not present during activity but return after, lasting up to 48 hr.

Phase 3: Stiffness or mild soreness before activity. Pain partially relieved by warm-up. Pain minimally present during activity but does not alter activity.

Phase 4: Pain more intense than phase 3. Performance of activity altered. Mild pain noticed with daily activities.

Phase 5: Significant (moderate or greater) pain before, during, and after activity, causing alteration of activity. Pain with daily activities but no major change.

Phase 6: Pain persists even with complete rest. Pain disrupts simple daily activities and prohibits doing household chores.

Phase 7: Phase 6 pain that also disrupts sleep consistently. Aching pain that intensifies with activity.

Exercise Prescription for Injured Clients

You must recognize the stages of healing and understand the characteristics of each. Only then will you be able to set appropriate objectives for range of motion, strength, and activity demands to progress from one phase of healing to the next.

Tissue damage can come from a macrotrauma or sudden onset (acute injury) or from microtrama or repeated abnormal stress (overuse injury). In most cases, it is easy to classify an injury as either acute or overuse. However, some injuries may have a sudden onset of symptoms, but they may have started much earlier with heavy training and little recovery. These should be treated as overuse injuries.

An important part of treating overuse injuries is preventing atrophy of the musculoskeletal system because of inactivity. Tendons, capsules, cartilage, and ligaments are just as affected by inactivity as muscles. It has been demonstrated that after 8 weeks of inactivity, 40% of strength

and 30% of stiffness in the tendons are lost (Bahr and Maehlum 2004).

Overuse injuries can be very discouraging to clients. Recurrent injury often results from incomplete rehabilitation. To optimize their quick (and permanent) return to their programs, encourage the following three-stage progression: (1) acute response (inflammation control), (2) recovery (repair), and (3) functional progression (remodeling) (figure 10.7).

Guidelines for Stage 1, Acute Response (Inflammation Control)

Goals: Control inflammation and manage pain. Prepare for new tissue formation during healing and avoid worsening the injury.

To achieve these goals, relative rest, anti-inflammatory treatment, and passive modalities including ice, compression, and elevation are the primary treatment options.

Inflammation can hamper reconditioning in many overuse injuries. Reduction and elimination of inflammation must be a priority of exercise prescriptions. To limit bleeding, relieve pain, decrease swelling, and improve healing, have the client begin effective PRICE (prevention, rest, ice, compression, elevation) treatment as soon as possible. Bleeding and plasma exudation continue for 48 hr after an acute soft tissue injury, so to be effective, PRICE treatment must continue for 2 to 3 days.

- Prevention and rest. With overuse injuries, the affected muscles must be allowed to rest, sometimes for several weeks depending on the pain. Andrish and Work (1990) suggested stopping the offending activity until the pain subsides, usually in about 1 to 2 weeks. Correct any biomechanical abnormality or training error that may have caused inflammation—such as work-related overuse, continuation of a sport while injured, or aggravation caused by poorly designed exercises.

- Ice. The use of cold (cryotherapy) is not only effective immediately after an injury or flare-up; it should be continued as long as inflammation persists. Ice causes local vasoconstriction and slows metabolic activity; it relieves pain and muscle spasm. When your client has joint pain, stop all painful activities immediately and ice the joint. Kaul and Herring (1994) reported that ice chips in a plastic bag were the most effective local application method, followed by use of frozen gel packs and endothermic chemical reaction packs. Frozen gel packs are convenient and reusable

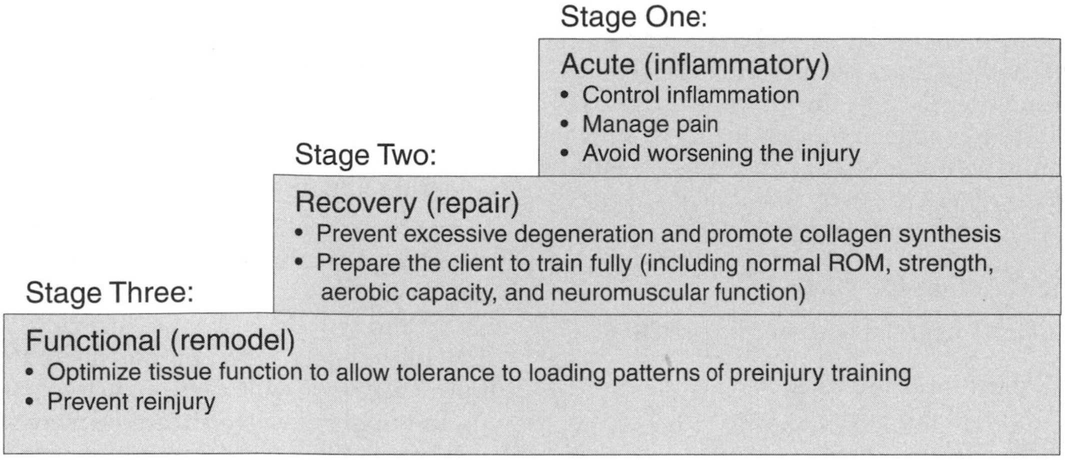

Stage One:

Acute (inflammatory)
- Control inflammation
- Manage pain
- Avoid worsening the injury

Stage Two:

Recovery (repair)
- Prevent excessive degeneration and promote collagen synthesis
- Prepare the client to train fully (including normal ROM, strength, aerobic capacity, and neuromuscular function)

Stage Three:

Functional (remodel)
- Optimize tissue function to allow tolerance to loading patterns of preinjury training
- Prevent reinjury

Figure 10.7   The three-stage progression to complete rehabilitation.

and require a thin insulating towel coverage to avoid nerve damage and frostbite. Ice massage with water frozen in a foam cup can be used to produce analgesia. Excess pressure should be avoided and sessions should be short (5-10 min). With acute tendinitis, ice should be applied at the end of every activity session.

• Compression. Compression with an elastic bandage will limit the development of hematoma. Reduced blood flow under the bandage can be significant and increases with the tightness of the fit. An ice bag under the compression bandage can increase local pressure over the injury site.

• Elevation. Elevation is recommended for the first 2 days whenever the client is lying down or sitting still. No reduction in blood flow occurs until the injured area is more than 30 cm (12 in.) above the level of the heart (Bahr and Maehlum 2004). Therefore, the injured limb should be propped up considerably, especially in bed at night.

• Medications. Pharmacological control of inflammation is often accomplished through NSAIDs (nonsteroidal anti-inflammatory drugs) such as aspirin (e.g., Bayer) and ibuprofen (e.g., Advil, Motrin). NSAIDs prevent plasma proteins (e.g., prostagladins) from acting by decreasing membrane permeability. They may also help ease symptoms such as pain and spasm. Ibuprofen has been shown to decrease muscle soreness induced after eccentric exercise (Tokmakidis et al. 2003).

When inflammation is acute, have your client take the medication regularly (without exceeding the label limit). Do not use NSAIDs to reduce pain to allow a more intense workout. Ensure that your client has no medical contraindications. If inflam-mation persists or worsens, your client should see a physician. Keep a proper perspective regarding the role of NSAIDs, especially given their risk of side effects and their potential to blunt the normal healing process (Stovitz and Johnson 2003).

Guidelines for Stage 2, Recovery (Repair)

Goals: Prevent excessive degeneration, promote collagen synthesis, and prepare the client to train fully (including normal ROM, strength, aerobic capacity, and neuromuscular function).

Initial Action for Stage 2

Pain and swelling are the main considerations when prescribing how much and what to do. Cryotherapy may continue to be useful, particularly after an exercise session. The client will begin with low-load stresses to promote increased collagen synthesis and prevent loss of joint motion. Relative rest is obviously protective.

Soon after an injury, exercise enhances tissue oxygenation, minimizes atrophy, and aligns collagenous fibers to increase tissue strength. At first, have your client

- limit excessive stretching of damaged tissue;
- do isometrics (progressing from submaximal) at different joint angles; and
- start with midrange isotonics (daily), completing about 30 repetitions in 2 or 3 sets (may start with no weight).

Design activities your clients can do to enhance healing and maintain fitness. For example, if your client has a running injury, running in water with a flotation belt can be an effective alternative. Healing also involves increased vascularization through rehabilitative exercise and cardiovascular conditioning. During this stage, your clients should limit the range of motion to that in which they remain pain-free. Pain can activate neural mechanisms within the body that inhibit strength, flexibility, and function (Ralston 2003).

Subsequent Action for Stage 2

As your clients heal, have them progress to

- full effort on isometrics;
- isotonics in full ROM—gradually increasing weight by 10% to 20% and reducing repetitions initially, and then gradually increasing them again; and
- a minimum frequency of three exercise sessions per week.

Stretching can be done two to three times per day, because increased joint ROM can be retained for 4 to 6 hr (Frontera 2003). As rehabilitation progresses, include strength exercises for muscle groups proximal and distal to the injured area. Use rubber tubing or elastic bands (if you deem them appropriate). Incorporate ROM exercises and moderate static stretching to regain muscle balance and to treat muscles that have tightened because of compensation. Prescribe light cardiovascular exercise that does not traumatize the injured tissue (e.g., aquafitness, hand ergometry, stationary bicycle).

At this point, your client may gradually resume training at about half the previous intensity and gradually increase the effort over 3 to 6 weeks. Returning too quickly is the most common reason injuries recur. Make sure that the warm-up and cool-down include complete stretching of the affected area.

Guidelines for Stage 3, Functional Progression (Remodeling)

Goals: Optimizing tissue function to allow tolerance to loading patterns of preinjury training. Prevent reinjury.

Functional progression is a planned, progressively difficult sequence of exercises that acclimatize the individual to training or competition demands or fitness needs (Ralston 2003). Thus, you must be able to evaluate exercises and categorize their levels of difficulty and appropriate applications.

With increased loading, the newly formed collagen fibers begin hypertrophy and align themselves along lines of stress (Earle and Baechle 2004). Prescribe functional activities using closed-chain, dynamic, multijoint exercises that closely mimic the demands and movements of preinjury endeavors.

General Guidelines

General body conditioning—including cardiovascular, strength and endurance, muscle balance, and flexibility—enhances rehabilitation of any injury and will decrease the chance of its recurring. Introducing exercises specific to the injury, however, can provide neurophysiological stimulus and help redevelop proprioceptive skills.

During stage 3, follow whichever of these guidelines are appropriate for your client:

- Include full ROM strengthening, reaching momentary failure at the end of each set.
- Insist on a minimum exercise frequency of two or three times per week.
- Select other resistance equipment (e.g., isokinetic, hydraulic, variable resistance).
- Use heavier or thicker tubing or bands to isolate movements and muscles.
- Include partner-resisted exercise and proprioceptive neuromuscular facilitation with client-specific static stretches.
- Add activities specific to the client's sport or usual training activities (e.g., interval training; muscle isolations; drills for agility, speed, and skill).
- If the client is involved in a power-oriented eccentric activity, progressively build the eccentric strength and power of the involved muscle groups (e.g., eccentric Achilles exercises, plyometrics).

Neuromuscular Concerns

Clients will continue to improve function by adding more advanced, activity-specific exercises. In addition, the client must regain normal neuromuscular function. If not, changes in recruitment patterns of muscles around the injured joint may alter technique and produce unfavorable loading. To avoid new injuries, training must include proprioceptive challenges, coordination, balance, and agility once the client has regained at least 85% of his original strength (Bahr and Maehlum 2004). Neuromuscular retraining contributes to the body's ability to maintain postural stability. Houglum (2001) identified a four-part progression to reestablish neuromuscular control:

1. Proprioceptive and kinesthetic awareness (joint position sense)
2. Dynamic joint stability (balance, agility, coactivation)
3. Reactive neuromuscular control (e.g., plyometrics)
4. Functional motor patterns (specific, complex, sportlike activities)

Too Painful to Jog

A 35-year-old woman approached you about some pain she had recently felt in her Achilles and just below her patella. She had been jogging 20 to 25 min/session, 2 or 3 days/week for the last 5 weeks and had been asymptomatic. Five days ago she participated in a 2 hr volleyball tryout after a regular jog. The pain escalated over the next 3 days to the point where it was too painful to jog.

The repetitive eccentric motion of the volleyball activity was sufficient to irritate the muscle–tendon unit of the Achilles and patellar areas. A normal initial inflammatory process had taken place; icing and rest were advised until the symptoms disappeared. In the interim, an aquafit program, upper-body resistance work with some tubing, and some therapeutic exercises for her lower legs would focus on some new and some parallel goals until she can resume jogging. Some counseling about overuse may be warranted.

This approach dealt with the extrinsic causes of the injury and could probably get the client back to jogging within a reasonable time. However, you have not yet addressed the potential for reinjury caused by a possible structural weakness (intrinsic). Once the discomfort has subsided, examine your client's muscle balance and alignment (chapters 4 and 8) to identify weak links and provide a basis for therapeutic exercise prescription.

You can combine these activity suggestions to correct intrinsic needs with guidelines emerging from the extrinsic causes of injury to design the core prescription for your client. From this point, progress with your client through the three stages of the overuse intervention progression: acute response, recovery, and functional progression.

Treating DOMS

DOMS is not as serious as the injuries discussed previously, but it is a lot more common. To reduce soreness and speed recovery, encourage the use of ice, gentle stretching, and massage. The use of a compressive sleeve can decrease perceived soreness, reduce swelling, and promote recovery of force production (Kraemer et al. 2001). Initially have the client avoid any vigorous activity. You may, however, work the unaffected areas of the body. If the client performs low-impact aerobic activity such as biking or walking, blood flow is increased to the affected muscles, which may reduce soreness. Also, NSAIDs such as aspirin or ibuprofen may temporarily help, although they won't speed healing. Of all the treatments, warm-up appears to be the most promising approach. Increasing muscle temperature reduces muscle and connective tissue viscosity, increases muscle elasticity, and increases resistance to tissue tearing (Szymanski 2001).

Start the client with a general warm-up designed to increase core body temperature (e.g., jogging, cycling, or aerobic activities for 5-10 min). Proceed to a specific warm-up including multijoint movements and skill application activity related to the activity (e.g., warm-up set on the weights; dynamic flexibility such as crossovers, lunges). Static stretching of the muscles used in the activity can be effective when it follows the low-impact aerobic activity. Encourage your client to cool down thoroughly after activity. With activities such as plyometrics, start with low-volume training. Progress the intensity of the workout (e.g., gradually increase intensity and duration for at least 2 weeks and incorporate some eccentric multijoint exercises).

Preventing Reinjury: Risk Control

Reexamine your client's history and assessment to uncover his unique combination of intrinsic and extrinsic risk factors for (re)injury. Controlling these forces is both an objective of Stage 3 and an ongoing preventive strategy. You must know the client's limitations, as well as the inherent demands of his training, and keep both extrinsic and intrinsic risks in mind at all times.

• Minimizing extrinsic risks. Avoiding training errors can be the single most effective way to minimize extrinsic risks. In a typical exercise prescription, the client follows a format that may start with a warm-up, lead into cardiovascular activity (balanced by some muscular conditioning), and finish with a cool-down. Review the discussion of training errors (p. 274) and copy and use the checklist on page 292 to ensure that each of these program segments is free of training errors.

• Minimizing intrinsic risks. As discussed, it is your job to assess the biomechanical or structural risks that each client brings to the initial exercise prescription. Always make it an objective of your prescription to correct malalignments, muscle imbalances, joint instability, and muscle tightness or weakness. A prescription must assess both initial and developing intrinsic risk to be truly client-centered. In addition to this chapter, review chapters 4 (assessment) and 8 (muscle balance) to ensure that you are well prepared for this task. Careful supervision and appropriate intervention or referral to a clinical specialist can minimize the effects of a client's intrinsic risk factors.

Highlights

1. **Describe the causes of soft tissue injury to ligaments, tendons, cartilage, and muscles.**

   The biomechanical causes of soft tissue injuries can be classified as intrinsic risk factors, extrinsic risk factors, or some combination of the two. The biological causes of overuse soft tissue injuries can be explained as repeated microinsult to the tissues. Intrinsic factors such as poor muscle strength or muscle imbalance, hypo- or hypermobility, excess weight, and malalignment all prevent the optimal distribution of loading. Subsequent exposure to extrinsic risk factors, such as type of training, equipment, or the environment, will affect those with a higher intrinsic risk more readily. Aside from the pain of a muscle or connective tissue injury, vigorous exercise can produce delayed-onset muscle soreness (DOMS). DOMS is thought to be a result of microscopic tearing of the muscle fibers or associated with damage to the connective tissue around the muscle.

2. **Describe the biomechanical characteristics of each kind of soft tissue that determine its vulnerabilities to injury.**

   Each type of tissue has different biological properties that influence its mechanism of injury and adaptation to training. The organization of the tough collagenous fibers in the ligament can be parallel, oblique, or even spiral (as in the anterior cruciate ligament). The fibers are arranged to provide the best stabilization for the joint. Ligaments contain slightly more elastic fibers than do tendons. As well, tendons have parallel collagen arrangement in successively larger bundles. Tendons vary in length and can be round, or, if the muscle is broad and flat, the specialized tendon (aponeuroses) also takes this shape. Muscle and tendon function as one unit. Injury may occur at any point along this muscle–tendon unit: in the muscle belly, in the tendon, at the musculotendinous junction, or at the tendon–bone attachment. Tissues such as ligaments, tendons, and muscles react to stresses such as stretching (tensile stress). Initially, the wavy configuration of the collagenous fibers in the connective tissue straightens out. If the change in length exceeds a "yield point," there is more permanent deformation (lengthening) and eventually collagen fibers start to rupture and injury occurs. The most common types of fitness injuries are caused by repetitive microtrauma in which soft tissue becomes inflamed or degenerates with damage that can be cumulative, resulting in ligament strains, joint synovitis, muscle myositis, or tendinitis.

3. **Describe the phases of injury healing.**

   All inflamed tissues (ligament, tendon, muscle, cartilage, and bone) follow the same basic pattern of healing (see table 10.2). The three phases of healing are inflammation, proliferation or repair, and remodeling. During inflammation, which generally lasts only a few days, the injury is stabilized and contained and debris is removed. Phase 1 (inflammation) needs to occur but should be minimized by applying ice, compression, elevation, and rest. Once the macrophages remove most of the debris from the area, the next step is the growth of new blood vessels and other tissue (Phase 2). With some overlap of phases, the remodeling begins as some of the fibroblasts become myofibroblasts to shrink the wound, which may cause adhesion formation and loss of motion at a joint. Remodeling of the scar tissue involves the formation of thicker collagen fibers with increased crosslinks. As the injured tissue is repaired, its tensile strength increases.

4. **Prescribe exercise appropriately for each healing stage.**

To optimize quick (and permanent) return to regular programs, follow a three-stage progression of exercise prescription: (1) acute response (inflammation control), (2) recovery (repair), and (3) functional progression (remodeling). Along with other health care professionals, you must provide specific objectives for range of motion, strength, and activity demands to allow the client to progress from one phase of healing to the next. Stage 1 must be used to control inflammation and manage pain and avoid worsening the injury by providing relative rest, anti-inflammatory treatment, and passive modalities including ice, compression, and elevation. Stage 2 must prevent excessive degeneration, promote collagen synthesis, and prepare the client to train fully (including normal ROM, strength, aerobic capacity, and neuromuscular function). During this stage, your clients should limit the range of motion to that in which they remain pain-free. As your clients heal, have them progress gradually over 3 to 6 weeks up to the resumption of training to about half the preinjury intensity. Stage 3 includes progressively more difficult sequences of exercises that facilitate acclimatization to the individual's competition demands or fitness needs.

5. **Describe how to minimize risk of injury or reinjury.**

The initial counseling session should establish past injuries, current pains, and potential causes of injury. You must know the client's limitations, as well as the inherent demands of his training, and keep both extrinsic and intrinsic risks in mind at all times. To prevent tissue degeneration and promote proper healing, you must interrupt the spiral of overuse (see figure 10.4). Watch for symptoms of overuse, and anticipate and intervene as necessary in these situations, which often lead to tissue damage. Recognize your areas of expertise and identify who is qualified to address the client's needs. Develop a network of credible exercise and medical health professionals to use as referrals.

Risk Control Checklist

Warm-Up

____ Use smooth, dynamic ROM movements—reaching as far as the muscle comfortably allows.

____ Avoid forced, prolonged, or rapid movements of the back.

____ Avoid hyperextension of the neck or lowering the head below the heart.

____ Avoid excessive reps with arms above shoulders; control arm speed.

____ Introduce and progress low-impact movements to raise temperature and heart rate.

____ After some warming, statically stretch the muscle groups to be used in the workout.

____ Add supplemental stretches if muscles are tight or sore or if expecting higher intensity than usual.

____ Progress to preaerobic level (lower end of target heart rate).

____ If workout is to be high eccentric, build eccentric overloading gradually.

Cardiovascular

This checklist is particularly relevant if your client is unconditioned, just returning from a layoff, or moving up to the next level.

____ Avoid excessive stress, especially to the lower body, by using intervals, pyramids up and down, split routines, or a circuit.

____ Help the client find the "stopping point," where the feeling of burn replaces momentary fatigue (especially in eccentric work).

____ Check for excessive pronation, forefoot weight bearing, turning with foot planted.

____ Minimize impact shock by encouraging light feet and resilient knees, providing low-impact alternatives, and ensuring that footwear and floor surface are appropriate.

____ Monitor intensity and duration, which are the training errors linked most closely to overuse injury. Look for signs of overtraining (e.g., decreased performance, lethargy, early fatigue, elevated heart rate).

____ Provide a few minutes of cardiovascular cool-down for circulatory adjustments and to gain flexibility—have client hold static stretches for up to 30 s.

Muscular Conditioning

____ In designing a program, consider previous injuries to structures providing joint stability (e.g., include avoidance or rehabilitation).

____ Contend with the forces of momentum and gravity.

____ Avoid excessive knee or back flexion, lifting arms with palms forward, and allowing hip extension to force the back into increased lumbar lordosis.

____ Remember that progression may be rapid initially and then level off.

____ Intervene with help or with an exercise alternative when technique or condition appears to be a problem.

____ Suggest beginning with a light set and following with static stretch of the muscles used (especially if used eccentrically).

____ Think muscle balance—remember, the cardiovascular activity has already worked selected muscles.

Cool-Down

____ Relieve anticipated muscle tightness that may result from eccentric work— for example, in quadriceps, calves, and erector spinae.

____ Stretch tight postural muscles—for example, anterior chest, hip flexors, hamstrings.

____ Be sure client is relaxed and cool before heading back to daily routine.

From *Client-Centered Exercise Prescription, Second Edition,* by John C. Griffin, 2006, Champaign, IL: Human Kinetics.

Exercise Prescription for Specific Injuries

Chapter Competencies

After completing this chapter, you will be able to demonstrate the following competencies:

1. Describe the functional anatomy and probable causes for each of the following conditions:
   - plantar fasciitis
   - Achilles tendinitis and tendinosis
   - shin splints (medial tibial stress syndrome)
   - patellofemoral syndrome
   - hamstring strain
   - low back pain
   - rotator cuff tendinitis (impingement syndrome)

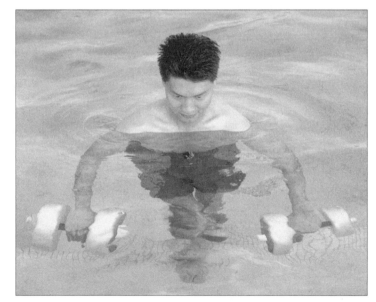

2. Describe preventive exercise strategies including precautions, beneficial activity indications, and inadvisable exercise contraindications.

3. Assist with the postrehabilitation treatment plan for a client to minimize risk of reinjury or to speed recovery by designing specific exercises and activities for stretching and for strengthening injured tissues.

This chapter should help anyone who works with clients recovering from, or having a history of, orthopedic injury. You will find a brief description and a background in functional anatomy for plantar fasciitis, Achilles tendinitis and tendinosis, shin splints (medial tibial stress syndrome), patellofemoral syndrome, hamstring strain, low back pain, and rotator cuff tendinitis (impingement syndrome). You will also find probable causes and strategies for prevention. Specific exercise designs for stretching and for strengthening injured tissues are grouped together near the end of each injury presentation. This convenient format will permit easy reproduction for practitioners wishing to provide visual aids for their clients. Although the exercises were designed for specific injuries, they can also serve as a glossary of exercises that may be selected for any of the prescription models outlined in earlier chapters.

The range of specific conditions discussed covers a sample of overuse injuries of tendons, muscles, and other connective tissue. They are common injuries seen in the fitness culture, but the chapter does not serve an exhaustive treatment of overuse injuries. More extensive coverage of athletic injuries and therapeutic exercise may be found in the Human Kinetics publications by Bahr and Maehlum (2004), *Clinical Guide to Sports Injuries,* and Houglum (2005), *Therapeutic Exercise for Musculoskeletal Injuries, Second Edition.*

The chapter emphasizes overuse injuries resulting from repeated abnormal stresses. As we saw in chapter 10, this microtrauma may be caused by extrinsic factors such as faulty equipment (e.g., worn shoes) or training errors (e.g., too little recovery) or intrinsic factors such as malalignment or muscle imbalance. The following section will examine the probable causes and strategies for prevention for overuse injuries of tendons (e.g., Achilles tendinitis), muscles (e.g.,

hamstring strain), and other connective tissue (e.g., plantar fasciitis and shin splints). Table 11.1 defines common injuries to muscle and connective tissues.

CPTs and Overuse Injuries

Understanding the injury and its potential cause can be the first step toward preventing it. The key to recovery is to recognize the problem and its causes in the early stages by monitoring symptoms carefully. Take time to listen to your client when you ask, "How are you feeling today?" You must understand preventive exercise strategies including **precautions,** beneficial activity **indications,** and inadvisable exercise **contraindications.** However, it is also your responsibility to recognize when you need to advise your client to seek medical assistance.

Plantar Fasciitis

Plantar fasciitis is inflammation of the strong tissue that runs along the bottom of the foot and connects the heel to the base of the toes. Along with the muscles and bones, this connective tissue, the plantar fascia, forms the arch of the foot (figure 11.1). The plantar fascia is multilayered fibrous connective tissue. It arises from the calcaneus and forms five divisions that insert on the ball of the foot. By tensing like a bowstring on the plantar surface of the feet, the plantar fascia helps to support the arch.

What starts as a slight pain in a client's heel may gradually build. It is usually worse the first step of the morning and can be quite intense when the area bears weight such as with walking or running.

Table 11.1 Common Injuries to Muscle and Connective Tissue

Injury	Description and definition
Ligament sprain	Trauma (often acute) to a ligament that compromises the stability of the joint. The injury can range from a first-degree sprain involving a partial tear and minor joint instability to a third-degree sprain involving a complete tear and full joint instability.
Tendinitis	Painful overuse tendon condition involving inflammation (Cook et al. 2000).
Tendinosis	Collagen degeneration rather than inflammation of a tendon (Cook et al. 2000). This tendinopathy often results from a lack of adequate repair of a tendinitis.
Muscle strain	Trauma to the muscle involving muscle fiber tearing. The injury can be a first-degree strain involving a partial tear, pain during muscle activity, but little loss in strength. A second-degree strain results in a loss of strength. A third-degree strain is a complete tear.

A sufferer may limp or bear weight on the lateral side of the foot to ease the pain.

Cause and Prevention

Plantar fasciitis is caused by overstretching the fascia. Alignment problems such as overpronation or low arches may contribute. Pressure on the fascia may be caused by weak foot muscles—including the small intrinsic muscles in the foot and other muscles in the lower leg such as the flexor digitorum and tibialis posterior. Tight gastrocnemius and soleus muscles can also cause fasciitis by keeping the Achilles tendon tight, thereby making the ankle less flexible and forcing the plantar fascia to absorb more weight. Any activity in which the weight is taken on the ball of the foot—such as high-impact aerobics, basketball, sprinting, tennis, or bounding—can create excessive pull on the fascia.

Massaging with ice for 5 to 7 min can be effective. Apply cold packs for up to 20 min (Rizzo 1991). Before advising clients to be fitted for an orthotic, help them look for good supportive footwear with distinct arch support, strong heel cup, and full sole cushioning. A heel lift may also be needed. Some clients may be helped with a heel cup, which forces more fat to remain below the heel. Even lacing shoes tightly can assist with medial support and reduce pronation. Although people with plantar fasciitis should avoid some high-trauma activities, other activities such as recline cycling, swimming, pool running, rowing machines, or circuit weight training should not produce discomfort. Anything that produces pain should be avoided. Walkers should decrease their mileage, avoid hills, and look for a softer surface.

Stretching Guidelines and Prescription

Gentle, prolonged stretching should be pain-free. Stretching exercises should focus on the Achilles tendon and the soleus and gastrocnemius muscles. Figure 11.2a shows a soleus stretch with the rear knee bent to further elongate the Achilles.

A simple wedged heel-cord box (figure 11.2b) can facilitate stretching. Your client can achieve more complete fiber elongation by using variations such as straight knees or toes inward or outward.

Massage and foot manipulation can help relax tight, rigid connective tissue in the foot itself and in the intrinsic muscles. Have your injured client stretch at least twice a day.

Strengthening Guidelines and Prescription

Weak foot muscles may not be able to support the dynamic structure of the foot. Strong muscles are required to help maintain a sound arch and withstand the sometimes three- to fivefold load increase placed on the plantar fascia when, for example, the foot is landing during a moderate downhill run (Batt and Tanji 1995). Once the foot is pain-free and flexibility is returning, your client should begin strengthening exercises. By using her toes to pull a towel (figure 11.3a) or to grasp a marble, your client can condition the intrinsic muscles of her foot and the toe flexors that help support the arch. Daily practice of this exercise may still take 6 weeks to improve the foot's configuration.

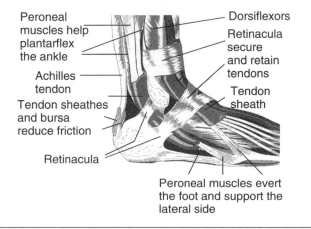

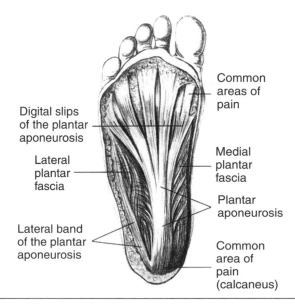

Figure 11.1   Anatomy of plantar fascia and Achilles tendon.

Adapted, by permission, from L. Jozsa and P. Kannus, 1997, *Human tendons* (Champaign, IL: Human Kinetics), 47.

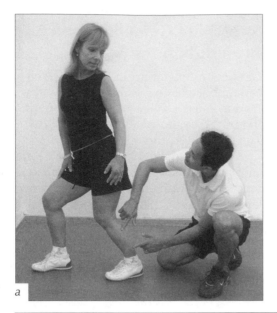
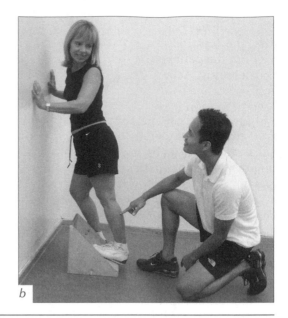

Figure 11.2   Achilles tendon stretches. *(a)* Slightly bend the knee with the heel on the floor for the soleus. *(b)* A straight-knee gastrocnemius stretch with a wedged box.

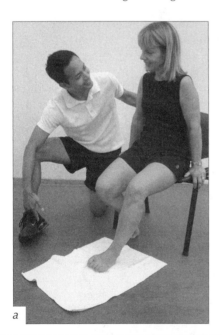
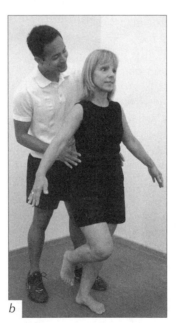
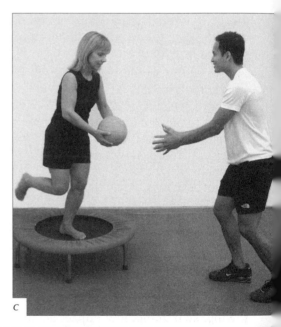

Figure 11.3   *(a)* Toe curls with towel. On a slippery surface, pull the towel in by curling the toes. *(b)* One-leg balance. Feel the muscles of the foot and lower leg working. Progress to eyes closed. *(c)* One-leg minitrampoline ball toss. While balancing on one leg on a minitramp, toss an appropriately weighted ball back and forth to a trainer.

Balancing on one leg will help strengthen and reacquaint the lower leg muscles with the proper support alignment (figure 11.3*b*). Many balance activities will train proprioceptive pathways that may have been damaged (Hanney 2000). The unilateral minitrampoline balance with ball toss (figure 11.3*c*) can be progressed with more difficult catches.

Before you permit resumption of full-intensity activity, prescribe a progression using closed kinetic chain (weight-bearing) exercises including the ankle, knee, and hip (chapter 7).

Achilles Tendinitis and Tendinosis

Achilles tendinitis is inflammation of the tendon, its sheath, or the bursae (figure 11.1). Your client may describe pain located 2 to 5 cm (0.78-2 in.)

above the calcaneus (Prentice 1994). In early, mild tendinitis, the foot loosens up at the beginning of activity but the pain gradually increases. More advanced, chronic **Achilles tendinosis** involves degenerative changes often attributable to uncorrected overpronation (Bahr and Maehlum 2004). This condition causes pain when your client climbs stairs or walks normally, it escalates with activity and subsides with rest, and it may be accompanied by weakness during plantar flexion. Morning stiffness, poor flexibility, and swelling or tightness of the calf muscles are common symptoms.

Cause and Prevention

Racket sports players and longer-distance runners are particularly susceptible to Achilles tendinitis. The combination of repetitive microtrauma from these activities and excessive pronation is particularly risky. Insufficient stretching or rapid overstretching can lead to damage. The injury is often slow to heal because of poor vascularization in the lower part of the tendon (Myerson and Biddinger 1995). Have your clients avoid repetitive, weight-bearing dorsiflexion, particularly during high-impact eccentric contractions of the calf muscles such as the push-offs required by many sports. Once you have established the cause, prescribe specific changes to prevent further aggravation. With Achilles tendinitis, use cryotherapy immediately after the injury or flare-up, as well as into the reconditioning and management stages (anti-inflammatory agents will not be as effective with tendinosis). Initial conservative management of mild to moderate Achilles tendinitis should involve a decrease in activity by at least 50%. Examine your client's running shoes for proper heel fit. If other biomechanical problems exist (chapters 4 and 10), consider adding a 1/4 to 1/2 in. heel lift or referring your client for orthotics. Low-impact activities such as cycling, rowing, swimming, low-impact aerobic dance, or most weight training—as long as they do not produce pain—can help your client maintain aerobic conditioning. Limit any toe push-offs.

Stretching Guidelines and Prescription

To avoid adhesions, your client should begin gentle, passive stretching as soon as pain allows. Have her stretch the Achilles tendon with a static dorsiflexion—knee straight (gastrocnemius) and bent (soleus) (figure 11.2). Turning the toes slightly inward during stretches shown in figure 11.2 will enhance the Achilles stretch.

If these stretches create pain, have your client use partial or non-weight-bearing ankle dorsiflexion stretches. Figure 11.4 shows a seated ankle dorsiflexion using tubing or Dynaband. This stretch may also be performed with a bent knee.

Strengthening Guidelines and Prescription

Begin with light progressive resistance exercises for the calf muscles. One easy method is to work against tubing or an elastic band by placing the foot in the loop and pressing down (starting position as in figure 11.4). Dynamic plantar flexion with weights or a machine may start in a seated position (figure 11.5). Single leg balancing (figure 11.3b) and standing toe raises are fully weight bearing with a closed kinetic chain.

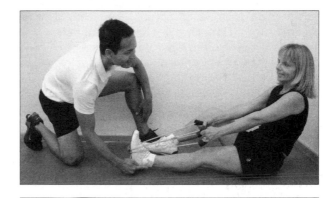

Figure 11.4   Seated tubing dorsiflexion. With tubing or Theraband securely wrapped around the ball of the foot with tension, have the client point her foot (plantar flex) and return slowly.

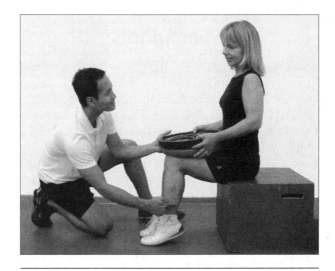

Figure 11.5   Seated heel lift. With a resistance on the thighs, the client presses up to the toes and returns slowly to a flat foot.

From *Client-Centered Exercise Prescription, Second Edition,* by John C. Griffin, 2006, Champaign, IL: Human Kinetics.

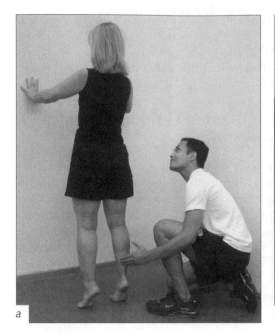
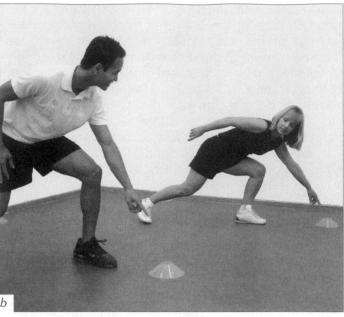

Figure 11.6 *(a)* Standing toe raises. While the client is standing (with some support, if needed), have her raise up onto her toes and slowly return down. *(b)* Four-corner plyometric drill. Set up four markers in a square, 3 m (10 ft) apart. From the center of the square, combine forward, backward, and lateral movements by touching various combinations of markers.

The final progressive stage before returning to activity should include progressive eccentric strengthening. This may be initiated with standing toe raises (figure 11.6*a*), moving rapidly into plantar flexion from a slow decent. A progression of this exercise involves performing it on the edge of a stair and allowing the heel to lower. Toor (2004) reported that clients in the final stage of recovery from Achilles tendinosis have responded well to regular progressive eccentric exercises such as the four-corner plyometric drill (figure 11.6*b*).

Shin Splints

Shin splints, or more precisely **medial tibial stress syndrome (MTSS),** is an inflammation of the fascia, tendon, periosteum, bone, or combination of these along the posterior medial border of the tibia (figure 11.7). The pain can range from a slightly uncomfortable dull ache to an intensity that makes weight bearing difficult. Shin splints account for an estimated 10% to 20% of all injuries in runners and up to 60% of all overuse injuries of the leg (Couture and Karlson 2002).

Sometimes referred to as **posterior shin splints,** MTSS is probably associated with fatigue tear of fibers of the soleus or tibialis posterior muscle at its insertion into the periosteum of the tibia (Korkola and Amendola 2001). Shin splints are an overuse condition common to people who start a

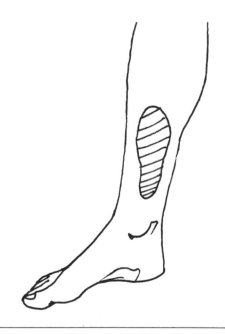

Figure 11.7 Pain location for shin splints (medial tibial stress syndrome).

weight-bearing training program too vigorously, to jumpers (e.g., volleyball, basketball, high-impact aerobics), and to runners logging more than 30 miles per week.

Occurring in the upper anterior shin, **anterior shin splints** are aggravated by overuse of the tibialis anterior and in some clients may reveal a stress fracture (Fick et al. 1992).

Cause and Prevention

MTSS pain is in the muscles that are active during the first 80% of the stance phase, such as the tibialis posterior and the flexors of the toes (Prentice 1994). The subtalar joint normally goes from a supinated position at heel strike to a pronated position during midstance and then returns to supination during push-off. Hyperpronation during midstance places these muscles under significant stress—they will contract eccentrically (lengthening) to try to stabilize, but eventually the point of attachment (origin) will become inflamed.

Other factors sometimes related to MTSS include a tight Achilles tendon, running on hard surfaces, progressing too rapidly in training, logging exceptionally long training hours, muscle imbalance between weak shin and strong calf muscles, and improper footwear. If a biomechanical abnormality or training error is the cause, it must first be corrected. Allow the affected muscles to rest, sometimes for several weeks depending on the pain. Use this time to ice (8-10 min, two or three times/day) and perhaps to investigate the need for orthotics or to ensure that the shoe is well-cushioned in the heel and insole. Andrish and Work (1990) suggested stopping the offending activity until the pain subsides (usually about 1-2 weeks), resuming training at about half the previous intensity, and gradually working up to previous levels over 3 to 6 weeks. Returning too quickly is the most common reason shin splints recur. Be sure your client pays close attention to warm-ups and cool-downs, ensuring complete stretching of the lower leg. Consider prescribing cross-training, particularly with non-weight-bearing exercise such as swimming, stair climbing, cycling, rowing, or low-impact aerobic classes. If your client is a die-hard jogger, direct her to the grass or flat bark-covered trails and increase mileage before increasing intensity throughout the recovery.

Stretching Guidelines and Prescription

Inflammation of the tibialis posterior and flexors of the toes causes tightness and decreased flexibility. After some rest and anti-inflammatory treatment, stretching exercises should target these muscles as well as the gastrocnemius, soleus, tibialis anterior, and peroneals. After some aerobic exercise to warm the muscles, your client should do static stretches several times, holding all the stretches at least 30 s and holding stretches for the Achilles tendon up to 60 s. The heel cord box

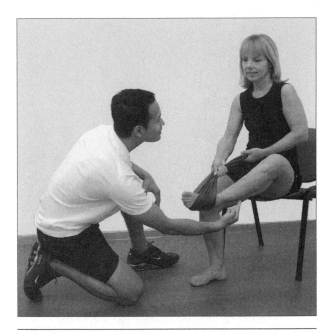

Figure 11.8 Dynaband peroneal stretch. With the client in a seated position, have her invert her foot and wrap a Theraband around the forefoot, placing tension on the band. She slowly everts her foot against this tension.

as shown in figure 11.2b is very effective. The bent-knee position aids in stretching the tibialis posterior as well as the soleus.

Figure 11.4 uses surgical tubing (or Dynaband) to stretch the calf muscles. The peroneal muscles on the lateral side of the calf are the ankle evertors and can be stretched by wrapping a Dynaband around the lateral side of the foot and pulling the ankle into inversion (figure 11.8). Your client should relax at the end of the range of motion to feel the stretch.

Using the Dynaband or a hand (figure 11.9), have the client pull the foot up behind, bringing the heel to the buttock. This shifts the stretch to the front of the shin to reach the tibialis anterior.

Strengthening Guidelines and Prescription

Start a strengthening program when the pain is minimal. The affected muscles in shin splints usually show signs of weakness and early fatigue. Toe curls with a towel (figure 11.3a) will strengthen the flexors of the toes and the tibialis posterior as well as strengthen the arch to minimize hyperpronation.

The anterior muscle groups are very often weak and out of balance with the posterior plantar flexors. Movements as simple as seated or standing toe lifts or drawing the alphabet with the feet usually

From *Client-Centered Exercise Prescription, Second Edition,* by John C. Griffin, 2006, Champaign, IL: Human Kinetics.

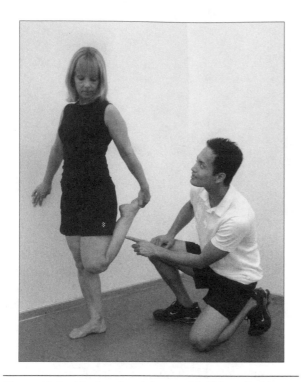

Figure 11.9   Heel to buttock stretch. Although this can stretch the quads, by grasping the instep (not the ankle) and pulling up on the foot, the shin receives an effective stretch.

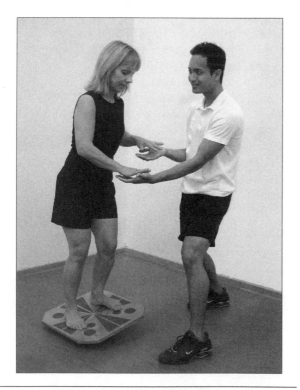

Figure 11.10   Wobbleboard inversion and eversion. In bare feet, the client rocks side to side on the wobbleboard in a controlled manner. Have her progress to keeping her balance on a multiplane wobbleboard.

present enough of an overload for the early stages of conditioning. The opposite foot, a partner's resistance, or surgical tubing can all be used to create added resistance to this dorsiflexion.

Clients with MTSS (posterior shin splints) should also strengthen their ankle evertors and invertors. A uniplane wobble board, which is simple to build (figure 11.10), can be used with the foot aligned with the half-cylinder keel under the board. Have your client rock back and forth in a controlled manner, touching the right edge and then the left edge. Although a well-cushioned shoe is mandatory for a return to training, most of the rehabilitation exercises will provide greater benefit if done with bare feet.

Patellofemoral Syndrome

The patella moves up and down within a groove at the front of the femur (figure 11.11). Deviation from this aligned tracking produces **patellofemoral pain,** resulting from irritation behind the patella and wearing of the articular cartilage.

Clients may complain of pain in the front of the knee when they sit in a car or at the movies, kneel or squat, get up from a chair and start walking, or go up or down stairs. The pain may appear at the beginning or end of a workout and may result in swelling or fullness in the knee. Other symptoms may include giving way, popping, catching, or locking (Doucette and Goble 1992). Patellofemoral syndrome is one of the most common knee complaints, accounting for 57.5% of the knee injuries in one group of runners (Taunton et al. 1987). It occurs most often in women, in the young, and in those who are active in running or in court sports such as basketball and tennis.

Cause and Prevention

Improper alignment and tracking of the patella are major causes of patellofemoral pain (figure 11.11c). Your clients may notice such pain especially as they run up hills or straighten their knees with weights. Causes of poor tracking include the following:

• **Deficiency of supporting and stabilizing muscles.** Kneecap motion is guided by the quadriceps, particularly the vastus medialis. This muscle may be less resistant to fatigue than the vastus lateralis, creating an uneven pull on the patella (Earle and Baechle 2004).

• **Tightness of supporting structures.** If the vastus lateralis or the lateral retinaculum (figure 11.11a) are tight, lateral tilting or tracking of the patella may occur. Because the iliotibial band is connected to the lateral retinaculum, its tightness may affect tracking during flexion. Both the hamstrings and the gastrocnemius cross the knee joint, and tightness can increase patellar pressure. Tight hamstrings increase knee flexion and can change lower leg mechanics. A tight gastrocnemius muscle can limit dorsiflexion and produce excessive subtalar motion (Galea and Albers 1994).

- **Structural alignments.** Wide hips and knock-knees may contribute to lateral tracking of the patella (Bahr and Maehlum 2004). An awareness of this alignment problem can help you direct your client to alternate activities or reduce the prescription load. Excessive pronation of the foot usually causes a rotation of the tibia, which may result in increased lateral pull on the patella. Orthotics may be appropriate.

Besides poor tracking, patellofemoral syndrome may be caused by acute trauma, chronic repetitive stress such as running, sudden increases in workloads or mileage, uneven or hilly terrain, or poor running shoes. In addition, deep squats and other closed kinetic chain exercises requiring knee flexion greater than 90° increase compression and tissue stress between the patella and the femur.

To avoid this syndrome, have your client replace running shoes that are older than a year, have more than 500 miles on them, or look worn out on the soles or broken down on the uppers. Ask at-risk clients if they have changed their intensity, distance, or terrain. Have them stay away from hills, switch to lower impact aerobic activities, or decrease mileage. DePalma and Perkins (2004) reported that the substantial forces generated in landing can be reduced by 60% through absorbed forces in the ankle and foot. When the knee and hip go through a wider range of flexion, another 25% of the force is reduced when combined with forefoot landing.

However, when a client already has knee pain, stop all painful activities for at least 2 to 4 weeks. Aspirin or ibuprofen may help ease symptoms, as may icing.

Stretching Guidelines and Prescription

Tightness in a number of muscles may contribute to patellofemoral pain: vastus lateralis, iliotibial band, hamstrings, and gastrocnemius. Stretching the quadriceps (including vastus lateralis) can decrease patellofemoral compression during dynamic activities. However, stretching this muscle may be contraindicated if pain exists past the 70° position of knee flexion. From a prone position, your client should flex one knee to the end of the active range of motion (ROM). If there is no pain, she should then reach back and grasp the ankle with the opposite hand and continue gently to increase the knee flexion (figure 11.12*a*). If she has difficulty reaching her ankle, you can passively assist the stretch.

To stretch the iliotibial band, your client stands with legs crossed. The affected leg is close to an adjacent wall or table and behind the other leg. She then moves her pelvis toward the table, keeping the back leg straight (figure 11.12*b*).

To stretch the hamstrings, your client places one leg on a table with knees straight. While holding her back straight, she bends forward from the hips to a point of tension. After about 20 s, she lowers slightly, tilting the pelvis forward and holding for another 10 to 15 s (figure 11.12*c*). The gastrocnemius can be stretched effectively with exercises shown in figures 11.2 and 11.4.

Strengthening Guidelines and Prescription

To guarantee a safe return to normal activities, your client must fully regain strength in the injured leg. Have her do the following exercises every second day, stopping if there is any pain or she is unable to do the exercise correctly. Most people do well by progressing from about 5 to 15 repetitions, then adding a second set and building from 10 to 15 reps. The client should allow a minute or two between sets, depending on her stage of recovery, eventually building to 4 or 5 sets. Exercises to strengthen the vastus medialis will promote a return to muscular balance and increase the medial stabilization of the patella.

Start with end range extensions, in which your client reclines with a firm pillow or rolled towel under her knee to create about 30° of flexion. With her hip slightly rotated laterally and the opposite knee flexed, she then straightens her knee and holds for 10 s. Small ankle weights can increase resistance.

Exercises with the foot in a fixed position on the ground (closed-chain exercises) are especially functional because they use common movement patterns and control the body's momentum (eccentric contractions) as well as teach kinesthetic awareness. Closed kinetic chain exercises are favored in therapeutic exercise prescription, particularly for the knee (Post 1998). Closed kinetic chain exercises include leg press, partial squats, stepping, stationary cycling, and plyo-metrics. Two specific examples of closed-chain exercises are forward lunges (figure 11.13a) and step-downs (figure 11.13b).

In a forward lunge, your client steps forward about 2 to 3 ft (0.60-0.91 m) from a standing posi-tion, keeping the knee over the foot and not allow-ing the front knee to flex more than 90°. At the same time, she lowers the back knee until it is 4 to 6 in. (10-15 cm) from the floor. She returns to an upright position and alternates legs. As her strength increases, she can hold small hand weights.

In a step-down, she stands sideways on a bottom step or aerobic step box with the injured leg nearest the stair. Slowly she bends the injured knee until the opposite foot lightly touches the ground and then slowly straightens it. As she progresses, she may add hand weights or use higher steps.

Working with a wobble board (figure 11.10) can strengthen supporting muscles of the lower leg. Open chain exercises (the foot is free), such as provided by isokinetic knee extension equipment, can isolate a muscle such as the vastus medialis by using ROM stops for the last 30° of extension. These exercises can also introduce higher speed contractions under stabilized conditions, which may be appropriate for athletes.

Rubber tubing or Dynabands can also be used, especially when knee movement is still painful. From a supine position, with the tubing around both legs just above the knee, your client performs straight leg raises to strengthen hip flexors (figure 11.13c).

Finally, because most of the vastus media-lis originates from the tendon of the adductor magnus (Doucette and Goble 1992), strengthen-ing the muscles of the inner thigh may help pull the kneecap into alignment. For the inner thigh pillow squeeze (figure 11.13d), have your client hold or pulse the squeeze for 15 to 20 s, repeating three to five times.

Hamstring Strain

The hamstring muscle, located on the posterior thigh, comprises the semimembranosus, semiten-dinosus, and biceps femoris (figure 11.14). The hamstrings are biarticular (two-joint) muscles producing extension of the hip and flexion of the knee. As with other frequently injured biarticu-lar muscles (e.g., rectus femoris or long head of the biceps brachii), the hamstrings are subject to stretching at more than one point. Injuries to this muscle complex usually affect the common origin on the ischial tuberosity and may affect the inser-tion behind the knee or the belly of the muscle.

As with most muscle strains, symptoms include tenderness and, usually, a large area of swelling. An injured person feels discomfort when gentle resistance is applied against knee flexion and hip extension.

Hamstring strains are described in three grades. Grade I sufferers complain of tightness at the end range of hip flexion and some pain or palpation. People with Grade II strains usually

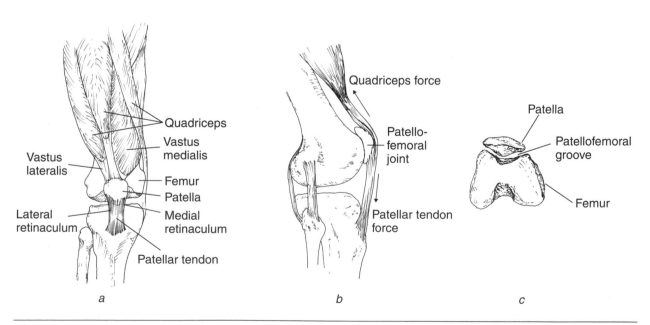

Figure 11.11 Anatomy of the patellofemoral joint with (a) anterior knee joint, (b) forces on the patellofemoral joint, and (c) patellofemoral tracking.

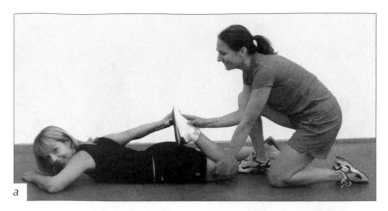

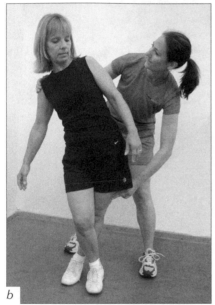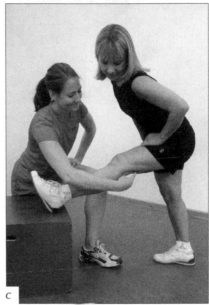

Figure 11.12   *(a)* Vastus lateralis stretch. From a prone position, the client flexes one knee and grasps the foot with the opposite hand, pulling gently if there is no pain. *(b)* Iliotibial band stretch. Standing (with support if needed), the client crosses the affected leg behind the other leg and pushes her hip in the opposite direction. *(c)* Hamstring stretch. The client lifts one leg onto a bench or table. She moves her pelvis and trunk as a unit, slowly lowering her abdomen toward her thigh.

have adjusted their gaits, perhaps landing flat-footed with limited swing-through. Knee flexion and hip extension may cause moderate to severe pain with noticeable weakness. Recovery takes between 1 and 3 weeks. Grade III hamstring strains usually require the use of crutches and require a 3- to 12-week rehabilitation period (De Palma 1994).

Cause and Prevention

Hamstring strains are common with sprinters, gymnasts, and athletes in soccer, football, lacrosse, and basketball. These strains can result from a quick, explosive contraction while the hip is in flexion and the knee is extending. For those cli-

ents involved in running activities, the hamstrings may simultaneously work concentrically at the hip and eccentrically at the knee (e.g., striding before foot strike). The hamstring muscles decelerate the forward swing of the tibia, thus opposing the activity of the quadriceps. The imbalance of an overly strong quadriceps may cause the injury. Other causes may be hamstring fatigue or weakness, tight hamstrings, imbalance between the medial and lateral hamstrings, or improper running style.

The strong tendency for hamstring injuries to recur makes a solid case for a supplemental exercise prescription including stretching, strengthening, and cardiovascular maintenance. Best and Garrett (1996) reported that following a hamstring

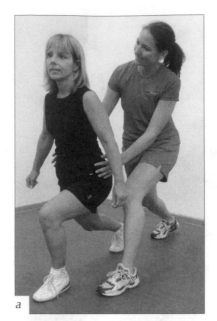
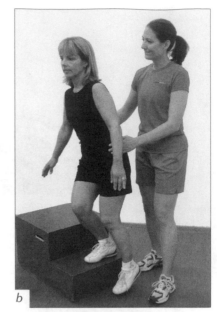
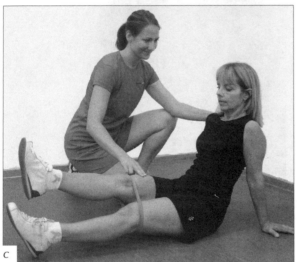
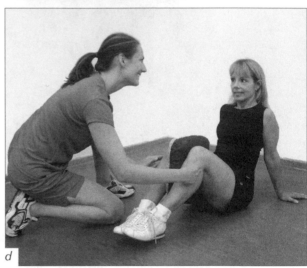

Figure 11.13 *(a)* Forward lunges. She steps forwards about 2 to 3 ft (0.60-0.91 m), lowering the body. Ensure the knee does not go beyond the front foot. *(b)* Step-downs. Standing sideways on a step with the injured side nearest the stair and supporting the weight as the knee bends, she allows the opposite foot to lower and return. *(c)* Straight-leg raises with tubing. With tubing around both legs just above the knees, she performs straight-leg raises. *(d)* Inner thigh pillow squeeze. From a recline position with knees bent and a pillow between them, she squeezes together or pulses.

injury, there is decreased flexibility and lower eccentric strength. Initial treatment typically consists of rest, ice, compression (elastic wrap), elevation, and pain relief (e.g., acetaminophen for 7-10 days). After the acute stages, heat (hot packs, whirlpool, or heating pad) may be used before the stretching exercises (DeLisa 1998). All activities should be followed by ice treatments to decrease inflammation and discomfort. Although someone with a Grade I hamstring strain may continue to be active, a supplementary prescription for extra stretching and strengthening should begin immediately to avoid further injury.

Stretching Guidelines and Prescription

In addition to predisposing your client to a hamstring strain, tight hamstrings may cause low back pain. Because hamstrings attach to the back of the pelvis (see figure 11.14), tight hamstrings can prevent the pelvis from tilting forward when the spine flexes, forcing all movement to come from the low back. Avoid stretches such as standing or sitting toe touches, where the lower body is static and the upper body is rounded and actively flexing.

The doorway hamstring stretch (figure 11.15a) promotes a static upper body with lower-body hip flexion. Your client lies on his back in a doorway with his buttocks close to the wall. One leg extends through the door while the other is raised up against the wall. The heel slides up the wall, gradually straightening the leg; after the client feels a comfortable, pleasant stretch, he holds his position for 30 to 60 s. This may also be performed as a self-administered PNF stretch (chapter 8).

The straddle hamstring stretch (figure 11.15b) uses a table or chair for support. With feet pointing forward and one foot 3 to 4 ft behind the another, your client bends forward at the hips (not the waist) while holding the table for support. As the front leg stretches, he must avoid hyperextending the knee. He holds for 30 s, lowers slightly, and holds for another 15 to 30 s. Maintaining the lumbar lordotic curve in the low back isolates the hamstrings and safeguards the back.

You may need to delay these stretches until the second week for Grade II hamstring strains. Active ROM movements in a prone or seated position can begin earlier or as soon as there is no pain (De Palma 1994). Work with a physician or physiotherapist for the timing on Grade III strains; your client should be pain-free.

Strengthening Guidelines and Prescription

You can begin resistance strengthening exercises immediately for a Grade I strain, after about 3 to 6 days for Grade II, and after 10 to 14 days for a Grade III strain (De Palma 1994).

Avoid resistance exercises using a machine (such as knee flexion in a prone position), because the hamstrings are less efficient in a shortened position. However, knee flexion from a seated position allows the hamstrings to start stretched at the buttocks, improving their mechanical advantage in working through a full ROM. An added advantage with some machines is the ability to change the lever arm and torque by adjusting the position of the lower leg pad. A straight-leg hip extension machine is also safe for strengthening hamstrings. If such a machine is not available, substitute elastic tubing or bands (figure 11.16a). Eccentric exercises such as the reverse curl (figure 11.16b) should be part of a preventive program. With ankles supported, the client leans forward in a smooth movement with core stabilized. He resists the fall as long as possible, then lowers onto his hands and pushes off immediately with his arms.

To simulate the function of the hamstrings during running, Santana (2000) suggested a challenging stability ball exercise that combines a bridge, a leg curl, and some alternate leg action (figure 11.16c). The leg pushes against the ball, lifting the hips upward as the opposite leg curls forward; the client then returns to the ball and repeats with the other leg.

Isokinetic exercises, such as with an electronic Cybex knee flexion machine, are effective in conjunction with isotonic and isometric exercises. Progressions to faster speeds may be more sport-specific for athletes.

In later phases of all three grades of hamstring strains, educate your clients to perform light-weight squats. Clients should do squats rather than leg curls, because in a squat, the feet are fixed on the ground and the lower body joints form a closed kinetic chain.

If your client is pain-free, have him swim or bike to maintain cardiovascular condition. Add jogging a few days later if appropriate. Simulate sport-specific activities for athletes, gradually introducing those skills that involve eccentric contraction of the hamstrings.

Low Back Pain

Low back pain in active clients is common and often recurs. Estimates of lifetime prevalence range from 60% to 90%, and the annual incidence is 5% (Drezner and Herring 2001). Back pain usually arises in the soft tissues such as ligaments, fascia, and muscle and with most clients should last no longer than 3 weeks. Ninety

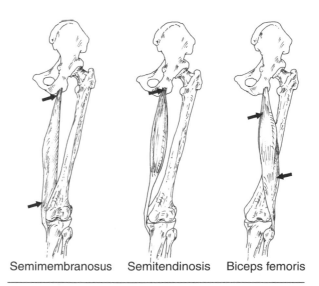

Semimembranosus   Semitendinosis   Biceps femoris

Figure 11.14 Anatomy of the hamstrings. Arrows indicate most common sites of injury.

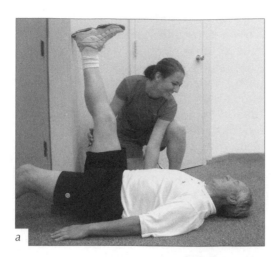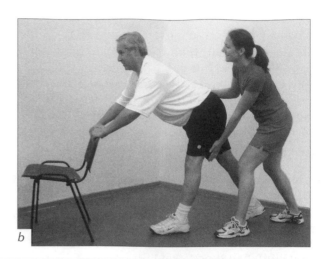

Figure 11.15 *(a)* Doorway hamstring stretch. The client lies on his back in a doorway with one leg through the door and the other leg raised up straight against the wall. He slowly moves his buttocks closer to the wall to increase the stretch. *(b)* Straddle hamstring stretch. Using a table or chair for support and one leg about 3 ft (0.91 m) in front of the other, the client bends forward at the hips, not the waist, feeling the stretch in the front leg hamstring.

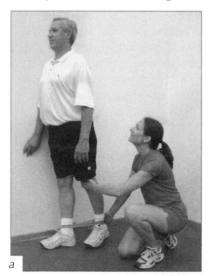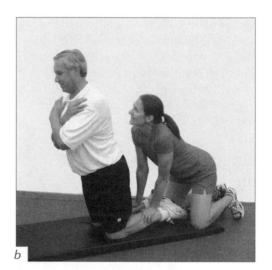

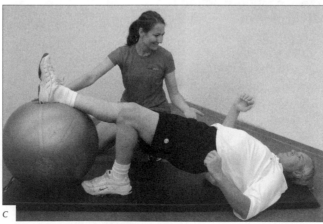

Figure 11.16 *(a)* Straight leg hip extension with tubing. With a band or tubing around both ankles, the client extends one leg straight backward. *(b)* Reverse curl. From a kneeling position with the ankles secured, the client slowly lowers his straight body down to a push-up position. *(c)* Stability ball simulated run. The client starts in a bridge position with one heel on the ball and the other leg on the ground flexed at the knee. He pushes downward with the heel on the ball, raising the hips and torso. He repeatedly raises and lowers the bent knee, building speed with recovery.

From *Client-Centered Exercise Prescription, Second Edition,* by John C. Griffin, 2006, Champaign, IL: Human Kinetics.

percent of clients with back pain should lose their symptoms within 6 weeks with or without intervention (Waddell 1987). People whose pain persists beyond 6 weeks, or who have exacerbated a previous injury, usually have not removed the stresses that created the original injury.

Cause and Prevention

Back pain is usually attributed to strain of the lumbar muscles, inflammation of the facet joints, or degeneration of the intervertebral discs. Knowledge of the individual sport or training regime can help us understand the injury mechanism. In skiing, throwing sports, weightlifting, and martial arts, the muscle–tendon insertions might become inflamed because of sudden or repeated loading. In football, the injury mechanism may be sudden loading (throwing), compression (falls or contact), or torsion (rapid turning). Dance and gymnastics involve increased lumbar lordosis and hyperextension, making them susceptible to facet joint inflammation.

Tight hip flexor muscles initiate a common muscle imbalance pattern that affects lumbar motion. The result is an excessive anterior pelvic tilt and lumbar lordosis. These factors lengthen the hip extensors (e.g., hamstrings), placing them at a mechanical disadvantage and causing early recruitment of the spinal extensors (e.g., erector spinae).

Deep posterior muscles (e.g., multifidus muscles) work together with the deep abdominal muscles (e.g., transversus abdominis), the diaphragm, and the pelvic floor muscles as a functional stabilizing unit. But recent studies have indicated that pain has a reflex effect on muscle activity by inhibiting the deep stabilizing musculature while activating muscles like the iliopsoas and the erector spinae, which increases the anterior tilt forces (Bahr and Machlum 2004).

Another common cause of back problems is simply aging. With increasing age, the nucleus pulposus decreases in volume and the vertebrae end up sitting closer to each other. The annulus fibrosus becomes more lax, and the increased play around the vertebral margins can cause osteophytes. These changes put more stress on the synovial facet joints and ligaments, leaving them inflamed and tender. Movements may become restricted and alignments altered (Liemohn 2001).

Long-term management consists of regaining muscle balance and joint ROM. Trunk muscles must be strengthened with exercises or swimming. You must also give each client personal counseling about suitable activities and advice on back care and lifting techniques. For example, Watkins (1999) showed a 33% reduction in the tension on the spinal extensor muscles when lifting from a squat rather than a stoop and a 50% reduction if core stability was maintained.

General Considerations for Prescription

Be aware of the stage of the injury. Gradually introduce appropriate exercises following the acute treatment stage (mainly modality treatment and pain relief). Be sure that your clients ask their therapists or physicians for any precautions or advice that will help you design a safe and effective exercise plan.

Base your exercise prescription goals for back rehabilitation on the specific diagnosis, history, and evaluation your client receives from his physician or therapist:

- Which structures and muscles need stretching?
- Which structures and muscles need strengthening?
- What deviations in posture, alignment, and stabilization need attention (see chapter 8)?
- What faults are present in movement mechanics in daily life, work environment, sport, or exercise routine (see chapters 5 and 10)?

A comprehensive approach to low back pain should include lumbar stabilization exercises; correction of muscle inflexibilities; strengthening of the lumbar spine, abdominal muscles, and kinetic chain; aerobic conditioning; and correction of faulty mechanics.

See the brief descriptions, with implications for exercise, in table 11.2. Then study figures 11.17 through 11.30 to learn a variety of exercises that will increase both the strength and the flexibility of the back. Remember, if your client has a back problem of any kind, she should consult a physician, physiotherapist, or chiropractor.

Prescribing for Core Stability

When teaching clients about how their backs work, I describe the structure as having three layers: deep, middle, and outer, each with its own function. The tiny muscles of the deep layer provide positional information to the brain. The middle layer provides a bulk of the routine stability and includes the quadratus lumborum, multifidus, and transversus abdominis (along with the

Table 11.2   Low Back Conditions and Exercise Implications

Condition	Description and cause	Exercise implication
Muscular strain	Clients report a history of sudden or chronic stress that initiates pain in a muscular area during the workout. Pain is provoked by contraction or stretching of the involved muscle. If an overuse injury, correct any improper posture or movement patterns.	Prescribe mild contraction followed with a stretch (figures 11.17-11.19). Progress with intensity. Include abdominal strengthening (figures 11.25, 11.28, 11.29) and active extension exercise (figures 11.23, 11.27, 11.30). At early stages of tissue healing, avoid direct contraction of the strained muscle (e.g., hyperextension) and passive lumbar flexion (e.g., knee to chest stretch) (Earle and Baechle 2004).
Piriformis or quadratus lumborum myofascial pain or strain	The piriformis muscle refers pain to the posterior sacroiliac region and buttocks. It is a deep ache that worsens when sitting with hips flexed or adducted or during weight-bearing hip rotation. Pain from the quadratus lumborum is an aching or sharp pain in the lateral back area and upper buttock. Pain is felt on moving from sitting to standing, during prolonged standing, or during sneezing.	Stretching is the main component in changing any myofascial pain. Exercises should include stretching exercises such as in figures 11.18, 11.19, and 11.22. They should also include strengthening exercises such as in figures 11.24, 11.26, 11.29, and 11.30.
Lumbar facet joint sprains	The client will report a specific event that caused the problem or a series of repetitive stresses that progressively got more painful. Pain gets sharper with certain movements. The pain feels deep and localized near the spinous process.	Stretching in all directions should be within a comfort range (figures 11.17, 11.18, 11.20). Exercises should involve joint mobility, trunk stabilization, and posture control. Pain-free abdominal and back strengthening is important (figures 11.23, 11.25, 11.27, 11.28).
Disc-related back problems	Pain is usually central but radiates across the back of one side. The client may describe a sudden or gradual onset after a workout that becomes more severe during resumption of activity. Forward bending and sitting increase pain, and a postural analysis may reveal a shifted hip and slightly flexed posture.	Unless working with a therapist, prescribe only gentle mobilization and postural exercises until the client is pain-free (figures 11.17, 11.20, 11.21). At this point, abdominal and back extensor strengthening should be emphasized with an eye to preventing reinjury (figures 11.23, 11.25, 11.26, 11.27). Avoid exercises involving significant lumbar flexion such as bent-over rowing, full sit-ups, deadlift, standing toe touch, spinal twists, and flexion-based movements in aerobic dance.
Sacroiliac (SI) joint dysfunction	The client will describe a dull, achy back pain near the bone prominences of the SI joint. The pain may radiate to the buttocks or thigh, particularly during hip flexion, during side bending to the painful side, or during the stance phase of walking. Pain may also be felt during trunk rotations, landing heavily on one leg, kicking, and jumping.	If one side of the back is tight, stretching is important (figures 11.18, 11.19, 11.22). Exercises that help (re)gain alignment and stability of the pelvis are important. Appropriate exercises may include those in figures 11.24 through 11.27.

diaphragm and pelvic floor muscles). The outer layer of thick, long muscles provides for more powerful movements and includes the erector spinae, obliques, and rectus abdominis. One or two exercises for each layer should be included in any well-balanced preventive program, as in the following example:

- **Deep layer (positional):** Ball sitting single foot contact—the client sits tall with low back in natural curve and adds arm movements (figure 11.31).

- **Middle layer (stabilization):** Belly blaster—the client lies on back with knees bent, pelvis tilted back, and abdominal core held tight. She

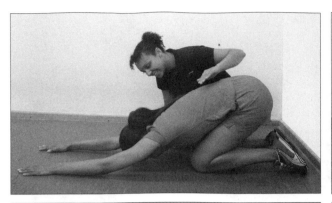

Figure 11.17 Kneeling back stretch. Have the client tuck head and reach forward, rounding the back and moving the chest toward the floor.

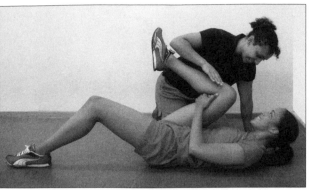

Figure 11.18 Single knee to chest. The client lies supine with low back pushed down. The client pulls one knee to the chest—enough to feel a comfortable stretch in the low back.

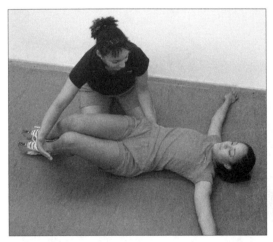

Figure 11.19 Lying knee rocking. The client lies supine with knees bent 90°. The knees slowly rock from side to side through a pain-free range of motion. The back will rotate slightly.

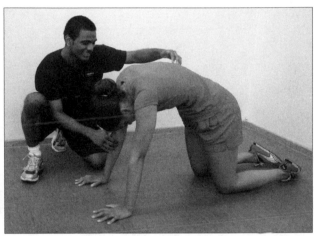

Figure 11.20 Mad cat stretch. The client arches the back while tucking the chin and tightening the stomach.

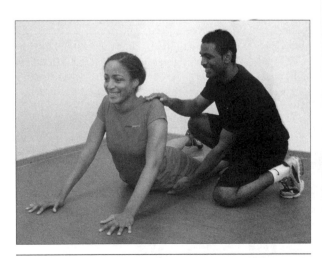

Figure 11.21 Prone press-up. From a prone position, the client extends elbows to raise upper body. Hips stay on the floor and the back is relaxed.

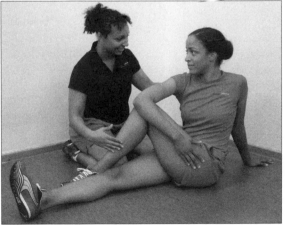

Figure 11.22 Spinal twist. The client sits with right leg straight and left leg bent and on the outside of the right knee. The right elbow is placed on the outside of the upper left thigh. The client slowly turns her head to look over her left shoulder.

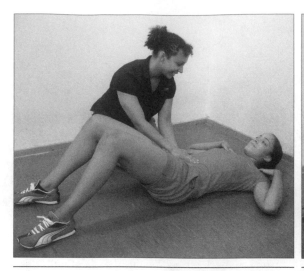

Figure 11.23 Back press. Lying on back with knees bent, the client tightens the stomach by pressing elbows to floor.

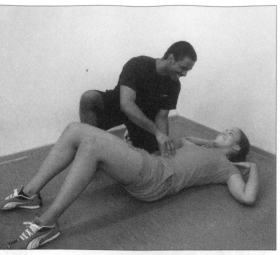

Figure 11.24 Diagonal curl-up. Lying on back with knees bent at 90° and pelvis stabilized, the client raises the head and shoulders while rotating to one side, reaching with arms at sides.

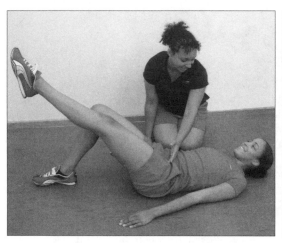

Figure 11.25 Hip lift bridge. Lying on back with both knees bent 90°, the client lifts the buttocks from the floor and extends one knee, keeping stomach tight.

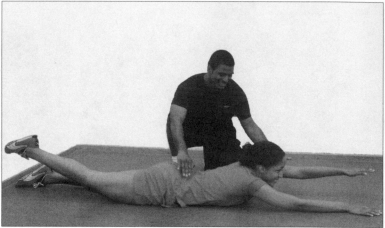

Figure 11.26 Opposite arm and leg lifts. From a prone position (or on all fours), the client raises the opposite arm and leg 4 to 6 in. (10-15 cm) from the floor. Firm pillows or rolled towels should be under the pelvis and forehead.

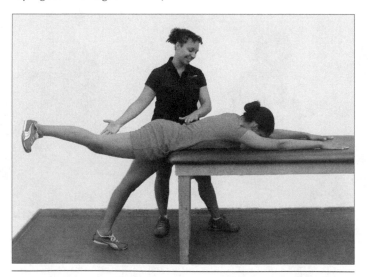

Figure 11.27 Supported hip extension. With the torso leaning flat over a table, the client raises legs alternately from the floor.

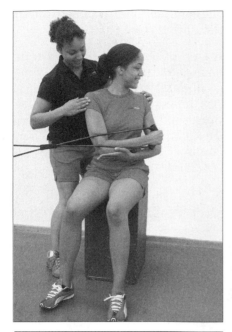

Figure 11.28 Seated trunk rotation with tubing. The client holds the band tight to chest (taut) and gently rotates away with pelvis and knees in place and back straight, exercising only within a pain-free range of motion.

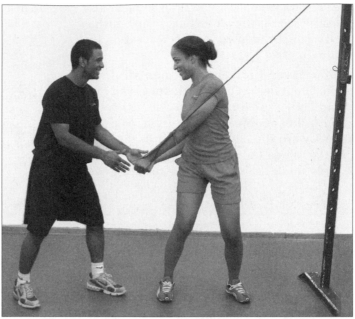

Figure 11.29 Diagonal downward rotation with tubing. Standing with feet shoulder-width apart, the client pulls tubing with both hands downward across the body.

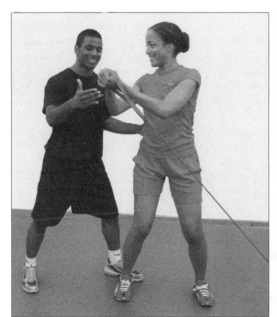

Figure 11.30 Diagonal upward rotation with tubing. Standing with feet shoulder-width apart, the client pulls tubing with both hands, straightening the body and rotating away from the door or anchor.

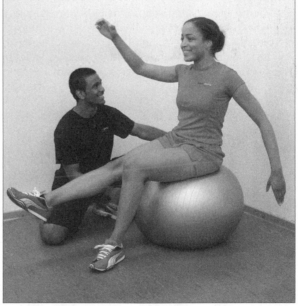

Figure 11.31 Deep layer (positional): ball sitting single foot contact. The client sits in the center of the ball with hips and knees at 90° and tightens core. She gradually straightens one leg, leaving one point of ground contact. Once stable, she mixes various arm movements (e.g., side, forward, alternating). She can progress by closing eyes.

lifts one leg with knee still bent. With shoulders on the mat, she extends the opposite arm and pushes the hand against the knee for 5 s. Repeat on the other side (figure 11.32).

• **Outer layer (power movements):** Dead bugs—the client lies on back with knees and hips at 90° and both arms directly up. She tilts pelvis back and holds abdominal core tight. She lifts one knee toward the chest and extends the other leg upward. When the one leg moves toward the chest, the arm on the same side is reaching over the head. She continues until a smooth alternating pace is difficult (figure 11.33).

Because lack of core stability can reinforce dysfunctional patterns of movement, you need to increase clients' awareness and conscious activation of the core stabilizers (figures 11.34-11.36). Proprioceptive (neuromuscular) training using closed kinetic chain exercises on a mobile surface is optimal for reactive stability (figures 11.37 and 11.38).

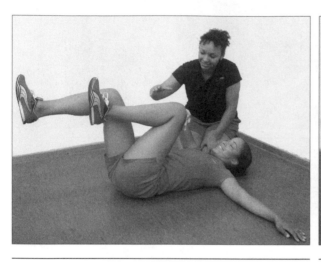

Figure 11.32 Middle layer (stabilization): belly blaster. Lying on the back with knees bent, the client presses low back into the mat and tightens core. She lifts one leg up with knee bent and then reaches across with the opposite hand and pushes against the knee. She holds for a count of 6 and repeats on the other side.

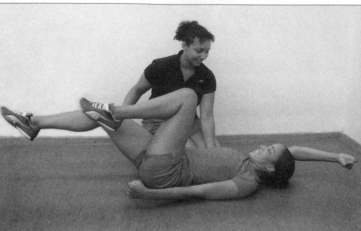

Figure 11.33 Outer layer (power movements): dead bug run. Lying on the back with knees bent, the client presses low back into the mat and tightens core. She extends arms straight up and lifts both legs up with knees bent. Keeping back flat against mat, she extends one leg out and then the other in a cycling motion. She progresses by adding an alternating pumping motion of the arms.

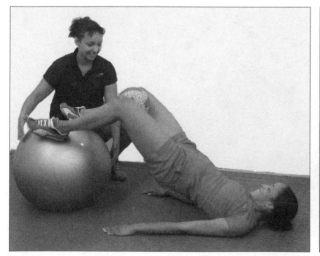

Figure 11.34 Buttocks curl. The client lies on her back with hips and knees at 90° and a small ball between her knees. She then tightens her core. She curls the pelvis and lifts the buttocks off the floor. Have her avoid using the momentum of her legs. She holds for 5 s and slowly lowers.

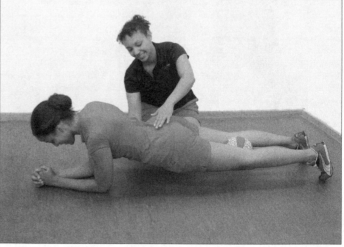

Figure 11.35 Plank. The client kneels with forearms resting on the floor and ball between the knees. She tightens her core. Have her lift knees and support the straightened body between her elbows and toes.

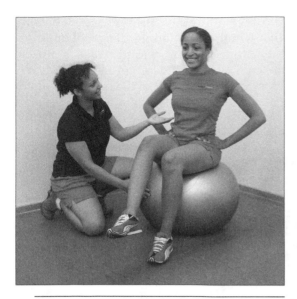

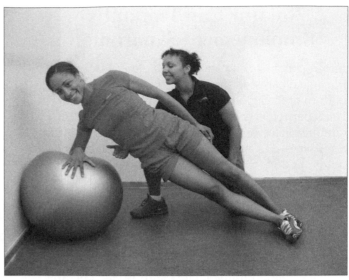

Figure 11.36 Sitting hip rib lift. The client sits in the center of the ball with hips and knees at 90°. She places her hands on the top of the pelvis with her fingers on her abdominals. Have her tighten core (feel it!) and keep the ribcage elevated. She lifts one foot off the ground without allowing the level of the pelvis to drop. Have her progress by reaching arms above her head.

Figure 11.37 Side bridge support on stability ball. The client performs a side support position from the knees with the forearm across the ball. Have her maintain a straight line between the knees, hips, and shoulders. Progression may involve a side bridge from the feet and the addition of a top leg lift.

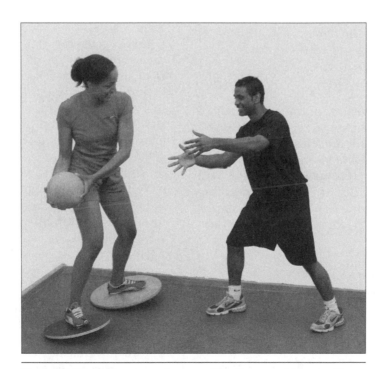

Figure 11.38 Neuromuscular core. Standing on rubber air pillows or wobble boards with tight core, the client performs tosses to their trainer in a cross-body, diagonal direction. Use the reverse movement when receiving the ball.

Rotator Cuff Tendinitis (Impingement Syndrome)

Impingement in the shoulder is common because the space between the top of the humerus and the bottom of the acromion (the "roof" of the shoulder) is not particularly large (figure 11.39). Under certain circumstances, any of the structures running through the space—the supraspinatus tendon, the infraspinatus tendon, the tendon of the long head of the biceps, or the subacromial bursa—can be impinged on. Impingement usually occurs between the greater tubercle and either the acromion or the shoulder ligaments. Impingement impairs the ability of the supraspinatus to depress the humeral head allowing the deltoid to pull the head up toward the acromion, worsening the impingement. Voluntary abduction ROM is reduced and painful, and scapulohumeral rhythm is altered (Bahr and Maehlum 2004).

Impingement syndrome often originates with soft tissue trauma that sets up a cycle of pain, biomechanical changes, and weakness. Swelling of the tissues makes the space even smaller, further irritating the tendons. There also may be reduced blood supply and the start of tendon degeneration. Pain may occur when the shoulder is abducted while internally (medially) rotated. Any movement that calls for raising the arm overhead while internally rotated has the potential to impinge on the tendons and bursa and cause injury.

Cause and Prevention

In clients without a history of trauma, repetitive overhead motion is usually the cause of impingement syndrome. As the muscles fatigue, tendon degeneration occurs. This is evident in activities with rapid eccentric contraction of the external (lateral) rotators such as throwing, swimming the butterfly, and serving in tennis. For example, someone doing an upright row exercise rotates

his shoulder internally as he raises it. Raising the elbows high magnifies the danger of impingement. Another cause of impingement is muscle imbalance. The potential for muscle imbalance is high: Major muscles such as the pectoralis major and latissimus dorsi rotate internally, countered only by small muscles such as the infraspinatus and teres major (chapter 5). Proper biomechanics requires a fine balance between joint mobility and stability. Overlooking such common causes may lead to progression of the impingement.

Modification of activities or of the workplace is critical for prevention and treatment. You can modify some activities to allow limited participation. It may be helpful to modify movements to be in the plane of the scapula, that is, with the humerus in abduction at about 30° of flexion anteriorly. Suggest swimming with fins and kicking only, or avoiding overhead serving when playing tennis or volleyball. Monitor your client's technique for faults such as upright rowing or lateral flies with the thumbs pointing down. To promote circulation in the shoulder area, prescribe upper-body aerobics such as cross-country skiing, rowing, or arm ergometry.

Stretching Guidelines and Prescription

After testing for postural alignment and muscle tightness (chapter 4), address muscle imbalance with static stretches or PNF stretches (chapter 8). Demonstrate proper execution of shoulder exercises, including ROM exercises as in figure 11.40. Be sure that your client performs stretches with relaxed shoulder girdles and proper alignment and with elbows below shoulder height to avoid entrapment of the supraspinatus tendon. Figures 11.41 and 11.42 illustrate specific stretches for internal and external rotators, designed to maintain muscle balance.

Overdevelopment or overtightness of the pectoralis major and anterior deltoid can force the shoulder into internal rotation. Figures 11.43 and 11.44 show exercises designed to stretch these muscles as well as the long head of the biceps.

Strengthening Guidelines and Prescription

Before progressing to specific shoulder joint resistive exercises, your clients should be able to lift their humerus (thumbs down) to 90° while maintaining the scapula stabilized in retraction (adduction). The exercise for this involves actively stabilizing the scapula in retraction while actively abducting the arms with elbows flexed. Figure

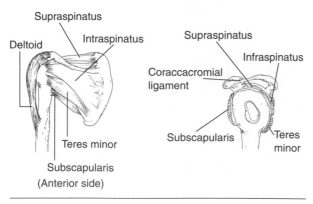

Figure 11.39   Anatomy of the shoulder rotator cuff.

11.45 illustrates another exercise for this training as well as for strengthening the scapular retractors. Emphasize good coordination between movements of the humerus and the scapula. To achieve optimal results, postural correction including scapular stabilization exercises should be done before a rotator cuff or deltoid strengthening program (DePalma and Johnson 2003).

A shoulder strengthening program for prevention or treatment of rotator cuff tendinitis centers around two activities: (1) strengthening the external rotators to maintain muscle balance and (2) strengthening the supraspinatus because of its role in impingement syndrome.

Figures 11.46 and 11.47 show resistance exercises for strengthening the external rotators.

Releasing and catching a small ball in front of the body will eccentrically train the external rotators (figure 11.48). Use of tubing or dumbbells can strengthen the supraspinatus and deltoids.

The strengthening program should progressively increase repetitions, and then resistance, to build a strength and endurance base. Free weight exercises and a modified push-up on a wobbleboard (figure 11.49) train proprioception and stabilization. Tubing, machines, and isokinetics help movement in various positions and speeds.

Always keep in mind the impingement zone and the stage of rehabilitation. Clients should continue on a maintenance program of core exercises several times per week and continue applying ice after workouts.

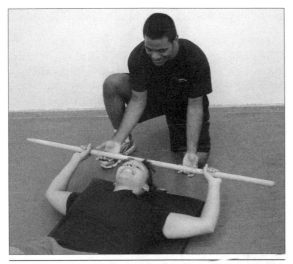

Figure 11.40 Lying wand shoulder rotations. Lying on table or floor, the client moves a wand toward the head and then down toward the waist through a pain-free range of motion.

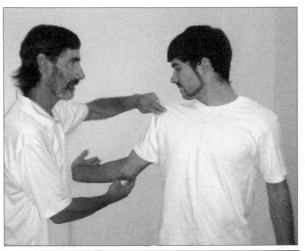

Figure 11.41 Doorway internal rotator stretch. With shoulder abducted 60° and externally rotated, the client turns his body gently away from doorway and holds.

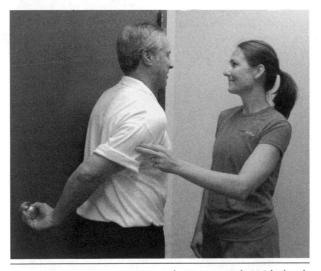

Figure 11.42 Doorway external rotator stretch. With shoulder abducted 60° and externally rotated, the client turns his body gently away from doorway and holds.

From *Client-Centered Exercise Prescription, Second Edition*, by John C. Griffin, 2006, Champaign, IL: Human Kinetics.

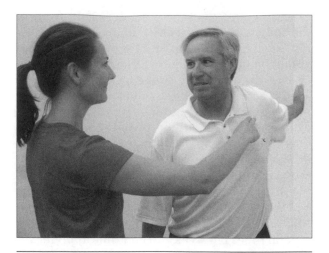

Figure 11.43 Wall pectoralis stretch. With the arm horizontally abducted against a wall, the client turns his body away from the wall. Repeat with elbow bent.

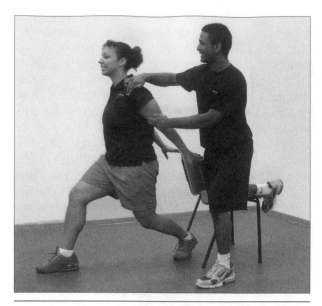

Figure 11.44 Anterior deltoid and biceps stretch. The client reaches behind with a straight arm and grasps the top of a chair. She moves her body forward and downward with arm directly back.

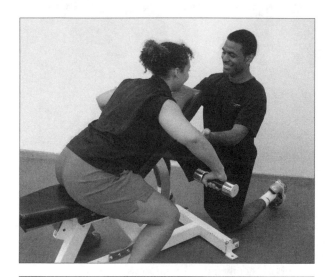

Figure 11.45 Scapular retraction with dumbbells. From a supported prone or incline position, the client lifts dumbbells toward chest with elbows bent and close to her side. Have her try to pinch the scapulae together.

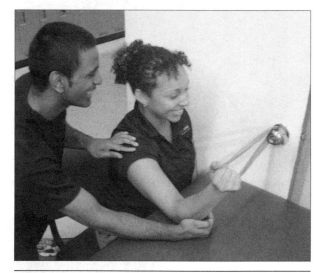

Figure 11.46 Shoulder external rotation with tubing. The client pulls tubing away from anchor point, keeping elbow bent at 90°.

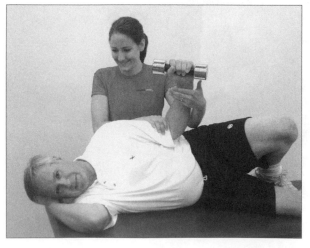

Figure 11.47 Side-lying flies with dumbbells. From a side-lying position, the client grasps a dumbbell or tubing with the top arm bent 90° at the elbow. He lifts the weight upward (keeping the elbow tight) and returns slowly.

 From *Client-Centered Exercise Prescription, Second Edition,* by John C. Griffin, 2006, Champaign, IL: Human Kinetics.

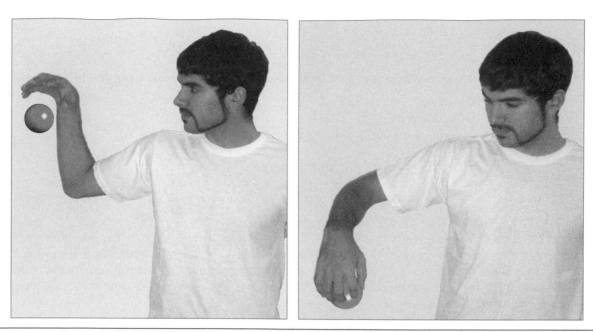

Figure 11.48 Eccentric ball catch. With the arm abducted 90° and elbow flexed, a ball is held in the up position. The ball is released and the hand comes down quickly to catch it. The upper arm remains abducted.

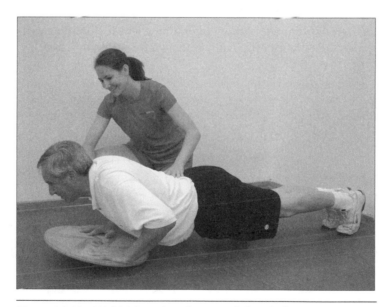

Figure 11.49 Wobbleboard push-up. With hands flat on the top of a wobbleboard, the client performs push-ups in a slow and controlled manner.

Highlights

1. **Describe the functional anatomy and probable causes for each of the following conditions:**
   - plantar fasciitis
   - Achilles tendinitis and tendinosis
   - shin splints (medial tibial stress syndrome)
   - patellofemoral syndrome
   - hamstring strain
   - low back pain
   - rotator cuff tendinitis (impingement syndrome)

   Probable causes for overuse injuries of tendons (e.g., Achilles tendinitis), muscles (e.g., hamstring strain), and other connective tissue (e.g., plantar fasciitis and shin splints) were illustrated and discussed. You must understand preventive exercise strategies including **precautions,** beneficial activity **indications,** and inadvisable exercise **contraindications.** Understanding the injury and its potential cause can be the first step toward preventing it.

2. **Describe preventive exercise strategies including precautions, beneficial activity indications, and inadvisable exercise contraindications.**

   Strategies for preventing overuse injuries of tendons (e.g., rotator cuff tendinitis), muscles (e.g., hamstring strain), and other connective tissue (e.g., shin splints) were outlined as well as specific exercise designs for stretching and for strengthening these injured tissues.

3. **Assist with the post-rehabilitation treatment plan for a client to minimize risk of reinjury or to speed recovery by designing specific exercises and activities for stretching and for strengthening injured tissues.**

   Specific exercise designs for stretching and strengthening injured tissues were grouped together near the end of each injury presentation. However, it is your responsibility to recognize the signs of overuse and the progression of symptoms as the time to refer your client to seek medical assistance.

Credits

Figure 7.3 part 7—Reprinted, by permission, from C. Norris, 2002, *Back stability* (Champaign, IL: Human Kinetics), 188.

Table 7.4 figure 1—Reprinted, by permission, from T.R. Baechle and R.W. Earle, 1995, *Fitness weight training* (Champaign, IL: Human Kinetics), 155.

Table 7.4 figure 2—Reprinted, by permission, from T.R. Baechle and R.W. Earle, 1995, *Fitness weight training* (Champaign, IL: Human Kinetics), 155.

Table 7.4 figure 3—Reprinted, by permission, from T.R. Baechle and R.W. Earle, 1995, *Fitness weight training* (Champaign, IL: Human Kinetics), 155.

Table 7.4 figure 4—Reprinted, by permission, from T.R. Baechle and R.W. Earle, 1995, *Fitness weight training* (Champaign, IL: Human Kinetics), 155.

Table 7.4 figure 5 —Reprinted, by permission, from B.B. Cook and G.W. Stewart, 1996, *Strength basics: Your guide to resistance training for health and optimal performance* (Champaign, IL: Human Kinetics), 112.

Table 7.4 figure 6—Reprinted, by permission, from B.B. Cook and G.W. Stewart, 1996, *Strength basics: Your guide to resistance training for health and optimal performance* (Champaign, IL: Human Kinetics), 112.

Table 7.4 figure 7—Reprinted, by permission, from B.B. Cook and G.W. Stewart, 1996, *Strength basics: Your guide to resistance training for health and optimal performance* (Champaign, IL: Human Kinetics), 113.

Table 7.4 figure 8—Reprinted, by permission, from B.B. Cook and G.W. Stewart, 1996, *Strength basics: Your guide to resistance training for health and optimal performance* (Champaign, IL: Human Kinetics), 113.

Table 7.4 figure 9—Reprinted, by permission, from T.R. Baechle and R.W. Earle, 1995, *Fitness weight training* (Champaign, IL: Human Kinetics), 150.

Table 7.4 figure 10—Reprinted, by permission, from T.R. Baechle and R.W. Earle, 1995, *Fitness weight training* (Champaign, IL: Human Kinetics), 150.

Table 7.4 figure 12—Reprinted, by permission, from T.R. Baechle and R.W. Earle, 1995, *Fitness weight training* (Champaign, IL: Human Kinetics), 157.

Table 7.4 figure 13—Reprinted, by permission, from T.R. Baechle and R.W. Earle, 1995, *Fitness weight training* (Champaign, IL: Human Kinetics), 157.

Table 7.4 figure 14—Reprinted, by permission, from T.R. Baechle and R.W. Earle, 1995, *Fitness weight training* (Champaign, IL: Human Kinetics), 148.

Table 7.4 figure 15—Reprinted, by permission, from T.R. Baechle and R.W. Earle, 1995, *Fitness weight training* (Champaign, IL: Human Kinetics), 148.

Table 7.4 figure 16—Reprinted, by permission, from T.R. Baechle and R.W. Earle, 1995, *Fitness weight training* (Champaign, IL: Human Kinetics), 152.

Table 7.4 figure 17—Reprinted, by permission, from T.R. Baechle and R.W. Earle, 1995, *Fitness weight training* (Champaign, IL: Human Kinetics), 152

Table 7.4 figure 20—Reprinted, by permission, from T.R. Baechle and R.W. Earle, 1995, *Fitness weight training* (Champaign, IL: Human Kinetics), 144.

Table 7.4 figure 21—Reprinted, by permission, from T.R. Baechle and R.W. Earle, 1995, *Fitness weight training* (Champaign, IL: Human Kinetics), 144.

Table 7.4 figure 22—Reprinted, by permission, from B.B. Cook and G.W. Stewart, 1996, *Strength basics: Your guide to resistance training for health and optimal performance* (Champaign, IL: Human Kinetics), 149.

Table 8.12 figure 1—Reprinted, by permission, from M. Alter, 1997, *Sport stretch* (Champaign, IL: Human Kinetics), 50. © Michael Richardson.

Table 8.12 figure 2—Reprinted, by permission, from M. Alter, 1997, *Sport stretch* (Champaign, IL: Human Kinetics), 38. © Michael Richardson.

Table 8.12 figure 3—Reprinted, by permission, from M. Alter, 1997, *Sport stretch* (Champaign, IL: Human Kinetics), 42. © Michael Richardson.

Table 8.12 figure 4—Reprinted, by permission, from M. Alter, 1997, *Sport stretch* (Champaign, IL: Human Kinetics), 129. © Michael Richardson.

References

Chapter 1

Clark, J., and S. Clark. 1993. *Prioritize Organize: The Art of Getting It Done.* Shawnee Mission, KS: National Press.

DeBusk, R.F., U. Stenestrand, and M. Sheehan. 1990. Training effects of long versus short bouts of exercise. *American Journal of Cardiology* 65(15):1010-1013.

Duffy, F.D., and L. Schnirring. 2000. How to counsel patients about exercise. *The Physician and Sports Medicine* 28 (10): 53-58.

Egan, G. 1990. *The Skilled Helper.* Pacific Grove, CA: Brooks/Cole.

Francis, L. 1990. Setting goals. *IDEA Today* (May): 8-10.

Goldfine, H., A. Ward, P. Taylor, D. Carlucci, and J.M. Rippe. 1991. Exercising to health—What's really in it for your patients? *The Physician and Sportsmedicine* 19 (6): 81-93.

Jones, A.P. 1991. Communication and teaching techniques. In *Program Design for Personal Trainers.* San Diego: IDEA.

Kimiecik, J. 2000. Bashing through barriers. *IDEA Health and Fitness Source* (March): 42-46.

Kyllo, L.B., and D.M. Landers. 1995. Goal setting in sport and exercise: A research synthesis to resolve the controversy. *Journal of Sport and Exercise Psychology* 17:117-137.

Orme, M. 1977. Teaching strategies and consultation skills: Probing techniques. In *Innovation in School Psychology,* ed. S. Miezitis and M. Orme, 70-83. Toronto: OISE.

Prochaska, J.O., C.C. DiClemente, and J.J. Norcross. 1992. In search of how people change: Applications to addictive behaviours. *American Psychologist* 47 (9).

Prochaska, J.O. 1994. Strong and weak principles for progressing from precontemplation to action on the basis of twelve problem behaviors. *Health Psychology* 13 (1): 47-51.

Prukop, N. 1997. Selling with style. *IDEA Personal Trainer* (November/December): 41-47.

Sotile, W.M. 1996. *Psychosocial Interventions for Cardiopulmonary Patients.* Champaign, IL: Human Kinetics.

Tod, D., and M. McGuigan. 2001. Maximizing strength training through goal setting. *Strength and Conditioning Journal* 23(4):22-26.

Trottier, M. 1988. Client-driven programming. Keynote address: Fit Rendezvous. Edmonton, Canada.

Weylman, C.R. 1995. *Reaching the Potential Client.* Atlanta: The Achievement Group.

Wheeler, G.D. 2000. Counselling and Behaviour Change. *Handout During PFLC Training.* Edmonton, Alberta.

Chapter 2

Annesi, J. 2000. Retention crisis? Exercise dropouts and adherents. *Fitness Business Canada* (July-August): 6-8.

Ball, D.R. 2001. Cognitive strategies. *IDEA Personal Trainer* (November-December): 22-29.

Brehm, B.A. 2003. Cognitive restructuring supports behavior-change efforts. *Fitness Management* (April): 22.

Canadian Society for Exercise Physiology. 2003. *The Canadian Physical Activity, Fitness, and Lifestyle Approach.* 3rd ed. Ottawa: CSEP.

Brooks, C.M. 2000. Marketing the active lifestyle. *Fitness Management* (July): 44-50.

Canadian Society for Exercise Physiology. 2003. *The Canadian Physical Activity, Fitness, and Lifestyle Approach.* 3rd ed. Ottawa: CSEP.

Cantwell, S. 2003. Lifestyle coaching. *Fitness Trainer Canada* (February-March): 10-15.

De Bourdeauhuij I., and J. Sallis. 2002. Relative contribution of psychosocial variables to the explanation of physical activity in three population-based adult samples. *Preventive Medicine* 34: 279-288.

Dishman, R.K. 1990. Determinants of participation in physical activity. *Journal of Applied Sport Sciences* 8:104-13.

Kimiecik, J.C. 1998. The path of the intrinsic exerciser. *IDEA Health and Fitness Source* (March): 34-42.

Patrick, K., B. Long, W. Wooten, and M. Pratt. 1994. A new tool for encouraging activity. Project PACE. *The Physician and Sportsmedicine* 22 (11): 45-55.

Pronk, N.P., R.R. Wing, and R.W. Jeffery. 1994. Effects of increased stimulus control for exercise through use of a personal trainer. *Annals of Behavioral Medicine* 16:SO77.

Wheeler, G.D. 2000. Counselling and Behavior Change. *Handout During PFLC Training.* Edmonton, Alberta.

Chapter 3

American College of Sports Medicine. 1990. The recommended quantity and quality of exercise for developing and maintaining fitness in healthy adults. *Medicine and Science in Sports and Exercise* 22: 265-274.

American College of Sports Medicine. 2000. *Guidelines for Exercise Testing and Prescription.* 6th ed. Philadelphia: Lea and Febiger.

Åstrand, P.O., and K. Rodahl, eds. 2003. *Textbook of Work Physiology.* 6th ed. New York: McGraw-Hill.

Blair, S.N., H.W. Kohl III, R.S. Paffenbarger Jr., D.G. Clark, K.H. Cooper, and L.W. Gibbons. 1989. Physical fitness and all-cause mortality: A prospective study of healthy men and women. *Journal of the American Medical Association* 262 (17): 2395-2401.

Bompa, T.O. 1999. *Periodization Theory and Methodology of Training.* 4th ed. Champaign, IL: Human Kinetics.

Bouchard, C. 1994. Physical activity, fitness, and health: Overview of the Consensus Symposium. In: *Toward Active Living,* ed. H.A. Quinney, L. Gauvin, and A.E.T. Wall. Champaign IL: Human Kinetics.

Burfoot, A. 1995. How much should you run? *Runner's World* (September): 66-67.

Canadian Society for Exercise Physiology. 2003. *The Canadian Physical Activity, Fitness, and Lifestyle Approach.* 3rd ed. Ottawa: CSEP.

De Busk, R.F., U. Stenestrand, and M. Sheehan. 1990. Training effects of long versus short bouts of exercise. *American Journal of Cardiology* 65 (15):1010-1013.

Ebisu, T. 1985. Splitting the distance of endurance running: On cardiovascular endurance and blood lipids. *Japanese Journal of Physical Education* 30 (1): 37-43.

Feigenbaum, M.S., and M.L. Pollock. 1997. Strength training: Rationale for current Guidelines for Adult Fitness Programs. *The Physician and Sports Medicine,* 25(2):44-64.

Getchell, B., and W. Anderson. 1982. *Being Fit: A Personal Guide.* NY: Wiley.

Gledhill, N., and V. Jamnik. 1996. Figure 4-1. In *The Canadian Physical Activity, Fitness, and Lifestyle Appraisal: CSEP's Plan for Healthy Active Living.* Ottawa: CSEP.

Goldfine, H., A. Ward, P. Taylor, D. Carlucci, and J.M. Rippe. 1991. Exercising to health—What's really in it for your patients? *The Physician and Sportsmedicine* 19(6):81-93.

Hagan, R.D. 1988. Benefits of aerobic conditioning and diet for overweight adults. *Sports Medicine* 5:144-155.

Haskell, W.L. 1985. Physical activity and health: Need to define the required stimulus. *American Journal of Cardiology* 55:4D-9D.

Haskell, W.L. 1995. Resolving the exercise debate: More vs. less. *IDEA Today* (October):40-47.

Hawley, C.J. and R.B. Schoene. 2003. Overtraining syndrome. A guide to diagnosis, treatment, and prevention. *The Physician and Sports Medicine* 31(6): 25-31.

Heyward, V.H. 2002. *Advanced Fitness Assessment and Exercise Prescription.* 4th ed. Champaign, IL: Human Kinetics.

Heyward V.H., and D. Wagner. 2004. *Applied Body Composition Assessment.* 2nd ed. Champaign, IL: Human Kinetics.

Hoeger, W. and S. Hoeger. 1999. *Principles and Labs for Fitness and Wellness.* 5th ed. Englewood, CA: Morton.

International Federation of Sports Medicine Position Statement. 1990. Physical exercise: An important factor for health. *The Physician and Sportsmedicine* 18 (3):155-156.

Katzmarzyk, P.T., and C.L. Craig. 2002. Musculoskeletal fitness and risk of mortality. *Medicine and Science in Sports and Exercise* 31(5): 740-744.

Kesaniemi, Y.I., et al. 2001. Dose-response issues concerning physical activity and health: An evidence-based symposium. *Medicine and Science in Sports and Exercise* 34(suppl.): S351-S358.

Kuipers, H., and Keizer, H.A. 1988. Overtraining in elite athletes. *Sports Medicine* 5:79-92.

La Forge, R. 2001. Exercise and health: Dose-response issues. *IDEA Health and Fitness Source* (September): 21-25.

Malkin, M. 2002. Exercise as preventive medicine. *Fitness Management* (February): 64-67.

Malkin, M. 2004. Warming up, cooling down and stretching. *Fitness Management* (January): 30-32.

Nieman, D.C. 1990. *Fitness and Sports Medicine: An Introduction.* Palo Alto: Bull Publishing.

NIH, NHLBI. 1998. *Clinical Guidelines on the Identification, Evaluation and Treatment of Overweight and Obesity in Adults.* NIH Publication No. 98-4083. www.nhlbi.nih.gov/guidelines/obesity/ob_home.htm

Paffenbarger, R.S. Jr., R.T. Hyde, A.L. Wing, and C. Hsieh. 1986. Physical activity, all-cause mortality, and longevity of college alumni. *New England Journal of Medicine* 314 (10): 605-613.

Payne, N., et al. 2000. Health implications of musculoskeletal fitness. *Canadian Journal of Applied Physiology* 25(2): 114-126.

Pate, R.R., M. Pratt, S.N. Blair, et al. 1995. Physical activity and public health: A recommendation from the Centers for Disease Control and Prevention and the American College of Sports Medicine. *Journal of the American Medical Association* 273(5): 402-407.

Quinney, H.A., L. Gauvin, and A.E.T. Wall, eds. 1994. *Toward Active Living.* Champaign IL: Human Kinetics.

Ross, R., I. Janssen, and A. Trembley. 2000. Obesity reduction through lifestyle modification. *Canadian Journal of Applied Physiology* 25(1):1-18.

Shephard, R.J. 1988. PAR-Q, Canadian home fitness test and exercise screening alternatives. *Sports Medicine* 5:185-195.

Shephard, R.J., and C. Bouchard. 1994. Population evaluations of health related fitness from perceptions of physical activity and fitness. *Canadian Journal of Applied Physiology* 19(2): 151-173.

Skinner, J.S. 1987. General principles of exercise prescription. In *Exercise Testing and Exercise Prescription for Special Cases,* ed. J.S. Skinner. Philadelphia: Lea and Febiger.

Stone, M.H., S.J. Fleck, N.T. Triplett, and W.J. Kraemer. 1991. Health- and performance-related potential of resistance training. *Sports Medicine* 11(4): 210-231.

Stone, M.H., R.E. Keith, J.T. Kearney, S.J. Fleck, G.T. Wilson, and N.T. Triplett. 1991. Overtraining: A review of the signs, symptoms and possible causes. *Journal of Applied Sports Science Research* 5(1): 35-50.

Tremblay, M. et al. 2001. Physical activity assessment options within the context of the Canadian Physical Activity, Fitness, and Lifestyle Appraisal. *Canadian Journal of Applied Physiology* 26 (4): 388-407.

Warburton, D., N. Gledhill, and A. Quinney. 2001. The effects of changes in musculoskeletal fitness on health. *Canadian Journal of Applied Physiology* 26(2): 161-216.

Wenger, H.A., and G.J. Bell. 1986. The interactions of intensity, frequency, and duration of exercise training in altering cardiorespiratory fitness. *Sports Medicine* 3: 346-356.

Westcott, W.L. 1989. When more isn't better. *IDEA Today* (February): 24.

Wilmore, J.H. 2003. Aerobic exercise and endurance improving fitness for health benefits. *The Physician and Sports Medicine* 31(5): 45-51.

Wilmore, J.H., and D.L. Costill. 2004. *Physiology of Sport and Exercise.* 3rd ed. Champaign, IL: Human Kinetics.

Wilson, D.M.C., and D. Ciliska. 1984. Lifestyle assessment: Development and the use of the FANTASTIC Checklist. *Canadian Family Physician* 30.

Chapter 4

Albert, W., J. Bonneau, J. Stevenson, and N. Gledhill. 2001. Back fitness and back health assessment considerations for the Canadian Physical Activity, Fitness, and Lifestyle Appraisal. *Canadian Journal of Applied Physiology* 26(3): 291-317.

Alter, M.J. 2004. *Science of Stretching.* 3rd ed. Champaign, IL: Human Kinetics.

American College of Sports Medicine. 2000. *Guidelines for Exercise Testing and Prescription.* 6th ed. Philadelphia: Lea and Febiger.

Anderson, G. 2003. Body composition: Weighing the options. *Unpublished paper.* University College Fraser Valley, British Columbia.

Baechle, T. and R. Earle. 2000. *Essentials of Strength Training and Conditioning.* Champaign, IL: Human Kinetics.

Canadian Society for Exercise Physiology. 2003. *The Canadian Physical Activity, Fitness, and Lifestyle Approach.* 3rd ed. Ottawa: CSEP.

DeLisa, J. ed. 1998. *Rehabilitation Medicine Principles and Practice.* Philadelphia: J.B. Lippincott.

Ellison, D. 1995. Beyond the sit-up. *IDEA Today* (September): 33-39.

Getchell, B., and W. Anderson. 1982. *Being Fit: A Personal Guide.* New York: Wiley.

Griffin, J.C. 1989. *All the Right Moves.* An unpublished manual.

Griffin, J.C. 1998. *Client-Centered Exercise Prescription.* Champaign, IL: Human Kinetics.

Heyward, V.H. 2002. *Advanced Fitness Assessment and Exercise Prescription.* 4th ed. Champaign, IL: Human Kinetics.

Hoeger, W., and S. Hoeger. 1999. *Principles and Labs for Fitness and Wellness.* 5th ed. Englewood, CA: Morton.

Imrie, D and L. Barbuto. 1988. *The Back Power Program.* Toronto, ON: Stoddard Pub.

Jackson, A.S., and M.L. Pollock. 1985. Practical assessment of body composition. *The Physician and Sportsmedicine* 13: 76-90.

Janssen, I., S. Heymsfield, and R. Ross. 2002. Application of simple anthropometry in the assessment of health risk: Implications for the Canadian Physical Activity, Fitness, and Lifestyle Appraisal. *Canadian Journal of Applied Physiology* 27(4): 396-414.

Kendall, F.P., McCreary, E.K., and Provance, P.G. 1993. *Muscles: Testing and Function.* Baltimore: Williams and Wilkins.

Kravitz, L., and V. Heyward. 1997. The many aspects of fitness assessment body composition-Skinfold technique. *IDEA Personal Trainer* (June): 19-23

Larsson, B., B. Svardsudd, L. Weilin, L. Wilhelmsen, P. Bjorntorp, and G. Tibbin. 1984. Abdominal adipose tissue distribution, obesity, and risk of cardiovascular disease and death: 13-year follow-up of participants in the study of men born in 1913. *British Medical Journal* 288:1401-1404.

Lean, M.E., T.S. Han, and J.C. Seidell. 1998. Impairment of health and quality of life in people with large waist circumference. *The Lancet* 351: 853-856.

Michaelson, F., and P. Gagne. 2002. Upper limb evaluation. *Fitness Trainer Canada* (February): 30-33.

Nieman, C. 2003. *Exercise Testing and Prescription: A Health-Related Approach.* 5th ed. Mountain View, CA: Mayfield.

NIH. NHLBI. 1998. *Clinical Guidelines on the Identification, Evaluation and Treatment of Overweight and Obesity in Adults.* NIH Publication No. 98-4083. www.nhlbi.nih.gov/guidelines/obesity/ob_home.htm

Nordvall, M., and K. Sullivan. 2002. Pre-preparation health and fitness assessments. *Fitness Management* (February): 44-49.

Norkin, C., and D.J. White. 1995. *Measurement of Joint Motion: A Guide to Goniometry* 2nd ed. Philadelphia: F.A. Davis.

Roskopf, G. 2001. When clients feel pain. *IDEA Personal Trainer* (February): 45-53.

Ross, R., Rissanen, J., and Hudson, R. 1996. Sensitivity associated with the identification of visceral adipose tissue levels using the waist cicumference in men and women: Effects of weight loss. *International Journal of Obesity* 20: 533-538.

Sale, D., and MacDougall, J.D. 1981. Specificity in strength training: A review for the coach and athlete. *Canadian Journal of Applied Sport Science* 6: 87-92.

Chapter 5

Baker, D. 2001. Science and practice of coaching a strength training program for novice and intermediate-level athletes. *Strength and Conditioning Journal* 23(2): 61-68.

Batman, P., and M. Van Capelle. 1992. *Exercise Analysis Made Simple.* 2nd ed. Arncliffe, NSW: F.I.A.

Cantwell, S. 1998. "On the Floor" communication skills. *IDEA Personal Trainer* (February): 34-39.

Edman, K.A.P. 1992. Contractile performance of skeletal muscle fibres. In *Strength and Power in Sport.* Boston: Blackwell Scientific.

Ellison, D. 1993. *Advanced ExerciseDesign for Lower Body.* San Diego: Movement That Matters.

Escamilla, J. et al. 1998. Biomechanics of the knee during closed kinetic chain and open kinetic chain exercises. *Medicine and Science in Sport and Exercise* 24(4): 556-569.

Griffin, J.C. 1986a. A system for: Exercise analysis. *Canadian Association for Health, Physical Education, and Recreation Journal* 52(1): 30-31.

Griffin, J.C. 1986b. A system for: Exercise design. *Canadian Association for Health, Physical Education, and Recreation Journal* 52(2): 38-39.

Hagan, M. 2000. Training tips for today's fitness professionals. *Fitness Business Canada.* (March-April): 38-39.

Hamill, J., and K.M. Knutzen. 1995. *Biomechanical Basis of Human Movement.* Media, PA: Williams and Wilkins.

Komi, P.V. 1992. Stretch-shortening cycle. In *Strength and Power in Sport.* Boston: Blackwell Scientific.

Lockwood, C.M. 1999. Troubleshooting: The most common training mistakes and how to fix them. Quads and Gluts. *Muscle and Fitness* (October): 76-79.

Lyons, P.M., and J.F. Orwin. 1998. Rotator cuff tendinopathy and subacromial impingement syndrome. *Medicine and Science in Sport and Exercise* 30(4): S12-S17.

Signorile, J.F., et al. 2002. A comparative electromyographical investigation of muscle utilization patterns using various hand positions during the lat pull-down. *Journal of Strength and Conditioning Research* 16(4): 539-546.

Tortora, G.J., and S.R. Grabowski. 2003. *Principles of Anatomy and Physiology.* 10th ed. New York: John Wiley and Sons, Inc.

Westcott, W., et al. 2003. Using performance feedback in strength training. *Fitness Management* (September): 28-33.

Wilmore, J.H., and D.L. Costill. 2004. *Physiology of Sport and Exercise.* 3rd ed. Champaign, IL: Human Kinetics.

Chapter 6

Allen, D., and L. Goldberg. 1986. Physiological comparison of two cross-country ski machines. Paper presented at the annual meeting of the American College of Sports Medicine, Indianapolis. May.

American College of Sports Medicine. 2000. *Guidelines for Exercise Testing and Prescription.* 6th ed. Philadelphia: Lea and Febiger.

Åstrand, P.-O., and K. Rodahl. 2003. *Textbook of Work Physiology.* 6th ed. New York: McGraw-Hill.

Baechle, T.R., and R.W. Earle, eds. 2000. *Essentials of Strength Training and Conditioning.* 2nd ed. Champaign, IL: Human Kinetics.

Black, S.A. 2001. Heart rate training: A valuable exercise barometer. *Fitness Management.* (August): 40-45.

Blair, S.N., H.W. Kohl, R.S. Paffenbarger, D.G. Clark, K.H. Cooper, and L.W. Gibbons. 1989. Physical fitness and all-cause mortality. *Journal of the American Medical Association* 262 (17): 2395-2401.

Brooks, and Copeland-Brooks. 1991. Are you ready for the next step in circuit training? *IDEA Today* (November-December): 34-39.

Brynteson, P., and W.E. Sinning. 1973. The effect of training frequencies on the retention of cardiovascular fitness. *Medicine and Science in Sports and Exercise* 5: 29-33.

Dishman, R.K. 1990. Determinants of participation in physical activity. *Journal of Applied Sports Science Research* 8:104-113.

Fair, E. 1992. Have equipment, will travel. *IDEA Today* (May): 57-61.

Fox, E.L. 1979. *Sports Physiology.* Philadelphia: Saunders.

Gaesser, G.A. 2003. On the Move: Pedometer based walking initiative encourages physical activity. *Sports Medicine Digest* 25(8): 90, 92.

Gettman, L.R., and M.L. Pollock. 1981. Circuit weight training: A critical review of its physiological benefits. *The Physician and Sports Medicine* 9: 44-60.

Haskell, W.L. 1985. Physical activity and health: Need to define the required stimulus. *American Journal of Cardiology* 55: 4D-9D.

Haskell, W.L. 1995. Resolving the exercise debate: More vs. less. *IDEA Today* (October): 40-47.

Heyward, V. 2002. *Advanced Fitness Assessment and Exercise Prescription*. 4th ed. Champaign, IL: Human Kinetics.

Horswill, C.A., C.L. Kien, and W.B. Zipf. 1995. Energy expenditure in adolescents during low intensity, leisure activities. *Medicine and Science in Sports and Exercise* 27(9):1311-1314.

Howard, M. 2003. Cardiovascular programming: Are we selling our clients short? A trainer's guide. *Fitness Trainer Canada* (February-March): 26-30.

Howley and Franks. 1997. Health and Fitness Instructor's Handbook. 3rd ed. Champaign, IL: Human Kinetics.

Iknoian, T. 1992. 10 equipment trends that changed fitness. *IDEA Today* (July-August): 33-36.

Karp, J.R. 2000. Interval Training. *Fitness Management*. (August): 46-48.

Kesaniemi, Y.A. et al. 2001. Dose-response issues concerning physical activity and health: An evidence-based symposium. *Medicine and Science in Sports and Exercise*. 34(suppl.): S351-S358.

Kosich, D. 1991. Exercise physiology 4(4). In *Personal Trainer Manual. San Diego: American Council on Exercise*.

Marion, A., G. Kenny, and J. Thoden. 1994. Heart rate response as a means of quantifying training loads: Practical considerations for coaches. *Sports* 14(2): Part 1.

McArdle, W., F. Katch, and V. Katch. 1991. *Exercise Physiology: Energy, Nutrition, and Human Performance*. 3rd ed. Philadelphia: Lea and Febiger.

Nieman, D.C. 1999. *Exercise Testing and Prescription: A Health-Related Approach*. 4th ed. Mountain View, CA: Mayfield.

Pollock, M., L. Gettman, C. Milesis, M. Bah, L. Durstine, and R. Johnson. 1977. Effects of frequency and duration of training on attrition and incidence of injury. *Medicine and Science in Sports and Exercise* 9: 31-36.

Porcari, J., C. Foster, and P. Schneider. 2000. Exercise response to elliptical trainers. *Fitness Management* (August): 50-53.

Powers, S.K., and E.T. Howley. 1990. *Exercise Physiology*. Dubuque, IA: Brown.

Schnirring, L. 2001. New formula estimates maximal heart rate. *The Physician and Sports Medicine* 29(7): 13-14.

Sharkey, B.J. 1984. *Physiology of Fitness*. 2nd ed. Champaign, IL: Human Kinetics.

Sillery, B. 1996. Essential technology guide to exercise and fitness. *Popular Science* (January): 65-68.

Stewart, G.W. 1995. *Active Living*. Champaign, IL: Human Kinetics.

Swain, D., B. Leutholtz, M. King, L. Haas, and D. Branch. 1998. Relationship between % heart rate reserve and % VO2 reserve in treadmill exercise. *Medicine and Science in Sports and Exercise* 30(2): 318-321.

Tanaka, H., K.D. Monahan, and D.R. Seals. 2001. Age-predicted maximum heart rate revisited. *Journal of American College of Cardiol*ogy 37(1):153-156.

Wilmore, J.H., and D.L. Costill. 2004. *Physiology of Sport and Exercise*. 3rd ed. Champaign, IL: Human Kinetics.

Yacenda, J. 1995. *Fitness Cross-Training*. Champaign, IL: Human Kinetics.

Chapter 7

American College of Sports Medicine. 2002. Position Stand: Progression models in resistance training for healthy adults. *Medicine and Science in Sport and Exercise* 34(2):364-380.

American College of Sports Medicine. 2000. *Guidelines for Exercise Testing and Prescription*. 6th ed. Philadelphia: Lea and Febiger.

Baechle, T.R., and R.W. Earle. ed. 2000. *Essentials of Strength Training and Conditioning*. 2nd ed. Champaign, IL: Human Kinetics.

Bompa, T.O. 1999. Periodization Theory and Methodology of Training. 4th ed. Champaign, IL: Human Kinetics.

Calder, A.W., P.D. Chilibeck, C.E. Webber, and D.G. Sale. 1994. Comparison of whole and split weight training routines in young women. *Canadian Journal of Applied Physiology* 19(2): 185-199.

Chu, D.A. 1992. *Jumping Into Plyometrics*. Champaign, IL: Leisure Press.

Fleck, S.J. 1999. Periodized strength training: A critical review. *Journal of Strength and Conditioning Research* 13(1): 82-89.

Fleck, S.J., and W.J. Kraemer. 2004. *Designing Resistance Training Programs*. 3rd ed. Champaign, IL: Human Kinetics.

Heyward, V. 2002. *Advanced Fitness Assessment and Exercise Prescription*. 4th ed. Champaign, IL: Human Kinetics.

Kraemer, W.J. 2003. Strength training basics designing workouts to meet patients' goals. *The Physician and Sports Medicine* 31(8): 39-45.

Larson, et al. 1997. A comparison of three different rest intervals between multiple squat bouts. *Journal of Strength and Conditioning Research* 11 (2):115-118.

Marx, J.O., et al. 2001. Low-volume circuit versus high-volume periodized resistance training in women. *Medicine and Science in Sport and Exercise*. 33(4): 635-643.

O'Hagan, F.T., T.G. Sale, J.D. MacDougall, and S.H. Garner. 1995. Comparative effectiveness of accomodating and weight resistance training modes.

Medicine and Science in Sports and Exercise 27(8): 1210-1219.

Riley, D.P. 1982. *Strength Training by the Experts.* Champaign, IL: Leisure Press.

Sorace, P., and T. LaFontaine. 2005. Resistance Training Muscle Power: Design Programs That Work! *ACSM's Health and Fitness Journal* 9(2):6-12.

Stone, M.H., et al. 1999. Periodization: Effects of manipulating volume and intensity. Part 1. *Strength and Conditioning Journal* 21 (2): 56-62.

Voight, M., and S. Tippett. 1994. Plyometric exercise in rehabilitation. In *Rehabilitation Techniques in Sports Medicine.* 2nd ed. W.E. Prentice, ed. St. Louis: Mosby.

Wolkodoff, N.E. 1989. Building strength. *IDEA Today* (July-August): 17-22.

Chapter 8

Alter, M.J. 2004. *Science of Stretching.* 3rd ed. Champaign, IL: Human Kinetics.

Bandy, W.D., J.M. Irion and M. Briggler. 1997. The effect of time and frequency of static sretching on flexibility of the hamstring muscles. *Physical Therapy* 77(10): 1090-1096.

Blievernicht, J. 2000. Round Shoulder Syndrome. *IDEA Health and Fitness Source.* (September): 44-53.

Brooks, D. 1993. Where does PNF fit into a training program? In *Program Design for Personal Trainers.* San Diego: IDEA.

Eitner, E. 1982. Loosening. In *Physical Therapy for Sports.* W. Kuprian, ed. Philadelphia: Saunders.

Germann, W.J., and C.L. Stanfield. 2002. *Principles of Human Physiology.* San Francisco, CA: Benjamin Cummings.

Hendrick, A. 2000. Dynamic flexibility training. *Strength and Conditioning Journal* 22(5): 33-38.

Heyward, V. 2002. *Advanced Fitness Assessment and Exercise Prescription.* 4th ed. Champaign, IL: Human Kinetics.

Holcomb, W.R. 2000. Improved stretching with proprioceptive neuromuscular facilitation. *Strength and Conditioning Journal* (February): 59-62.

Kendall F.P., E.K. McCreary, and P.G. Provance. 1993. *Muscles: Testing and Function.* Baltimore: Williams and Wilkins.

Knudson, D.V., P. Magnusson, and M. McHugh. 2000. Current issues in flexibility fitness. President's Council on Physical Fitness and Sports. *Research Digest.* 3(10): 1-8.

Kuprian, W., ed. 1982. *Physical Therapy for Sports.* Philadelphia: Saunders.

McAtee, R.E., and J. Charland. 1999. *Facilitated Stretching.* 2nd ed. Champaign, IL: Human Kinetics.

Ninos, J. 2001a. A chain reaction: The hip rotators. *Strength and Conditioning Journal.* (April): 26-27.

Ninos, J. 2001b. Chain reaction: A tight gastroc-soleus group. *Stength and Conditioning Journal* (February): 60-61.

Nordin, M., and V. Frankel. 2001. *Basic Biomechanics of the Musculoskeletal System.* 3rd ed. Baltimore: Lippincott Williams and Wilkins.

Norris, C.M. 2000. *Back Stability.* Champaign: Human Kinetics.

Osternig, L.R., R.N. Robertson, R.K. Troxel, and P. Hanson. 1990. Differential responses to PNF stretching techniques. *Medicine and Science in Sports and Exercise* 22:106-111.

Roskopf, G. 2001. When clients feel pain. *IDEA Personal Trainer* (February): 45-53.

Sapega, A.A., T.C. Quendenfeld, R.A. Moyer, and R.A. Butler. 1991. Biophysical factors in range of motion exercise. *The Physician and Sportsmedicine* 9(12): 57-65.

Shrier, I., and K. Gossal. 2000. Myths and truths of stretching individualized recommendations for healthy muscles. *The Physician and Sportsmedicine.* 28(8): 57-63.

Voss, D., M. Ionta, and B. Myers. 1985. *Proprioceptive Neuromuscular Facilitation: Patterns and Techniques.* 3rd ed. Philadelphia: Harper and Row.

Chapter 9

Ainsworth, B., et al. 2000. Compendium of physical activities: An update of activity codes and MET intensities. *Medicine and Science in Sports and Exercise* 32 (supplement): S498-S516.

American College of Sports Medicine. 2000. *Guidelines for Exercise Testing and Prescription.* 6th ed. Philadelphia: Lea and Febiger.

Andersen, R., and J. Jakicic. 2003. Physical activity and weight management. Building the case for exercise. *The Physician and Sports Medicine* 31(11): 39-45.

Bartlett, S. 2003. Motivating patients toward weight loss practical srategies for addressing overweight and obesity. *The Physician and Sports Medicine* 31(11): 29-36.

Bean, A. 1996. The truth about fat-burning. *Runner's World* (September): 46-50.

Blackburn, G.L., G.T. Wilson, B.S. Kanders, L.J. Stein, and P.T. Lavin. 1989. Weight cycling: The experience of human dieters. *American Journal of Clinical Nutrition* 49:1105-1109.

Brehm, B.A. 1996. Fat-burning: Getting down to the basics. *Fitness Management* (March): 25-26.

Campbell, W.W., M.C. Crim, V.R. Young, and W.J. Evans. 1994. Increased energy requirements and changes in body composition with resistance training in older adults. *American Journal of Clinical Nutrition* 60: 167-175.

Canadian Society for Exercise Physiology. 2003. *The Canadian Physical Activity, Fitness, and Lifestyle Approach.* 3rd ed. Ottawa: CSEP.

Clark, N. 2003. *Sports Nutrition Guidebook.* 3rd ed. Champaign, IL: Human Kinetics.

Cullinen, K., and M. Caldwell. 1998. Weight training increases fat-free mass and strength in untrained young women. *Journal of the American Dietetic Association* 98(4): 414-418.

Dattilio, A. 1992. Dietary fat and its relationship to body weight. *Nutrition Today* 27:13-19.

Dietitians of Canada. 2005. Keep an Eye on Your Proportion Size. www.dietitians.ca

Garfinkel, P., and D. Coscina. 1990. Discussion: Exercise and obesity. In *Exercise, Fitness and Health,* ed. C. Bouchard, R.J. Shephard, T. Stephens, J.R. Sutton, and B.D. McPherson. Champaign, IL: Human Kinetics.

Health and Human Services (HHS) and Department of Agriculture (USDA). 2005. *Dietary Guidelines for Americans.* 6th ed.

Heyward, V.H. 2002. *Advanced Fitness Assessment and Exercise Prescription.* 4th ed. Champaign, IL: Human Kinetics.

Hodgetts, V., et al. 1991. Factors controlling fat metabolism from human subcutaneous adipose tissue during exercise. *Journal of Applied Physiology* 71:445-451.

Hoeger, W., and S. Hoeger. 1999. *Principles and Labs for Fitness and Wellness.* 5th ed. Englewood, CA: Morton.

Klesges, R., et al. 1993. Effects of television on metabolic rate: Potential implications for childhood obesity. *Pediatrics* 91: 281-286.

Marks, B.L., A. Ward, D.H. Morris, J. Castellani, and J.M. Rippe. 1995. Fat-free mass is maintained in women following a moderate diet and exercise program. *Medicine and Science in Sports and Exercise* 27 (9): 1243-1251.

McArdle, W.D., F.I. Katch, and V.L. Katch. 1991. *Exercise Physiology: Energy, Nutrition, and Human Performance.* Philadelphia: Lea and Febiger.

Miller, W.C. 1991. Diet composition, energy intake and nutritional status in relation to obesity in men and women. *Medicine and Science in Sports and Exercise* 23(3): 280-284.

National Heart, Lung, and Blood Institute: Clinical Guidelines on the Identification, Evaluation, and Treatment of Overweight and Obesity in Adults: Executive Summary. National Institutes of Health publication no. 00-4084, Rockville, MD, October 2000.

Nieman, D.C. 1990. *Fitness and Sports Medicine: An Introduction.* Palo Alto, CA: Bull Publishing.

Peterson, et al. 2004. Comparison of caloric expenditure in intermittent and continuous walking bouts. *Journal of Strength and Conditioning Research* 18(2): 373-376.

Romijn, J., et al. 1993. Regulation of endogenous fat and carbohydrate metabolism in relation to exercise intensity and duration. *American Journal of Physiology* 265: E380-E391.

Sharkey, B. 1978. *Physiological Fitness and Weight Control.* Missoula: Mountain Press.

Simopoulos, A., ed. 1992. *Metabolic Control of Eating, Energy Expenditure and the Bioenergetics of Obesity.* Basel, Switzerland: Karger.

Tremblay, A., et al. 1989. Impact of dietary fat content and fat oxidation on energy intake in humans. *American Journal of Clinical Nutrition* 47: 799-805.

Walberg, J.L. 1989. Aerobic exercise and resistance weight training during weight reduction. *Sports Medicine* 47:343-356.

Williams, M.H. 1995. *Nutrition for Fitness and Sport.* 4th ed. Dubuque, IA: Brown and Benchmark.

Chapter 10

Andrish, J., and J.A. Work. 1990. How I manage shin splints. *The Physician and Sportsmedicine* 18 (12): 113-114.

Bahr, R., and S. Maehlum. 2004. *Clinical Guide to Sports Injuries.* Champaign, IL: Human Kinetics.

Clement, D.B., J.E. Taunton, and G.W. Smart. 1984. Achilles tendinitis and peritendinitis: Etiology and treatment. *American Journal of Sports Medicine* 12 (3):179-184.

Earle, R.W., and T.R. Baechle. 2004. *NSCA's Essentials of Personal Training.* Champaign, IL: Human Kinetics.

Frontera, W.R. 2003. Exercise and musculoskeletal rehabilitation. *The Physician and Sports Medicine.* 31(12): 39-45.

Germann, W.J., and C.L. Stanfield. 2002. *Principles of Human Physiology.* San Francisco, CA: Benjamin Cummings.

Griffin, J.C. 1987. Fitness injury survey: Fitness assessors and programmers. *Canadian Association for Health, Physical Education and Recreation Journal.* 53(1): 15-17.

Hess, G.P., W.L. Cappiello, R.M. Poole, and S.C. Hunter. 1989. Prevention and treatment of overuse tendon injuries. *Sports Medicine* 8(6): 371-384.

Houglum, P. 2001. *Therapeutic Exercise for Athletic Injuries.* Champaign, IL:Human Kinetics.

Kahn, K.M., et al. 2000. Overuse tendinosis, not tendinitis. *Physician and Sports Medicine* 28(5): 38-48.

Kaul, M.P., and S.A. Herring. 1994. Superficial heat and cold. *The Physician and Sports Medicine* 22(12): 65-72.

Kraemer, W., et al. 2001. Influence of compression therapy on symptoms following soft tissue injury from maximal eccentric exercise. *Journal of Orthopaedic and Sports Physical Therapy* 31(6): 282-298.

Nirschl, P.R. 1988. Prevention and treatment of elbow and shoulder injuries in the tennis player. *Clinical Sports Medicine* 7(2): 289-308.

O'Connor, F.G., J.R. Sobel, and R.P. Nirschl. 1992. Five-step treatment for overuse injuries. *The Physician and Sportsmedicine* 20 (10): 128-142.

Ralston, D.J. 2003. The RAMP System: A template for the progression of athletic-injury rehabilitation. *Journal of Sports Rehabilitation* 12: 280-290.

Ross, M. 1999. Delayed-onset muscle soreness. *The Physician and Sports Medicine* 27(1):107-108.

Stovitz S.D. and R.J. Johnson. 2003 .NSAIDs and musculoskeletal treatment. *The Physician and Sports Medicine* 31(1):35-52.

Styf, J. 1988. Diagnosis of exercise-induced pain in the anterior aspect of the lower leg. *American Journal of Sports Medicine* 16(2): 165-171.

Szymanski, D.J. 2001. Recommendations for the avoidance of delayed-onset muscle soreness. *Strength and Conditioning Journal* 23(4): 7-13.

Tokmakidis, S.P., E.A. Kokkinidid, I. Smilios and H. Douda. 2003. The effects of ibuprofen on delayed muscle soreness and muscular performance after eccentric exercise. *Journal of Strength and Conditioning Research* 17(1): 53-59.

Chapter 11

Andrish, J., and J.A. Work. 1990. How I manage shin splints. *The Physician and Sportsmedicine* 18 (12): 113-114.

Bahr, R., and S. Maehlum 2004. *Clinical Guide to Sports Injuries*. Champaign, IL: Human Kinetics.

Batt, M.E., and J.L. Tanji. 1995. Management options for plantar fasciitis. *The Physician and Sportsmedicine* 23 (6): 77-86.

Best, T.M., and W.E. Garrett. 1996. Hamstring strains. Expediting return to play. *The Physician and Sportsmedicine* 24 (8): 37-44.

Cook, J.L., et al. 2000. Overuse tendinosis, not tendinitis. *The Physician and Sports Medicine* 28(6): 31-46.

Couture, C.J., and K.A. Karlson. 2002. Tibial stress injuries. *The Physician and Sports Medicine* 30(6): 29-36.

DeLisa, J.A. 1998. *Rehabilitation Medicine Principles and Practices*. Philadelphia: Lippincott-Raven.

DePalma, M.J., and R.H. Perkins. 2004. Patellar tendinosis. *The Physician and Sports Medicine* 32(5): 41-45.

DePalma, M.J., and E.W. Johnson. 2003. Detecting and treating shoulder impingement syndrome. *The Physician and Sports Medicine* 31(7): 25-32.

De Palma, B. 1994. Rehabilitation of hip and thigh injuries. In *Rehabilitation Techniques in Sports Medicine*. 2nd ed. W.E. Prentice, ed. St. Louis: Mosby.

Doucette, S.A., and E.M. Goble. 1992. The effect of exercise on patellar tracking in lateral patellar compression syndrome. *American Journal of Sports Medicine* 20 (4): 434-440.

Drezner, J.A., and S.A. Herring. 2001. Managing low-back pain. *The Physician and Sports Medicine* 29(8): 37-43.

Earle, R.W., and T.R. Baechle 2004. *NSCA's Essentials of Personal Training*. Champaign, IL: Human Kinetics.

Fick, D.S., J.P. Albright, and B.P. Murray. 1992. Relieving painful "shin splints." *The Physician and Sportsmedicine* 20(12): 105-113.

Galea, A.M. and J.M. Albers. 1994. Patellofemoral pain. Beyond empirical diagnosis. *The Physician and Sportsmedicine* 22 (4): 48-58.

Hanney, W.J. 2000. Proprioceptive training for ankle instability. *Strength and Conditioning Journal* 22(5): 63-68.

Houglum, P. 2005. *Therapeutic Exercise for Musculoskeletal Injuries* 2nd ed. Champaign, IL:Human Kinetics.

Korkola, M., and A. Amendola. 2001. Exercise-induced leg pain. *The Physician and Sports Medicine* 29(6): 35-50.

Liemohn, W. 2001. *Exercise Prescription and the Back*. New York: McGraw-Hill.

Myerson, M.S., and K. Biddinger. 1995. Achilles tendon disorders. Practical management strategies. *The Physician and Sportsmedicine* 23 (12):47-54.

Post, W.R. 1998. Patellofemoral pain. *The Physician and Sports Medicine* 26(1): 68-78.

Prentice, W.E. 1994. *Rehabilitation Techniques in Sports Medicine*. 2nd ed. St. Louis: Mosby.

Rizzo, T.D. 1991. Plantar fasciitis. Overcoming a nagging pain in the arch. *The Physician and Sportsmedicine* 19(4):129-130.

Santana, J.C. 2000. Hamstrings of steel: Preventing the pull, Part ll – Training the triple threat. *Strength and Conditioning Journal* 23(1):18-20.

Tauton, J.E., D.B. Clement, G.W. Smart, and K.L. McNicol. 1987. Non-surgical management of overuse knee injuries in runners. *Canadian Journal of Sports Science* 12 (1): 11-18.

Toor, H. 2004. Calf pain. Common causes, treatment and preventive measures. *Fitness Trainer Canada* (February-March): 20-23.

Waddell, G. 1987. A new clinical model for the treatment of low back pain. *Spine* 12 (7): 632-644.

Watkins, J. 1999. *The Structure and Function of the Musculoskeletal System*. Champaign, IL: Human Kinetics.

Index

Note: Page numbers followed by an italicized *f* or *t* refer to the figure or table on that page, respectively.

1RM test 92, 94*f*

A

abdominal
  strength and core stability 96*f*
  strength testing 93, 94, 96
abdominal exercises 133
  curl ups 121*f*
  theraball crunch 140
abdominal girth measurement 88–89
abduction
  definition 120
  of scapula 120
  at specific joints 119*f*
absorbed strain 281
Achilles tendon
  and plantar fasciitis 295
  tendinitis 275*t*
  tendinitis and tendinosis 296–298
ACSM. *See* American College of Sports Medicine
action-oriented objectives 34
actions of joints 119*f*
action stage 20, 24
  counseling strategies 43*t*
  matching strategies for 25
active and fit client 69
active listening skills 9
active living 54–55, 168
  intensity of exercise 167*t*
active loosening 223–224
active static stretching 225
activities and energy requirements 254–255
activity counseling ix
activity counseling model
  communication and rapport 8–10
  description 5
  gathering information 10–19
  goals and objectives 23–38
  learning style of client 17–19
  lifestyle/activity preferences 17, 21, 22
  needs of client 12–13
  personality of client 17–19
  questioning skills 16–17
  rapport 6–7
  stages of change 19, 23–26
  strategies for change 28–29, 30, 31
  wants of client 13
activity preferences 13, 17
  questionnaire 18, 21

adduction
  definition 120
  of scapula 120
  at specific joints 119*f*
adductor brevis 146*t*
adductor longus 136*f*
  actions 146*t*
adductor magnus 146*t*
adherence
  and motivation 42
  and problem solving 50–52
aerobic conditioning. *See also* cardiovascular exercise
  and body composition 252
  as part of balanced exercise program 77
  safety 138*t*
  for weight management 259
aerobic energy system 161
aging, and muscle imbalance 216
agonists 231–232*t*
air displacement plethysmography 87
alcohol intake 62
alignment
  of foot 105
  and force application 133
  and injury risk 274
  of joints and muscle balance 217*f*
  and patellofemoral syndrome 301
  of spine 104–105
  and stretch quality 222
American College of Sports Medicine (ACSM)
  cardiovascular endurance activity groups 160
  interval training 259
  interval training recommendations 162
  leg ergometer equation 170
  muscular fitness guidelines 195
  recommended kilocalories burned 74
  running equation 170
  Web site 73
anaerobic energy system 160
anaerobic threshold 161, 179
analysis of exercise 116, 117
  about 117–118
  active muscles 123–124
  biomechanics 125–134
  contraction types 121–122
  effectiveness 125
  joints and movements 118, 120–121
  phases 118

purpose 124, 125*t*
  risk 125
anatomical position 118
Andersen, R. 248, 252
ankle
  actions 119*f*
  flexibility evaluation 99, 100
  joint-action-muscle chart 147*t*
  range of motion 99, 101*f*
  resisted toe points 121*f*
Annessi, J. 42
antagonists 231–232*t*
anterior deltoid 145*t*
anterior shin splints 298
anthropometric measures 88–89
aponeuroses 279
appeal of workout 44
arches of foot 110
arm, as lever system 130*f*
arm ergometer protocol 85*t*
assertive personality 20
assessment
  body mass index 63
  cardiovascular 85–87
  cardiovascular exercise prescription without 187–188
  client reluctance for 4
  economy of test protocol 67
  FANTASTIC lifestyle checklist 61
  fitness test item selection 67
  flexibility 96–101
  health appraisal 60
  laboratory and field-based tests 67, 68*t*
  lifestyle appraisal 60, 61
  of muscle balance 220
  musculoskeletal test selection 90–92
  PAR-Q 64, 66
  as part of prescription model xi
  Physical Activity Index (PAI) 65
  posture (case study) 234
  reliability 67
  resources 84
  retesting as motivation 50
  RISK-I 63
  strength testing 92–96
  use of observation 64
  validity 67
assessment forms
  flexibility and muscle tightness 98–99
  injury risk control checklist 292
  joint stress questionnaire 221
  pain questionnaire 285

segmental postural assessment 107–109
strength and endurance testing 93
ATP (adenosine triphosphate) 160
atrophy 286
attainable objectives 34
attendance 4. *See* compliance
attrition. *See* adherence
autogenic inhibition 226

B
back assessment 98
back pain 305, 307
Biering-Sorenson back endurance test 92, 94
conditions and exercises 308*t*
core stability exercises 307–313
and muscle tightness 111
upper back tension 137*f*
Baechle, T.R. 84
balanced exercise prescription 77–78
Balke protocol 259
Ball, D.R. 47
ballistic stretching 226
Bandy, W.D. 225
barbell curl, common faults 140*t*
barbells 196
barriers to exercise 14–16
eliminating through problem solving 50–52
internal 15*t*
obstacle management 44
baseball, and muscle imbalance 216
behavioral changes
and activity counseling model 5
and counseling interventions 5
Bell, G.J. 74
bench press
analysis of exercise 123*t*
force application and alignment 131
bench step 159
intensity of exercise 167*t*
Best, T.M. 303
biarticular muscle action 126–127
biceps brachii 136*f*
actions 145*t*
biceps curl mechanics 219
biceps femoris 136*f*
actions 146*t*
bicycle ergometry protocols 85
Biering-Sorenson back endurance test 92, 94
bioelectric impedance 87
biomechanics of exercise
alignment of external resistance 132–133
arm raises 133–134
biarticular muscle action 126–127
composition of forces 128–129
direction of force application 130–131
isolating one-joint muscles 126–127
lever systems 129–130
muscle length and force 125–126
sticking point 125–126

biomechanics of injury 274–275
terms 281
body composition
and aerobic conditioning 252
assessment 87–89
and balanced exercise program 77
case histories 89
comparison of measuring methods 87*t*
as part of physical fitness 69
tests 68*t*
body fat. *See* body composition
and client goals 70
distribution and disease risk 88
recommended values 88
body mass index (BMI) 63, 88
body weight
and body mass index 88
and injury risk 274
and musculoskeletal testing 91
use for resistance training 195–196
boredom 14
Borg scale of RPE 172*t*, 173
Bouchard, C. 70
brachialis 136*f*
actions 145*t*
brachioradialis 136*f*
actions 145*t*
breaking down exercises 116
building exercises 116

C
cable machines 196–197
calcium 247*t*
Calder, A.W. 201
calisthenic training circuit 165–166
calories 247*t*
energy deficit point system 253–256
and weight management 250
Canada's Food Guide to Healthy Eating 62
Canadian Society for Exercise Physiology
exercise testing resources 84
PARmed-X 64
personal training certification xi
physical activity, fitness, and lifestyle approach 5
carbohydrate
caloric value 250
as energy source 249
recommended daily intake 247*t*
cardiovascular exercise prescription 187–188. *See also* cardiovascular fitness
active living 168
case studies 182–183, 187–189
circuit training 165
continuous training 161–162
cool-down 181–182
cross-training 166
duration of exercise 174–175
energy systems used 160–161
exercise diary 178
Fartlek training 166

FITT (frequency, intensity, time, type) 166
frequency of exercise 175–176
injury risk control 292
intensity calculations 169–172
intensity groups 160
interval training 162–165
metabolic calculations 170
METs 169–170
monitoring 177, 179, 181
and objectives 177*t*
prescription card (blank) 191–192
prescription card (sample) 184–185
progression of exercise 176–177
recording data 177
selecting activities 154, 156–157
selecting equipment 156–160
steps 155–156*t*
using client goals and needs 154
volume of exercise 174–176
warm-up 181
cardiovascular fitness
assessment methods 85–87
description 68–69
field-based tests 86–87
and intensity of exercise 74
laboratory tests 85–86
submaximal vs. maximal tests 86
tests 68*t*
care
and client rapport 7
helping relationships 43
cartilage 280–281
case studies/examples
circuit training 165–166
circuit weight training 202*f*
client with weight loss objective 89
compliance and convenience 14
developing options (post MI) 10
failure vs. success 4
general fitness prescription 74–75
health-related fitness prescription 72–74, 261*t*
impatient client 55–56
interval training 164–165
male sprinter 188–189
motivating a new client 52–54
motivating an intermittent exerciser 54–55
muscle balance prescription 233–237
overtraining 32
overweight client 89
performance related fitness prescription 75–77
plyometrics 201*f*
prescription without cardiovascular assessment 187–188
resistance training prescription 208–211
superset program 199*t*
weekend warrior 237–241
weight management prescription 262–266

case studies/examples *(continued)*
　　well-conditioned woman 182–183
　　woman with pain while jogging
　　　289
certification, personal training xi
cervical spine
　　joint-action-muscle chart 147*t*
　　muscle imbalance 218
　　range of motion 98
　　rotation 101
challenging objectives 44
change. *See also* stages of change
　　and counseling skills 6*t*
　　for health vs. fitness 71
　　as motivation 48
　　strategies for 29
change process 43–44
Charland, J. 227
chest muscles
　　assessment of tightness 235*t*
　　flexibility assessment 98
　　PNF stretch 227*f*
　　tests for muscle tightness 101–102
cholesterol 247*t*
chronic overwork overtraining 76
circuit training 165
circuit weight training 200–201
circumduction
　　definition 120
　　at shoulder 119*f*
clarifying techniques 26–27
Clark, Nancy 245
Clement, D.B. 274
client-centered, definition ix, xi
client trial (of exercise) 139
　　and connecting with client 144
closed kinetic chain exercises 127,
　　　132, 194
closed questions 16
collagen 282
commitment. *See also* stages of
　　　change
　　and activity counseling model 5
　　adherence rates 42
　　determining ix, xi
　　and motivation 44–48
　　potential pitfalls 28
　　pros and cons of activity 31*f*
　　and self-talk 44
communication. *See also* sample
　　　dialogues
　　accuracy and clarity 9
　　active listening skills 9
　　and client rapport 6
　　conversation during training 17
　　nonverbal 8
　　sample dialogue for rapport 7–8
　　self-talk 44
　　SOLER acronym 8
　　supportive 9–10
compliance
　　and barriers to exercise 14–16
　　and intensity of exercise 73
compound set system 200
compression 281, 287
computerized resistance machines 197

concentric contractions 118, 121–
　　122, 194
connective tissue
　　common injuries 294*t*
　　stretching 220
consciousness raising 43
constant resistance machines 196–197
contemplation stage 20, 23
　　counseling strategies 43*t*
contingency management 43
contraction types 121–122
contract-relax antagonist-contract
　　　PNF stretching 227
contract-relax PNF stretching 227
contracts
　　and client commitment 44
　　self-contract 45
contracture 218
contraindications 294
convenience 14
conversation during training 17
cool-down
　　for cardiovascular exercise 181–
　　　182, 183*t*
　　injury risk control 292
　　and muscle balance prescription
　　　229
　　as part of balanced exercise pro-
　　　gram 77
　　for resistance training program 207
　　safety 79, 138*t*
　　and weight management prescrip-
　　　tion 262
core stability 307–313
　　and lower abdominal strength 96*f*
coronary artery disease (CAD) 60, 71
Costill, D.L. 169
counseling
　　importance of ix
　　as part of prescription model x
　　skills and tools 6*t*
counseling styles 10
counselor counseling style 10
counterconditioning 43
creatine kinase 206
credibility 7
creep 220
crepitus 284
crossovers 132*f*
　　common faults 140*t*
　　force application and alignment
　　　131
cross-training 166
curl-ups 121*f*
Cybex 197
cycling
　　intensity of exercise 167*t*
　　stationary bicycles 157
　　submaximal vs. maximal tests 86

D
damping 281
David (machines) 197
decision balance summary 31*f*
defensive avoidance 28
delayed-onset muscle soreness
　　　(DOMS) 278

treating 289
deltoid 136*f*
　　actions 145*t*
　　exercises targeting 117*f*
demonstration ix, x, xi
　　as art 143–144
　　checklist 139, 141
　　and connecting with client 144
　　experiential approach 139, 141
　　modifying exercise during 116
　　psychosocial aspects 144*t*
　　science of 141–142
DePalma, M.J. 301
depression of scapula 120
design. *See* exercise design
director counseling style 10
disc injuries 307
Dishman, R.K. 47
dorsiflexion
　　at ankle 119*f*
　　definition 121
　　evaluation 100
dose of exercise
　　for health-related fitness 72
　　and response 73*f*
downward rotation of scapula 120
dumbbells 196
dumbell press 140*t*
duration of exercise
　　and cardiovascular exercise pre-
　　　scription 174
　　for general fitness prescription 74
　　for stretching exercises 222, 223
　　and weight management 247–248
Dynaband 197–198
　　peroneal stretch 299
　　straight-leg raises 302
dynamic stretching 226
dynamometers 197
E
Eagle (machines) 197
eating behaviors 244–245
eccentric contractions 121–122, 194
　　ball catch 317*f*
　　and muscular force 278
economy of test protocol 67
educational needs 12
educator counseling style 10
elastic deformation 220, 223
elasticity 281
elastic tubing 197–198
elastic zone 281
elastin 282
elbow
　　actions 119*f*
　　joint-action-muscle chart 145*t*
　　opposing muscles 232*t*
electronic resistance machines 197
elevation 287
elevation of scapula 120
elliptical trainers 158*t*, 159
emotion
　　clarifying 9
　　and self-efficacy 47
empathy 9
encouragement 44

endorphines 72
endotendineum 280
endurance. *See* cardiovascular fitness; muscular endurance
energy expenditure
    resting metabolic rate 248
    thermic effect of exercise 248
    thermic effect of food 248
energy systems 160–161
    and interval training exercise prescription 163*t*
    for sports 163*t*
enthusiasm 6–7
environment
    and injury risk 274
    welcoming 7
epitendineum 280
equipment
    and injury risk 274
    as limit to program design xv
    for musculoskeletal testing 91
    for resistance training 195–198
    selecting for cardiovascular exercise 156–160
    selecting for resistance training prescription 205
    and special design needs 13
erector spinae group
    actions 147*t*
    strength testing 93
error in musculoskeletal testing 91
eversion
    at ankle 119*f*
    definition 121
    exercises 300*f*
examples. *See* case studies/examples
exercise
    biochemical changes after 71
    design criteria 116
    METs 170*t*
    thermic effect 248
exercise analysis. *See* analysis of exercise
exercise design
    common faults 139, 140*t*
    criteria 116
    determining joint movements/ position 135
    identifying component and training method 135
    modifying 136–137
    safety 137, 138*t*
    targeting muscles 135
exercise prescription. *See also* cardiovascular exercise prescription; muscle balance prescription; resistance training prescription
    based on outcomes 68
    benefits of features 28*t*
    creating balance 77–78
    for health 261*t*
    for health-related fitness 72–73
    for injured clients 282–289
    interrelationships of activity, fitness and health 70*f*

introductory workout sample 57*f*
    safety for impatient client 56
    safety issues 78–79
    selecting appropriate exercises xi
exercise prescription forms
    heart rate recovery 180
    multipurpose exercise diary 178
exercises
    bench press 123*t*
    calf raises 127*f*
    common faults 140*t*
    curl ups 121*t*
    dorsiflexion 297*f*
    forward lunges 304*f*
    for hamstring strain 306*f*
    heel lifts 297*f*
    iliotibial band stretch 303*f*
    inversion/eversion 300*f*
    lateral arm raises 122*t*, 134*t*
    leg flexion 127*f*
    for lower back problems 309–313
    peroneal stretch 299*f*
    resisted toe points 121*t*
    scapular retraction (prone) 121*t*
    shin stretch 300*f*
    squats (partial) 124*t*
    step-downs 304*f*
    straight-leg raises 304*f*
    toe curls 296*f*
    toe raises 298*f*
    triceps kickbacks 276
    vastus lateralis stretch 303*f*
exhaustion set system 201–202
expectations
    and client wants 13
    impatient client 55–56
    questions for determining 21
    realistic 12
extension
    definition 120
    at specific joints 119*f*
extensor digitorum longus 147*t*
extensor hallucis longus 147*t*
external obliques 147*t*
extracellular matrix 282
extrinsic motivators 48–49
extrinsic risk factors 274–275
    minimizing 289–290
eye contact 8
F
failure
    avoiding 1
    reasons for 2
FANTASTIC lifestyle checklist 60, 61
Fartlek training 166
fat. *See also* body fat
    caloric value 250
    in fast food 246
    metabolic rate 248
    metabolism and exercise 249
    recommended daily intake 247*t*
fat-free weight 195
fatigue
    and eccentric contraction patterns 278
    and muscle imbalance 216

feedback
    and exercise demonstration 139
    and exercise design 116
    as part of counseling ix
    and quality of stretching exercises 223
    and stages of prescription model xi
fiber 247*t*
fibrocartilage 280
field-based tests
    body composition 88–89
    cardiovascular fitness 86–87
    flexibility and muscle tightness 96–97, 98–99, 100–103
    musculoskeletal assessment 92
    musculoskeletal system 90*t*
fitness. *See* physical fitness
fitness needs 12
fitness tests. *See also* assessment
    item selection 67
    laboratory and field-based 67, 68*t*
FITT (frequency, intensity, time, type) 166
Fleck, S.J. 200
flexibility. *See also* muscle tightness
    assessment 220
    evaluation form 98–99
    field-based tests 96–97, 100–103
    and injury risk 274
    and muscle imbalance 217–218
    as part of balanced exercise program 77
    as part of physical fitness 69
    sit-and-reach test 97
    stretching mechanisms 220
    stretch quality 222–223
flexibility prescription
    active loosening 223–224
    duration of exercise 223
    dynamic stretching 226
    proprioceptive neuromuscular facilitation (PNF) 226–228
    static stretching 224–226
    stretching techniques 224*t*
    stretch quality 222–223
flexion
    definition 118
    at specific joints 119*f*
flexometers 96
flexor digitorum longus 147*t*
flexor hallucis longus 147*t*
follow-through phase 118
follow-up 139, 144
food labels 244, 245*f*
foot
    actions 119*f*, 121
    alignment 105, 110
    opposing muscles 231*t*
    plantar fasciitis 294–296
force
    direction of application 132–133
    of eccentric contractions 278
    and lever system 130
    and muscular strength 194

force *(continued)*
  and power phase of exercise 118
  and proper alignment 133
  resultant 128*f*
  result on muscle 222*f*
  and variable resistance machines 197
force arm 130
forced repetition system 202
forms. *See* assessment forms; exercise prescription forms
Francis, L. 34
free fatty acids 249
free weights
  about 196
  advantages and disadvantages 196*t*
frequency of training
  and cardiovascular exercise prescription 175–176
  for general fitness prescription 74
  for stretching exercises 222
fulcrum 130

G
Garrett, W.E. 303
gastrocnemius 136*f*
  actions 146*t*, 147*t*
  isolating 127
  muscle imbalance 219
  resultant force 129*f*
genu valgum 107
genu varum 107
Gettman, L.F. 165
gluteus maximus 136*f*
  actions 146*t*
  joint movement 135
  strengthening exercises 137*f*
gluteus medius 146*t*
gluteus minimus 146*t*
goals
  and activity counseling model 5
  benefits of goal-setting 32–33
  and cardiovascular exercise prescription 154, 174
  and client needs 69
  and establishing strategies for change 35–37
  identifying 4
  as internal barrier to exercise 14
  as motivation 50
  and resistance training prescription 203
  short-term 15
  types of 33
  and weight management 256
  writing 36
golfer's elbow 275*t*
Golgi tendon organs (GTOs) 224, 226
goniometers 96
good health, definition 68
gracilis 136*f*
  actions 146*t*
graph method of metabolic calculations 170–171
Gravitron 196
gravity
  and eccentric contractions 121
  and resistance training 195
groin pull 275*t*

H
habits
  and counterconditioning 43
  developing 1
  and self-talk 46
hack squat 140*t*
hamstring curl
  common faults 140*t*
  and muscle imbalance 218–219
hamstrings
  anatomy 305*f*
  leg curl machines and force 133
  muscle length assessment 104*f*
  strain 302–305
  stretching 126, 306*f*
  test of muscle tightness 102
Hawley, C.J. 75
healing phases 282–283
health
  benefits of exercise 71
  as client goal 69
  exercise prescription targeting 73, 261*t*
health appraisal 60–67
health history 64
health issues 12
  definition of good health 68
  overtraining 32
health-related fitness components 69–70
  exercise prescription targeting 72–73
health-related fitness prescription 261*t*
heart rate
  and exercise intensity 172*t*
  and progression of cardiovascular exercise 179*f*
  recovery chart 180
  and submaximal vs. maximal tests 86
  target heart rate 161–162
  variations with exercise 179
heart rate reserve 173*f*
heart rate reserve (HRR) 172
heavy-to-light system 198
Herring, S.A. 286
Heyward, V.H. 84, 173, 252
high risk needs 12
hip
  actions 119*f*
  assessment of tightness 238*t*
  flexibility assessment 99
  joint-action-muscle chart 145*t*, 146*t*
  opposing muscles 231*t*
  range of motion 99, 101
hip flexors
  and back pain 218
  muscle length assessment 104*f*
  test of muscle tightness 102
histamine 282
history
  as counseling skill 6*t*
  as part of activity counseling model 5
Hoeger, W. 84

hold-relax PNF stretching 227
horizontal abduction
  definition 120
  at shoulder 119*f*
horizontal adduction
  definition 120
  at shoulder 119*f*
Horswill, C.A. 168
Howard, M. 179
hyaline cartilage 280
Hydra-Gym 197
hydraulic machines 197
hyperextension of spine 119*f*
hypertrophy 194
  training principles for 194
  and volume of exercise 206*t*

I
ice 286
iliacus 146*t*
iliotibial band stretch 301, 303*f*
imaging experiences 47
impatient client 55–56
impingement syndrome 314
inactivity
  effect of exercise 69
  and exercise prescription 32
indications of injury 294
inflammation phase 282
  exercise prescription 286
informational needs 12
information gathering 6*t*
  determining wants, needs, lifestyle 19
  questioning skills 16–17
  strategies 10–13
informed consent 64
infraspinatus 136*f*
  actions 145*t*
  exercises targeting 117*f*
initial fitness level 75
injuries
  Achilles tendonitis/tendinosis 296–298
  chronic microtrauma 276*f*
  common 294*t*
  eccentric contraction patterns 278
  healing phases 282–283
  momentum 275–276
  and muscle imbalance 104
  pain questionnaire 285
  plantar fasciitis 294–296
  preventing reinjury 289–290
  PRICE treatment 286
  recognizing overuse 284
  risk control checklist 292
  risk factors 274–275
  shin splints 298–300
  tissue types 279–281
injury exercise prescription 286–289
intensity of exercise
  calculation 180
  client-centered 173*t*
  and fat metabolism 249
  for general fitness prescription 74
  graph method 170–171
  guidelines for cardiovascular exercise 172–174

metabolic calculations 170
METs 169–170
moderate 72
and modifying the lever system 130
monitoring 181*t*
and other prescription factors 174
as percent of maximum heart rate 171–172
for resistance training 194
for resistance training prescription 206, 206*t*
for sedentary clients 32
for stretching exercises 222
for weight management 259
internal barriers 14
internal obliques 147*t*
interpreting, avoiding 9
interval training 162–165
guidelines for prescriptions 163*t*
samples 164–165
steps for prescriptions 164
intervertebral disc injury 307
intimidation 7
intrinsic aspects of activity 12
intrinsic motivators 50
intrinsic risk factors 274
minimizing 290
inversion
at ankle 119*f*
definition 121
exercises 300*f*
isokinetic machines 197
isometric contraction 122, 194
isometric stretching 227
isotonic contraction 194

J
Jackson, A.S. 165
Jakicic 248, 252
JAM charts
about 123–124
ankle 147
elbow 145
foot 147
hip 146
knee 146
radioulnar joint 145
shoulder 145*t*
spine 147
jogging
calculating intensity 170
intensity of exercise 167*t*
pain during 289
joint-muscle relationships 90
joints
actions at specific joints 119*f*
momentum and injury risk 275
multi-joint movements 118
and muscle imbalance 216–217
stop point 278
joint stress cycle 219–220
joint stress questionnaire 221
judgment, avoiding 10
jumper's knee 275*t*
jump rope 160
K
Kaul, M.P. 286

Keaemer, W.J. 200
Keiser equipment 197
Kendall, F.P. 84
kilocalories 74
for activities 254–255
Kin-Com 197
kinetic chain 194
and muscle imbalance 219
Klesges, R. 248
knee
actions 119*f*
assessment of tightness 238*t*
flexibility assessment 99
joint-action-muscle chart 146*t*
opposing muscles 231*t*
patellar pressure 130*f*
patellofemoral joint anatomy 302*f*
patellofemoral syndrome 300–302
range of motion 99
shear force on machines 133
knowledge, as motivation 50
Kosich, D. 166
kyphosis 106*f*
L
laboratory tests
cardiovascular fitness 85–86
musculoskeletal system 90*t*
lactic acid system 160
lateral arm raises
analysis of exercise 122*t*
biomechanical analysis 133–134
lateral lift test 96, 97*f*
lateral pull-down 140*t*
lateral rotation
definition 120
at specific joints 119*f*
latissimus dorsi 136*f*
actions 145*t*
learning style 19
about 17
leg press 140*t*
Leighton flexometer 96
levator scapulae
actions 145*t*
joint movement 135
levers 129–130
lifestyle
appraisal 60
definition 11
FANTASTIC lifestyle checklist 61
preferences 17
questionnaire 18
setting priorities 29
targeting 22
lifestyle appraisal
FANTASTIC Lifestyle Checklist 60, 61
observation 64
PAR-Q 64, 66
Physical Activity Index (PAI) 60, 65
RISK-I 60, 63
lifestyle coaching 48
ligaments 279
light-to-heavy system 198
limitations 86

lipoproteins 71
listening
active listening skills 9
and client rapport 1, 6
as critical component to exercise prescription xv
as part of counseling ix
lordosis 106*f*
and muscle imbalance 218
low back
case study 237–241
conditions and exercises 308*t*
core stability exercises 307–313
problems and muscle tightness 111
spasms and muscle imbalance 218
low back pain 305, 307
lower body
alignment 107
muscle balance prescription 220, 231*t*
muscle length assessment 104*f*
strength assessments 220
LSD (long, slow distance) training 161
lumbar spine
joint-action-muscle chart 147*t*
range of motion 98
rotation 101
lymph vessels 282
M
machines (for resistance training) 196–197
path of motion 132
macrophages 282
maintenance stage 20, 24
counseling strategies 43*t*
matching strategies for 25
manual resistance 198
maximal fitness tests 86
Mayer, Jean 247
McAtee, R.E. 227
measurable objectives 34
medial rotation
definition 120
at specific joints 119*f*
medial tibial stress syndrome (MTSS) 298–300
medical history 64
medical needs 12
medications 287, 289
metabolic calculations 170
metabolism
effect of dieting 250–251
energy systems 160–161
resting metabolic rate 248
METs
for activities 254–255
and exercise intensity 169–170
for sports and activities 170*t*
microtrauma 276*f*
middle deltoid 145*t*
Miller, W.C. 246
mode of activity 74
moderate exercise
benefits 72–74

moderate exercise *(continued)*
   motivating an intermittent exerciser 54–55
momentum
   and injury risk 275
   quiz 276–277
monitoring
   for muscle balance 229
   and overtraining 76
   and program safety 78
   of resistance training program 207
monotonous program overtraining 76
motivation
   and adherence 42
   and commitment 44–48
   extrinsic motivators 48–49
   and goal-setting 33
   impatient client case study 55–56
   intermittent exerciser case study 54–55
   intrinsic motivators 50
   and needs determination 12
   new client case study 52–54
   and overtraining 75
   and self-esteem 13
   and stages of change 42–44
   strategies 37
   and trust 1
multifidus 307
muscle balance
   importance of 216
   and low back injury 307
   and program safety 78
muscle balance assessment 102–111, 220
muscle balance prescription 238*t*
   case studies 233–236, 237–241
   lower body 231*t*
   precautions 228
   prescription card (blank) 230
   principles 228
   steps 228–229
muscle imbalance
   assessment 220
   causes and results 216–219
   detecting 219–220
   and injury risk 274
muscle-joint relationships 90
muscles
   active during exercise 123–124
   anterior and posterior view 136*f*
   autogenic inhibition 226
   biarticular 126–127
   common injuries 294*t*
   contraction types 121–122
   elastic properties 220
   length-tension relationship 125–126
   opposing 231–232*t*
   phasic mobilizers 217
   postural stabilizers 217
   relaxation techniques 223
   response to constant force 222*f*
   stiffness 220
   synergists 122
   targeting through exercise 135

muscle spindles 224
muscle tightness. *See also* flexibility
   and muscle imbalance 217–218
   tests 101–102
muscular endurance
   of back extensors 94
   definition 194
   evaluation form 93
   five-level sit-up test 94, 95*f*
   measuring 92
   as part of physical fitness 69
musculoskeletal assessment
   alignment 107–109
   and client strength level 90
   field-based tests 92
   flexibility tests 96–101
   foot alignment 105
   limitations of specific tests 91–92
   muscle tightness tests 102–103
   normative values 91
   postural assessment 104–105
   specificity, validity, reliability of tests 91
   test selection 90–92
   tightness and weakness 111
   using maximal effort 90
musculoskeletal system
   benefits of moderate exercise 72
   risk assessment 60
music
   and motivation 160
   as motivation 48
myosin 220

N
National Institutes for Health 89
Nautilus 197
needs
   and cardiovascular exercise prescription 154
   and client goals 69
   definition 11
   dynamic nature of 70
   and exercise design 116
   lifestyle 18
   and muscle balance prescription 228
   and resistance training prescription 203
   setting priorities 29
   types of 12
   and weight management 256
needs assessment ix
neural imbalance 218
neuromuscular retraining 288
neutrophils 282
Nieman, C. 84
Nirschl, P.R. 284
nonverbal communication 8
Norkin, C. 84
NSAIDs 287, 289
nutrition. *See also* weight management
   balanced diet 62
   basics 244–245
   fast food and fat 246

   healthy eating resources 246
   recommended daily intake 247*t*

O
obesity. *See* body composition
objectives
   and commitment 44
   creating 33
   and establishing strategies for change 35–37
   and exercise prescription 70
   identifying 5
   SMART objectives 34
   worksheet 38
   writing 36
observation 64
obstacle management 44
Omni-tron 197
open-ended questions 16
open kinetic chain exercises 132
options 27–28
   and client commitment 44
order of exercises 205
Orthotron 197
outcome goals 33
overreaching 75, 76
overtraining
   and client type 69
   example 32
   in runners 76
   types of 75–76
overuse injuries 279*f*
   and client goals 69
   common sites 275*t*
   pain scale 286
   prevention 294
   recognizing 284
   risk factors 274–275
   treating and preventing 283–285
oxygen system 161
oxygen transport system 68

P
Paffenbarger, R.S. 72
pain
   jogging example 289
   medications 287
   and muscle imbalance 218
   and overuse injuries 284, 286
   and phases of healing 282
   questionnaire 285
PARmed-X 64
PAR-Q 64, 66
partner-assisted stretching 226
partners (for workout) 50
passive static stretch 225–226
patella, resultant force 130*f*
patellofemoral syndrome 274, 300–302
pec decks
   path of motion 132
   pivot points 133
pectineus 146*t*
pectoralis major 136*f*
   actions 145*t*
   exercises targeting 117*f*
   stretching 316*f*
   test of muscle tightness 102

pectoralis minor
    actions 145*t*
    exercises targeting 117*f*
    test of muscle tightness 101
pedometers 179
pelvic girdle
    motions 120
    opposing muscles 232*t*
pelvic tilt 106*f*, 120
    and muscle imbalance 218
performance accomplishment 47
performance, as client goal 69
performance goals 33
performance-related fitness 75–76
periodization 75, 202–203, 206
Perkins, R.H. 301
peroneus 136*f*
    stretching 299*f*
peroneus brevis 147*t*
peroneus longus 147*t*
peroneus tertius 147*t*
personality style 17, 19
    identifying 20
    impatient client 55–56
personalized prescription x
personal trainers and adherence 42
personal training certification xi
Peterson et al. 259
phasic muscles 217
phosphocreatine 160
Physical Activity Index (PAI) 60, 65
physical fitness
    benefits of exercise 71
    as client goal 69
    components 68–69
    definition 68
    exercise prescription targeting 74
    performance-related components
        69–70
physiological state 47
piriformis 308
plantar fasciitis 294–296
plantar flexion
    at ankle 119*f*
    definition 121
    evaluation 100
plastic deformation 222
plasticity 281
plyometrics 200, 201*f*
pneumatic machines 197
Pochaska, J.O. 19
point system for weight management
    253–256
Polaris 197
Pollock, M.L. 165
popliteus 146*t*
portion sizes 244, 245*t*
posterior deltoid 145*t*
posterior shin splints 298
posture
    alignment when standing 104–
        105
    assessment 220
    assessment (case study) 234
    assessment form 107–109
    common faults 106*f*
    ideal alignment 106*f*

lower body assessment form 107
    and muscle balance prescription
        233
    and muscle imbalance 218–219
    muscle stabilizers 217
    upper body assessment form 108
power 194
power phase 118
preacher counseling style 10
precautions (injury) 294
precontemplation stage 20
    counseling strategies 43*t*
    matching strategies for 24
predemonstration 139
    and connecting with client 144
preferences. *See also* wants
    lifestyle and activity 17
    and order of exercises 77
    questionnaire 18, 21
preparation stage 20, 23
    counseling strategies 43*t*
    matching strategies for 25
preparatory phase 118
prescription card (blank)
    for cardiovascular exercise 191–
        192
    for muscle balance prescription
        230
    for resistance training 213
    for weight management 264
prestretching 126–127
PRICE treatment 286
priorities 29
    and exercise prescription 70
probing strategies 16
process goals 33
program demonstration. *See* dem-
        onstration
progression of exercise
    for cardiovascular exercise pre-
        scription 176–177
    for general fitness prescription
        74–75, 74–75
    for muscle balance 229
    and program safety 78
    for resistance training 207
progressive overload 207*t*
proliferation phase 282
pronation
    alignment 107
    definition 120
pronator quadratus 145*t*
pronator teres 145*t*
proprioceptive neuromuscular facili-
        tation (PNF) 226–228
protein 247*t*
    caloric value 250
psoas 146*t*, 147*t*
pull-down exercises 131
push-ups
    limitations as testing tool 91
    as musculoskeletal test 96, 97*f*
    using wobble board 317*f*
pyramid system 198

Q
quadratus lumborum 96
    actions 147*t*

    and core stability 307
    and low back injury 308
    strength testing 93
quadriceps, resultant force 129*f*
questioning
    and client rapport 1
    and information gathering 10–11,
        16–17
questionnaire
    joint stress 221
    lifestyle and activity preferences
        18
    pain 285
    relapse planning 49
    stages of change 30
    wants of client 21

R
radioulnar joint
    joint-action-muscle chart 145*t*
    opposing muscles 232*t*
range of motion
    active and passive 225
    causes of limitations 220
    and flexibility 111
    limiting factors 96
    and low back injury 307
    and muscle imbalance 217
    for shoulder 98
    of shoulder 100
    stop point 278
rapport 1
    and activity counseling model 5
    as counseling skill 6*t*
    and exercise demonstration 144
    sample dialog 7–8
    skills and tools 8–9
    strategies for establishing 6–7
rating of perceived exertion (RPE) 173
    and monitoring cardiovascular
        exercise 179
readiness of client. *See also* stages
        of change
    and success of program 1
realistic objectives 34
    for aerobic exercise 175
receptiveness 6–7
recovery
    heart rate chart 180
    and overtraining 76
rectus abdominis 136*f*
    actions 147*t*
    strength testing 93
rectus femoris 136*f*, 146*t*
    actions 146*t*
referral
    based on health history 64
    and client goals 69
reflex inhibition 220
reframing 47
rehabilitation, as client goal 69
reinforcement 44
relapse
    high-risk situations 47–48
    planning questionnaire 49
    preparing for 42
relaxation of muscle 223
reliability 67, 91

relief interval 162
remodeling phase 283
    exercise prescription 288
repair phase 287–288
repetition
    for interval training 162
    for resistance training 194
    for stretching exercises 222
repetition maximum 202
resilience 281
resistance arm 130
    adjusting 131*t*
resistance training
    alignment of external resistance 132–133
    equipment 195–198
    general conditioning prescription 195
    general fitness prescription 75
    general principles 194
    and lever system 130
    machines 196–197
    as part of balanced exercise program 77
    repetition maximum 202
    safety 78, 138*t*
    specificity principle 194
    superset system 199*t*
    and weight management 251–252
resistance training prescription
    case studies 208–211
    circuit training 200–201
    compound set system 200
    cool-down 207
    exercise selection 205
    exhaustion set system 201–202
    forced repetition system 202
    for hypertrophy vs. strength 206*t*
    injury risk control 292
    intensity of exercise 206
    length of workout 207
    methods 198–203, 205
    monitoring 207
    needs and goals 203
    order of exercises 205
    periodization 202–203
    plyometrics 200
    prescription card (blank) 213
    progression of exercise 207
    pyramid system 198
    sample prescription card 208–210
    selecting equipment 205
    split routine system 201
    standard set system 198
    steps 203–204*t*
    strengthening movement patterns 232–233
    superset system 198–199
    tri-set system 200
    volume of exercise 206
    warm-up 207
    and weight management 261–262
resources
    assessment methods 84
    scarcity for client-centered prescription xi

rest
    and injury treatment 286
    and interval training 163
    and resistance training 206
resultant force 128*f*
rhomboids
    actions 145*t*
    exercises targeting 117*f*
risk 12
risk assessment
    FANTASTIC lifestyle checklist 60–61
    injury risk control checklist 292
PAR-Q 64
    as part of exercise analysis 125
    Physical Activity Index (PAI) 60
    RISK-I 60, 63
RISK-I 60, 63
Rockport walking test 87
rope skipping 160
Roskopf, C. 228
rotation
    definition 120
    of hip 101
    range of motion of spine 98
    of shoulder 101*f*
    at specific joints 119*f*
    of spine 101
rotator cuff tendinitis 275*t*, 314–317
rowing
    common faults 140*t*
    force application and alignment 132
rowing machines 158*t*, 159
running
    ACSM equation for intensity 170
    avoiding overtraining 76
    case study 188–189
    eccentric contractions 278*f*
    and foot pronation 110
    injury risk 274
    intensity of exercise 167*t*
    overpronation and injury 274
    pain while jogging 289
    and patellofemoral syndrome 301

S
sacroiliac joint dysfunction 308
safe sex 62
safety
    of cardiovascular exercise equipment 157–158
    and exercise demonstration 142
    and exercise design 137
    and muscle balance prescription 229
    as part of balanced exercise program 78–79
sample dialogues
    barriers to exercise 15
    clarifying needs and wants 13
    contemplation stage client 23
    establishing rapport 7–8
    establishing strategies for change 35
    precontemplation stage client 20, 23
    summarizing tools for change 26–27

Santana, J.C. 305
sartorius 136*f*
    actions 146*t*
scaleni group 147*t*
scapula motions 120
    retraction 121*f*, 316*f*
Schoene, R.B. 75
scoliosis 109
screening 64. *See also* assessment; lifestyle appraisal
    and injury risk 274
seated row 140*t*
sedentary clients
    cardiovascular exercise prescription 161
    integrating activity 247–248
    intensity of exercise 32
self-efficacy 43
    promoting 47
self-esteem needs 12
selfishness 46
self-liberation 43
self-talk 44
semimembranosus 136*f*
    actions 146*t*
semitendinosus 146*t*
semitendionsus 136*f*
    actions 146*t*
serratus anterior 96
    actions 145*t*
    exercises targeting 117*f*
    strength testing 93
set
    for interval training 162
    for resistance training 194
sex, safe 62
Sharkey, B.J. 176
shear 281
shin splints 275*t*, 298–300
shoulder 316*f*
    actions 119*f*
    alignment 110–112
    assessment case study 235*t*
    clock test 111*f*
    dynamic alignment 110–111
    flexibility evaluation 98, 100
    joint-action-muscle chart 145*t*
    manual isometric stretch 227*f*
    movements 120
    muscle imbalance 216
    muscle length assessment 103*f*
    opposing muscles 232*t*
    rotation 101*f*
    rotator cuff tendinitis 314–317
side leg raise 118*f*
sit-and-reach test 97, 100*f*
    limitations 92
sit-ups
    five-level test 94, 95*f*
    limitations as testing tool 91
skinfold measures 88
Skinner, J.S. 69
slide (equipment) 159
SMART objectives 34, 36
    worksheet 38
smoking 63
sociable personality 20

sodium 247t
soft tissue
    biomechanics 281
    types of 279–281
soleus 136f
    actions 147t
    isolating 127
spasms 218
special interests 13
    questions for determining 21
specificity of testing 91
specificity principle 194, 195t
specific objectives 34
speed, and power 194
spine
    actions 119f
    flexibility test 101, 102f
    joint-action-muscle chart 147t
    postural assessment (case study)
        234t, 237t
    postural assessment form 109
    postural awareness 233
    range of motion 98, 101
split routine system 201
sports
    energy systems 163t
    equipment and cardiovascular
        exercise 158
    intensity of exercise 167t
    METs 170t
sport skill analysis 117
spotting 141–142, 143t
sprains 294t
    lower back 308
squats
    common faults 140t
    machines and biomechanics 133
stabilization of joint 122
stages of change
    characteristics 24t
    and counseling skill 6t
    counseling strategies 43t
    matching strategies for 24–25, 35
    and motivation 42–44
    questionnaire 30
    working with 19–20, 25–28
stages of prescription model x
stages of training ix
stair climbers 158t, 159
standard set system 198
static stretching 224–226
    and DOMS 289
stationary bicycles 157t, 159
    intensity of exercise 167t
step test protocols 85
sternocleidomastoid 147t
Stewart, Gord 168
sticking point 125–126, 196
stimulus control 44
stop point 278
strain (biomechanical) 281
strains 294t
    hamstrings 302–305
    to lower back 308
strategies for change
    as counseling skill 6t

setting priorities 29
skills and tools for establishing
    35–37
strength
    of agonists and antagonists 103
    assessment 220
    definition 194
    evaluation form 93
    five-level sit-up test 94, 95f
    and lever system 129–130
    and muscle imbalance 218
    as part of physical fitness 69
    tests 92, 96
    of tissues 281
    training principles for 194
    and volume of exercise 206t
strengthening exercises
    and Achilles tendonitis/tendinosis
        297
    and hamstring strain 305
    and patellofemoral syndrome
        301–302
    and plantar fasciitis 295–296
    and rotator cuff tendinitis 314–
        317
    and shin splints 299–300
strength training. See resistance
        training
stress
    and client commitment 46
    on tissues 281
stress-relaxation 220
stress-strain curve 281f
stretching. See also flexibility
    and Achilles tendonitis/tendinosis
        297
    dynamic 226
    factors affecting quality 222
    and hamstring strain 304–305
    manual isometric stretch 227
    mechanisms 220
    as part of balanced exercise pro-
        gram 78
    and patellofemoral syndrome 301
    and plantar fasciitis 295
    proprioceptive neuromuscular
        facilitation (PNF) 226–228
    and rotator cuff tendinitis 314,
        315–316
    and shin splints 299
    static 224–226
    techniques 224t
    and upper back tension 137f
    vastus lateralis 303f
submaximal fitness tests
    for cardiovascular fitness 86
    for muscular endurance 92
subscapularis 145t
substitution patterns 219
success
    and activity, fitness, and health 70
    and client-centered approach 4
    defining 14
    and needs, wants, lifestyle overlap
        11
    and stages of change progression 42

summarizing techniques 26–27
supercompensation response 75
superset system 198–199
supervision, as motivation 50
supination
    alignment 107
    definition 120
supinator 145t
supraspinatus 145t
swimmer's shoulder 275t
swimming
    intensity of exercise 167t
    use of home pool 159
synergists 122
    and muscle balance 104
    muscle imbalance among 219
T
talk test 179
target heart rate 161–162
    calculating 171–172
technical personality 20
temperature and stretch quality 222
tendinitis 280, 294t
    Achilles tendon 296–298
    rotator cuff 314–317
tendinosis 280, 294t
    Achilles tendon 296–298
tendons
    description 279–280
    overuse injuries 275t
    structure 280f
tennis elbow 275t
tensile 281
tensor fascia latae 146t
teres major 136f
    actions 145t
teres minor
    actions 145t
    exercises targeting 117f
tests. See assessment
Theraball 8
    core exercises 57
theraball crunch 140t
thermic effect of exercise 248
thermic effect of food 248
thoracic spine
    joint-action-muscle chart 147t
    rotation 101
tibialis anterior 136f
    actions 147t
tibialis posterior 147t
time 54–55
    length of resistance training work-
        out 207
time commitments
    dealing with 54–55
    as internal barrier to exercise 14
tissues
    biomechanical properties 281
    structural strength 281
    types 279–280
titin 220
touching 143
training distance 162
training time 162
transversus abdominis 307

trapezius 136*f*
  actions 145*t*
  exercises targeting 117*f*
  joint movement 135
treadmill protocols 85
treadmills 157*t*, 159
  submaximal vs. maximal tests 86
triceps brachii
  actions 145*t*
  kickback exercise 140*t*, 276
triglycerides 71
tri-set system 200
trunk
  flexibility testing 92
  muscle balance assessment 220
  opposing muscles 231*t*
  strength assessments 220
trust 4
  and establishing rapport 8
  and recognizing stages of change 25
  and supportive communication 9

U
underwater weighing 87
upper back tension 137*f*
upper body
  muscle balance assessment 220
  segment alignment 108
  strength assessments 220
upward rotation of scapula 120
U.S. My Pyramid 244

V
validity 67, 91
value 27–28
variable resistance machines 197
variety of workout
  as motivation 48
  and overtraining 76
vastus intermedius 146*t*
vastus lateralis 136*f*
  actions 146*t*
  stretching 303*f*
vastus medialis 136*f*
  actions 146*t*
  and patellofemoral syndrome 302
Venn diagram, needs, wants, lifestyle overlap 11
verbal persuasion 47
vicarious experience 47

videos 159
viscoelasticity of muscle 220
V̇O$_2$max 169
volume of exercise
  determining correctly 70–71
  dose-response relationship 73*f*
  for hypertrophy vs. strength 206*t*
  matching to client goals 70–71
  moderate 72
  overtraining 75–77
  and overuse injuries 274–275
  for resistance training prescription 206

W
waist (abdomen) girth 88–89
Walberg, J.L. 250
walking
  field test protocols 86–87
  intensity of exercise 167*t*
  pedometers 179
  Zen quality 259
walk-run field test protocols 86–87
wants
  and body image 256
  definition 11, 13
  questionnaire 21
  setting priorities 29
warm-up
  for cardiovascular exercise 181, 182*t*
  and DOMS 289
  for Fartlek training 166
  injury risk control 292
  and muscle balance prescription 229
  as part of balanced exercise program 77
  for resistance training program 207
  safety 78, 138*t*
  and weight management prescription 262
water, and resistance training 198
Web sites
  American College of Sports Medicine (ACSM) 73
  healthy eating resources 246
weekend warriors 139
  case study 237–241

weight management
  aerobic program design 259–260
  body composition assessment 87–89
  and body image 256
  calories 250
  case study 262–263, 265–266
  cool-down 262
  diet vs. exercise 250–251
  eating behaviors 244–245
  energy deficit point system 253–256
  exercise prescription 267*t*
  general guidelines 252–253
  integrating activity 247–248
  plan for 1 lb./week loss 251*t*
  prescription model 256
  prescription steps 257–258
  reasons for eating 246–247
  resistance training prescription 261–262
  role of exercise 252–256
  role of resistance training 251–252
  strategies for change 247
  warm-up 262
weight training. *See* resistance training
welcoming environment 7
wellness 70
Wenger, H.A. 74
Wilmore, J.H. 169
work, and cardiovascular exercise prescription 174
work interval 162
work-relief ratio 162
work task analysis 117
wrist
  actions 119*f*
  muscle actions 145*t*
  opposing muscles 232*t*

Y
yield point 281

Z
Zen of walking 259
Z line 220

About the Author

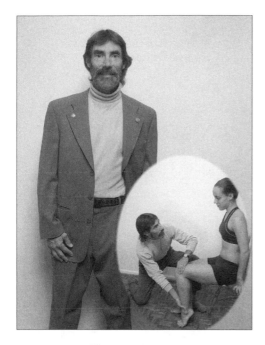

John C. Griffin, MSc, is coordinator of the Fitness and Lifestyle Management Program at George Brown College in Toronto. As a private consultant, speaker, and writer for public- and private-sector organizations, Griffin has authored more than 60 publications, including the first edition of *Client-Centered Exercise Prescription.* Working with the National Fitness Leadership Advisory Council (NFLAC), Griffin coauthored the first national standards for exercise leaders. After serving on the board of directors for Ontario Association of Sport and Exercise Sciences (OASES), Griffin worked with the Canadian Society for Exercise Physiology on a national certification for personal fitness trainers.

A professor, personal trainer, and coach for more than 30 years, Griffin has designed curricula for numerous courses in exercise prescription, personal training, musculoskeletal assessment and rehabilitation, biomechanics, and exercise and training techniques. He has received awards from NFLAC, OASES, the Ontario Fitness Council, George Brown College, the Province of Ontario, and the Australian Sport and Fitness Council. He has lectured in Sweden, Australia, Finland, many American cities, and all across Canada.

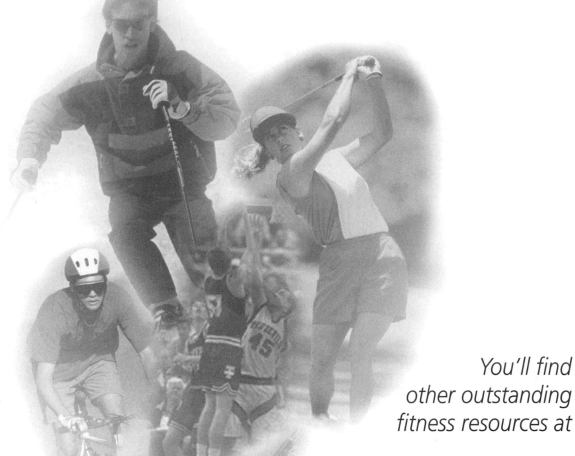